Ancestors and
Antiretrovirals

Ancestors and Antiretrovirals

The Biopolitics of HIV/AIDS in Post-Apartheid South Africa

CLAIRE LAURIER DECOTEAU

The University of Chicago Press   Chicago and London

CLAIRE LAURIER DECOTEAU is assistant professor of
sociology at the University of Illinois at Chicago, where she teaches
courses in social theory, the sociology of knowledge, and health
and medicine. She is also a research associate in the Department of
Sociology at the University of the Witwatersrand in Johannesburg,
South Africa.

The University of Chicago Press, Chicago 60637
The University of Chicago Press, Ltd., London
© 2013 by The University of Chicago
All rights reserved. Published 2013.
Printed in the United States of America

22 21 20 19 18 17 16 15 14 13   1 2 3 4 5

ISBN-13: 978-0-226-06445-1 (cloth)
ISBN-13: 978-0-226-06459-8 (paper)
ISBN-13: 978-0-226-06462-8 (e-book)
DOI: 10.7208/chicago/9780226064628.001.0001

Library of Congress Cataloging-in-Publication Data

Decoteau, Claire Laurier, author.
    Ancestors and antiretrovirals : the biopolitics of HIV/AIDS in
post-apartheid South Africa / Claire Laurier Decoteau.
        pages   cm
    Includes bibliographical references and index.
    ISBN 978-0-226-06445-1 (cloth : alkaline paper)
    ISBN 978-0-226-06459-8 (paperback : alkaline paper)
    ISBN 978-0-226-06462-8 (e-book)
    1. AIDS (Disease)—Social aspects—South Africa. 2. AIDS
(Disease)—Political aspects—South Africa. 3. HIV-positive
persons—South Africa. 4. Health services accessibility—
South Africa. 5. South Africans—Medicine. I. Title.
RA643.86.G4D43 2013
362.19697'9200967—dc23

                                        2013008863

♾ This paper meets the requirements of ANSI/NISO Z39.48-1992
(Permanence of Paper).

*In loving memory of Thulani Skhosana (October 18, 1976–
April 14, 2012)—who died, as he lived, struggling against the
injustices of poverty and AIDS.* Hamba kahle, *comrade.*

Contents

Acknowledgments

This book seeks to break the silence that shrouds the lives of so many people living with AIDS by including the stories of their lives in the way they saw fit to tell them. Because stigma still enigmatically cloaks this disease in shame and secrecy (even in communities where it has become the norm), I cannot properly thank all those who have helped me over the years. Even braver, therefore, are the decisions made by this book's two main characters, Pheello Limapo and Thulani Skhosana, who opened up their homes and shared some of their most intimate fears, bodily failings, and heartrending pain with me. They did this in an effort to challenge the ways in which so many people with HIV/AIDS have been forgotten and abandoned by the state, the health system, and the world at large. Over the years I have been welcomed as an honorary member of their families and communities, and I cannot begin to express the courage they inspire in me and the countless others whose lives they touch. They have both fought for so long—for proper housing, for the dignity of work, for the right to health care, and for life itself—a battle Thulani finally lost on April 14, 2012. The world is a sadder place without him.

There are countless people who have contributed to this project over the years, and I only hope the book contributes in some small way to their daily struggles for survival and dignity. First, I must thank my research assistant, Torong L. D. Ramela, whose boundless energy and extraordinary skill in translation and interpretation were essential to the success of this research. Torong also introduced me into the world of indigenous healing. Healers of all types and backgrounds in the Johannesburg region trusted him because he had worked as a facilitator in a series of workshops and forums set up to interface between healers and government health officials. It was in one of those moments of dumb luck, which are so often the trademark of successful ethnographies, that I happened to meet Torong, first as an activist, and only second as a researcher. Torong not only vouched for me and introduced me to indigenous healers all over the city, but he also opened the door to a whole different world, or rather, an entirely new way of seeing and interpreting the social world we inhabit.

Torong also introduced me to indigenous doctors Martha Mongoya and Robert Tshabalala, who not only patiently explained, step-by-step, certain tenets of the indigenous knowledge system (and endured my incessant interruptions and questions), but also introduced me to members of the organizations they lead and encouraged member participation. I have the utmost respect for their commitment to the struggle against HIV/AIDS and their dedication to their communities.

Through my involvement in certain activist organizations, including the Anti-Privatisation Forum and the Landless People's Movement, I met a whole host of activist scholars who became my intellectual and emotional support system during the thirty-two months I spent living and working in Johannesburg, between the years of 2002 and 2012. They include Ahmed Veriava, Prishani Naidoo, Salim Vally, Nicolas Dieltiens, Dale McKinley, Pier Paulo Frassenelli, Antina von Schnitzler, Ann Eveleth, Makoma Lekalakala, and Nerisha Baldevu. It cannot be overstated how rare and important it is to find people with whom one shares not only a common vision of struggle but also an epistemological orientation and theoretical commitment. I would also like to thank South African academics Achille Mbembe, Leah Gilbert, and Robert Thornton as well as the University of the Witwatersrand Department of Sociology and Institute for Social and Economic Research (WISER) for research support along the way.

I greatly appreciate the years of staunch support from three of my most significant intellectual mentors, George Steinmetz, Tobin Siebers, and Mamadou Diouf, whose own work has been a source of tremendous inspiration to me. I must also thank those who set aside their busy lives to read drafts of my chapters: Lorena Garcia, Laurie Schaffner, Andy Clarno, Anna Guevarra, Jennifer Brier, Barbara Risman, Sean Jacobs, Raka Ray, Fraser G. McNeill, Monika Krause, and Isaac Reed. Sandy Sufian and Sydney Halpern also provided constructive advice. Many of you really pushed me to deepen my analysis. The book is much better for it. The Great Cities Institute at the University of Illinois at Chicago provided me with an invaluable year of fellowship, which greatly enabled the writing of the manuscript. Thanks to Rachel Weber, Dennis Judd, and the rest of the 2010–11 cohort. I also benefited greatly from the support provided by my writing accountability group. The warm support and sound advice provided by Lorena Garcia, Anna Guevarra, Ayesha Hardison, and Andy Clarno served me well through the protracted and often alienating process of writing. In addition, my friends, colleagues, and mentors in the Future of Minority Studies community have provided me years of guidance, inspiration, and laughter.

I owe a debt of gratitude to Douglas Mitchell at the University of Chicago Press. I greatly enjoyed the production and editing process because of his unwavering commitment to good theoretical and ethnographic work, his willingness to engage in invigorating intellectual debate, and his enthusiastic support. I do not think most first authors are lucky enough to get such an incredible experience. I must also thank Tim McGovern for his meticulous and timely guidance through the review and editing process, as well as the entire editing, design, production, and marketing team at the University of Chicago Press.

Kelly Underman undertook the arduous and monotonous task of transcribing many of my interviews, running statistical analyses of the survey data, and checking historical and archival facts. Her eye for detail and willingness to put up with my compulsiveness are much appreciated. I must also thank Carly Siuta for the data entry work, and Jan Williams, who did a tremendous job with the index.

Although academics are too often encouraged to disavow their emotions for the sake of science, I would certainly not have survived or succeeded without the unwavering support and love of my family. This includes two of my most cherished long-term friends, Anna Zogas and Cedric de Leon, as well as the entire Decoteau and Clarno clans. Words cannot capture the depths of my appreciation. I'd like to thank Pam and Jack, in particular, for their persistent encouragement and pride, which never ceases to boost my spirits and keep me going.

My final and most heartfelt gratitude is reserved for my partner, Andy Clarno, whose tireless support, careful criticism, and revolutionary passion has been a bulwark. Without him, the years and struggles that went into conducting this research and writing this book would have been far more grueling and much less enjoyable. Shukran katir, habibi.

Note on Terminology

Language is always a political matter, and this is particularly true in a country with such a racially complex history. Therefore, it is essential that I explain some of the semiotic choices I made in representing South African society. First and foremost, the terms I use for racial demarcations themselves must be contextualized. Under apartheid, there were four legal racial categories: African (approximately 75 percent of the population), White (13 percent), "Coloured" (9 percent), and "Indian" (3 percent). The African population was further divided into ethnic categories that were used to segregate rural areas into "homelands" and urban townships by neighborhood. In an attempt to counter these racial categorizations and the division they sought to inculcate, the Black Consciousness Movement utilized the term "Black" to demarcate everyone who was denied privileges by whites, thereby forging a united cross-racial sensibility. Following this political trend, I use the term "Black" to refer to all nonwhite peoples of contemporary South Africa, but utilize the term "African" to refer to those populations of African descent (who make up the majority of the research participants of this study). This is not an uncontroversial compromise, but one to which I am committed, given the added confusion wrought by the post-apartheid commitment to "nonracialism" despite the continued exacerbation of racial inequalities.

I have chosen to use the term "indigenous healing" in the place of "traditional healing" despite the fact that "traditional healing" has become a commonplace and even institutionalized nomenclature for all indigenous forms of healing, and healers themselves choose to represent their own organizations and profession using the term. Most Africans also use the term "traditional healing" to refer to the various practices *izangoma* and *izinyanga* perform. However, I hold that the term "traditional healing" is problematic since it buttresses the false but prevalent assumption that indigenous healing is timeless, rigid, and static. It also contributes to the false binary this project is attempting to dismantle between the reified constructs of "traditionalism" and "modernity." Therefore, in my own analysis, I use the term "indigenous healing," but when quoting others, I have left the term "traditional" intact.

I used an interpreter for the interviews and focus group discussions I held with African populations. Although I took courses in isiZulu, which helped me follow conversations in isiZulu, the complexity and the sensitivity of the issues being discussed necessitated interpretation. In addition, many of the participants in this research did not speak isiZulu. Some were migrants from other regions of South Africa and preferred to speak in isiXhosa or seSotho, or more rarely, isiNdebele, tshiVenda, or seTswana. Many, who grew up in Soweto, spoke the slang often referred to as isiCamtho or Tsotsitaal, which are hybrid dialects that combine and creolize several African languages (most notably seSotho, isiZulu, and English). Torong Ramela, my interpreter, was fluent in all eleven South African languages and enjoyed conversing with people in their preferred tongue. As such, all quotes are interpretations of the original.

From this point on, I will avoid the use of prefixes and suffixes for African words. For example, the Zulu language is referred to as isiZulu, and the people amaZulu (or in the singular, umZulu); however, I will simply refer to both the language and the people as "Zulu" to avoid confusion for non-African-language speakers. Similarly, I refer to diviners as *sangomas*, as opposed to *izangoma*, and herbalists as *inyangas* in the place of *izinyanga*.

Abbreviations

3TC	Lamivudine (an antiretroviral drug)
ACT UP	AIDS Coalition to Unleash Power (US-based treatment activist organization)
AIDS	Acquired Immune Deficiency Syndrome
ALP	AIDS Law Project (has been incorporated into a new NGO titled Section 27)
ANC	African National Congress
APF	Anti-Privatisation Forum
ART	Antiretroviral therapy
ARVs	Antiretrovirals
AZT	Zidovudine (an antiretroviral drug)
BEE	Black Economic Empowerment
BI	Boehringher Ingelheim (the pharmaceutical company that patented nevirapine)
BIG	Basic Income Grant
CD4	Measurement of white blood cell count, also referred to as T-cell
COSATU	Congress of South African Trade Unions
DOH	Department of Health
DOT	Directly Observed Therapy
DRD	Durban Roodepoort Deep (often used as a moniker for Sol Plaatjie)
FDA	Food and Drug Administration (US)
FGD	Focus group discussion
GATT	General Agreement on Tariffs and Trade
GEAR	Growth, Employment, and Redistribution Macroeconomic Strategy
GSK	GlaxoSmithKline (the pharmaceutical company that patented AZT and 3TC)
HAART	Highly Active Antiretroviral Therapy
HBC	Home-based care

HIV   Human Immunodeficiency Virus
HSRC   Human Sciences Research Council
IMF   International Monetary Fund
IPR   Intellectual property right
LPM   Landless People's Movement
MCC   Medicines Control Council
MEC   Member of the Executive Council
MRC   Medical Research Council
MSF   Médecins sans Frontières, Doctors without Borders
MTCTP   Mother-to-Child-Transmission-Prevention
NAPWA   National Association of People with AIDS
OI   Opportunistic infection
PMA   Pharmaceutical Manufacturer's Association
RDP   Reconstruction and Development Programme
SANAC   South African National AIDS Council
STI   Sexually transmitted infection
TAC   Treatment Action Campaign
TB   Tuberculosis
THO   Traditional Healers Organization
TRIPS   Agreement on Trade-Related Intellectual Property Rights
UNGASS   United Nations General Assembly Special Session (on HIV)
USAID   United States Agency for International Development
WHO   World Health Organization
WTO   World Trade Organization
ZCC   Zion Christian Church

They told us to wait. So we waited. We saw apartheid criminals go free and men who called themselves leaders become rich. We saw them give up their red t-shirts for silk suits made in Italy. We watched as their bellies swelled and their voices thinned in their new accents of the market and the state. Still we waited. Fifteen years now we have been waiting, here in this place they call Orange Farm—a farm where nothing grows.

Fifteen years ago, hope brought us to this place. Some came here fleeing the violence of those who killed in the name of party and power, others came when they closed the factories where we once worked, or to escape the misery of life in the overcrowded backyard shacks in every Gauteng township. But we all came here because we hoped for more—for ourselves, and our children. Then, the world around us was changing, "Freedom is coming," they said, and all we had to do was wait. "Just wait, and don't forget to vote." So we waited, and we voted. We waited while they went fishing with Roelf Meyer, had tea with Verwoerd, and mourned Harry Oppenheimer. We waited while they cut our electricity and installed prepaid meters. We waited as HIV/AIDS killed our friends and relatives. We waited in darkness and rain. . . . We waited and nothing happened. No roads. No toilets, no houses and no jobs. Nothing . . . or what might as well have been.

So, we are not waiting anymore. None of us were born here. Still, each day, we bury our children here. Perhaps they thought we were waiting to die or maybe they simply forgot that we were alive. But we are not waiting, now we are . . . saying, "give us, or we take."

There will be no peace without development.

THE ORANGE FARM WATER CRISIS COMMITTEE, OCTOBER 2006

Postcolonial Paradox

Thulani Skhosana[1] grew up living in a squatter camp in the Orlando neighborhood of Soweto,[2] the largest township in apartheid South Africa. Although originally referred to as Forty-Seven, the camp was dubbed Mandelaville when Nelson Mandela was released from prison in 1990.[3] Thulani was born in the 1970s, a radical time to live in Soweto—a time when the struggles against the apartheid regime were at their peak, which were led, for the most part, by South Africa's youth. Thulani spent a lot of time going back and forth between his grandmother's four-room house and the shack where his older brother, Sibusiso, lived in Mandelaville. By the time he was in high school, he lived full time in the camp.

We used to be ashamed of ourselves, ashamed of where we come from . . . because we lived in informal settlements.[4] We would go with friends from the township, and we were ashamed . . . because we were poorer than everyone else . . . [quietly] . . . but it builds you as well. To be poor, it builds you, to be strong. Because I'm stronger than people who were rich before, or not people who were rich, but my friends who were better than me, you know. And I'm naturally stronger than them [laughs] because I was not born with a silver spoon in my mouth.[5]

Activists and guerilla fighters with the African National Congress (ANC) used the squatter camp to hide from the police. Some of Thulani's earliest memories were of the combined fear and excitement involved in hiding the soldiers of his country's revolution in his home while the police were shooting in the streets outside. "We helped to hide activists, and because of this, the police would come and raid us. They would come at any time. Everyone had to get up and be counted—if you didn't have a permit,[6] you would be arrested. We resisted the apartheid government—they tried to evict us and were unable to."[7]

It was a constant struggle for the residents of Mandelaville to remain in the area. Although they lived in shacks and didn't have water, electricity, or sanitation services, they were in a prime location—close to opportunities for work, as well as the local clinic, schools, parks, and grocery stores. Many, like Thulani, had family in the area. Residents were evicted on a regular basis, and so the population of Mandelaville was in a constant state of flux. Rates of crime and violence were also incredibly high.[8]

From the time Mandela was released from Robben Island in 1990 to the first democratic elections held in 1994, a palpable euphoria overcame the Black populations of South Africa. Finally, they could glimpse their hard-won freedom and the end to the brutal years of racism, oppression, and violence. They were convinced that the world and their own opportunities for success would suddenly and radically change forever. Despite the expedited and comprehensive nature of the *political* changes in South Africa (from the unbanning of anti-apartheid movements, to rapid democratization, voter franchise, the adoption of the constitution, and the Truth and Reconciliation Commission), the lives of most working-class and poor Africans either failed to improve or got progressively more and more difficult in the early years of democracy.

CD: Were there any significant changes in 1994/1995 with the political transition?
Environmentally, there was no significant changes . . . We continued to struggle with our daily struggles. Mainly, you know, the issue of shacks . . . electricity . . . toilets. People were facing a very serious challenge of crime in the area. . . . One thing is that . . . there were also divisions and then different, I mean, hopes for the community. Because as the time goes on, the struggles changed, you know, its form or shape. . . . To say that now we need a better place than this one that we are staying in. And other people, you know, they wanted to stay where they were, in Mandelaville . . . there was an announcement that the government has found a place for us, you know, we were all going to be relocated . . . this was in 1999. The new government proposed that we be removed to Cosmo City—which is in the northern part of Gauteng, far away from the city. . . . The leadership in Mandelaville refused.[9]

In December 2001, the community was once again told that it was going to be relocated, but no one believed it—most of the residents had been successfully fighting eviction their whole lives. Not this time. On January 7, 2002, the eviction squad showed up with trucks, bulldozers, and guns. "We were forcibly evicted. My kids still ask me about January 7th. We were held at gunpoint. Those who resisted were arrested."[10] Shacks were razed to the ground; people struggled to hold onto their household goods and keep their families together. Residents were loaded onto trucks that were piled high with belongings shoved quickly into plastic bags and any pieces of zinc they could manage to grab from the rubble the bulldozers left. The community was dropped off in a disused mining compound called Sol Plaatjie that none had ever before laid eyes on. When asked what he thought of his new home when he first saw it, Bongani Sibeko said: "Yeah, I saw that it's like we were—I need an appropriate word—like, condemned."[11] People struggled to build homes on this new land, still devoid of electricity, water, and sanitation, and much farther removed from job opportunities and social services.

Adding insult to injury, the residents later discovered that the city had sold the land in Soweto on which they had been squatting to a private housing developer. The land remains empty to this day. According to Thulani:

When we were evicted in 2002, it was because the government didn't want Mandelaville to be seen—it was an eyesore that showed the lies of the "new" South Africa . . . but now in Sol Plaatjie, people are tired . . . they adapt slowly to their conditions. They stop fighting and just accept what they have.[12]

In 2004, Thulani fell ill and told no one. At the time, he was working two small jobs and trying to attend an evening business school to get a certificate to improve his employment opportunities in the future. But he kept getting sick and missing work, or school, or both. He finally told his boss he had been diagnosed with HIV.

That's where I messed up . . . because people started talking about me. And I didn't feel safe. I didn't feel okay. And I had a lot of stress . . . I finally just gave up . . . Gave up, because I was running four feet behind, yeah. I can't . . . can't make it to school. I can't . . . I have no money, and, you know . . . I . . . [could have] cope[d] if I had . . . other revenues. . . . Because with that money I had to buy food, I had to look after my kids as well, you know. I have to travel, and that . . . I had to take a train and it takes time and money . . . I gave up.[13]

3

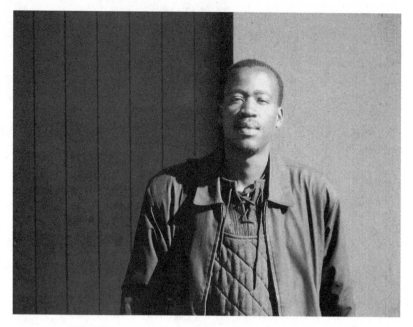

FIGURE 1.   Thulani Skhosana. Photo taken by the author in June 2005.

Thulani was hospitalized. "I think it was because of . . . [*pause*] . . . insecurity."[14] He stayed in the hospital for two months, and he returned home to find he had lost his job and his wife. He has never again worked formally. "I wish I could work . . . I don't like having to ask people for things . . . it's just . . . so unfair that I'm forced to in order to just survive."[15]

Thulani's story is not unique. The life histories of people living in South Africa's contemporary squatter camps are filled with accounts of bitter remorse and profound disappointment. A recent BBC article covered the story of veterans of the anti-apartheid struggle who never received compensation for their services, including health care and pension funds, despite promises the ANC made. As one man put it: "The government is forgetting that the same people who feel neglected and marginalised now are the same people who set the townships on fire in the 80s and brought the apartheid government to its knees" (Fihlani 2011).

After fighting apartheid, people expected that their lives would improve. But many live in worse material conditions than they did under apartheid and now face a disease that is devastating their communities at apocalyptic rates.

Nothing has changed with this new government. It is the same horse. It is only the jockey who has changed. The jockey is now Black. Apartheid has never changed. . . . We are still discriminated against. Now, it's even worse.[16]

How did this crisis of liberation come to pass?

The Postcolonial Paradox

Practically overnight, the ANC was forced to transform from a militant revolutionary movement into a reputable governing body. In the 1990s it faced a legacy of immense inequality, international pressure to abandon social democratic ideals in exchange for market competitiveness, and a disease that would become an epidemic of unparalleled proportions. The confluence of crises that marked the transition from apartheid to democracy has initiated a whole host of compromises. In 1996 the ANC unequivocally adopted a neoliberal macroeconomic strategy for development, which undermined the social democratic promises under which it had been voted into power. Many have argued that the entrenched inequalities of apartheid have been exacerbated by the adoption of neoliberalism (Bond 2000; Marais 2001). Seekings and Nattrass (2006) find that while there have been some changes in the racial dynamics of inequality, income distribution has only widened since the end of apartheid. Unemployment rose steadily in the first decade after apartheid and has plateaued at approximately 25 percent; however, it reaches 37.7 percent when discouraged work-seekers are included (Statistics South Africa 2011). Steinberg notes that of those who turned ten in the year South Africa achieved its freedom, only half would ever work a day in their lives by the time they turn twenty-five (Steinberg 2009). According to the United Nations, from 2000 to 2006, 26.2 percent of South Africa's population lived on less than $1.25 per day and 42.9 percent lived on less than $2 per day (UNDP 2007). One of my primary arguments is that it would be impossible to understand the emergence and history of AIDS in South Africa without paying heed to the impact of neoliberal economic restructuring and the country's often-contradictory relationship to globalizing forces.

It is clear that when the ANC took power, many of its leaders were aware of the risk HIV/AIDS posed if left unaddressed. Predictions of its scope were included in the 1994 National Health Plan for South Africa, and the National AIDS Convention of South Africa drafted a national

AIDS plan, which the Government of National Unity adopted as policy in 1994 (Heywood 2004b, 2–3).[17] And yet the business of "reconstruction and development," as well as undergoing a Truth and Reconciliation process, took up most of the ANC's time and energy in the first few years of democracy. As such, these predictions of the silent devastation being insidiously wrought by the hidden virus were all but ignored for several years. HIV/AIDS had grown into an epidemic by the time the government finally faced it head on.[18] Nelson Mandela, the first president of the "new" South Africa[19] hardly mentioned AIDS during his presidency and only broke this silence when one of his sons died of the disease five years after he left office (Thornton 2008, 11). In a BBC interview held in 2003, Mandela admitted: "I wanted to win and I didn't talk about AIDS," and then once president, he "had not the time to concentrate on the issue" (Heywood 2004b, 3n1). Despite his importance in South Africa's transition to democracy and his image as father of the nation, he will not figure prominently in this narrative because he has been so peripheral to South Africa's AIDS politics.

In 1993, the prevalence rate among pregnant women attending antenatal (prenatal) clinics was 4 percent, and by 2008 (a mere fifteen years later), this rate had climbed to 29.3 percent (South African Institute of Race Relations, SAIRR, 2010b).[20] The annual number of deaths rose by a massive 93 percent between 1997 and 2006, and among those aged twenty-five to forty-nine years, the rise was 173 percent in the same nine-year period (Statistics South Africa 2008a). As of 2010, almost six million people (5,813,088) had been infected with HIV (SAIRR 2010b).

HIV/AIDS is not indiscriminate in its impact: age, gender, race, and socioeconomic status all play a major role in its distribution. The more marginalized, the higher the infection rate. Archbishop Desmond Tutu once described AIDS as South Africa's new apartheid (*Independent Online* 2001). The prevalence rate among women of all age groups is higher than men (peaking at women, aged twenty-five to twenty-nine, who have a 32.7 percent prevalence rate, twice as high as that of men of the same age) (HSRC 2008a, 30). HIV prevalence in South Africa's African population is substantially greater (at 13.6 percent) than in any other racial group (ibid., 79). And HIV *incidence*[21] in the African population is nine times higher than in any other racial group (Rehle et al. 2007, 196). Similarly, people living in urban informal settlements have a 25.8 percent HIV prevalence rate, higher than rural informal settlements (17.3 percent), rural formal settlements (13.9 percent), and urban formal settlements (13.9 percent) (HSRC 2008a, 40).

The political transition from apartheid to democracy was marked by an ambiguous volleying, on the part of the state elite, between different ideological positions. On the one hand, the ANC promotes a pan-Africanist renaissance that incorporates a biting critique of Western cultural imperialism. On the other, the adoption of economic liberalism has wrenched open South Africa's national borders to the onslaught of international capital and its accompanying ideologies. The dilemma that all postcolonial states face of attempting to sustain a national identity in the face of the deterritorializing forces of globalization is heightened in South Africa for several reasons: its late transition from colonialism, its efforts to maintain its position as an economic leader on the African continent, and its need to deal successfully with the mutual pandemics of AIDS and poverty. AIDS and debates over healing, then, become overdetermined sites for working through what I refer to as the *postcolonial paradox*, which entails a simultaneous need to respect the demands of neoliberal capital in order to compete successfully on the world market *and* a responsibility to redress entrenched inequality, secure legitimacy from the poor, and forge a national imaginary. South Africa is heralded for adopting one of the most progressive constitutions in the world, and it provides substantial social service provisions for the poor and sick. It is also one of the wealthiest countries on the continent. And yet South Africa still maintains the noteworthy distinction of having the highest rates of HIV prevalence in the world, and ranks among the most unequal countries in the world in terms of its income and wealth distribution (UNDP 2009 and 2010).[22] Throughout the book, I show how the battle to resolve the paradoxes of postcolonialism is waged on the terrain of AIDS politics.

Whereas many have argued that the African postcolony is characterized by a particular "banality of power" (Mbembe 2001), this book takes seriously the real contestations the postcolonial state confronts in a neoliberal era—highlighting not only the economic but also the cultural and social stakes at play. In the years since apartheid, the South African public sphere has become a laboratory for a vociferous symbolic struggle over the signification of AIDS, taking place among developmental state actors, biomedical proponents, and indigenous healers. These symbolic struggles have proven to be fertile ground on which to resuscitate the idealized colonial constructs of "tradition" and "modernity," which the apartheid state utilized to implement and justify indirect rule (Mamdani 1996) and are now being rearticulated in the post-apartheid era in an attempt to resolve the postcolonial paradox. "Modernity" and "traditionalism" are binary constructs that serve to order and discipline the social, but as idealized tropes, they are malleable, and as discourses, they can be used strategically to mobilize power. Because they help to define the national body politic, they are often utilized to reconfigure the symbolism of and relationship between race, class, gender, and sexuality. They are also often used, in the context of HIV/AIDS, to construct and sustain what I refer to as a "myth of incommensurability"—the ideology that indigenous (read "traditional") and biomedical (read "modern") forms of healing are irreconcilably incompatible.

There are many constitutive elements of the postcolonial paradox. In the rest of this chapter, I discuss South Africa's adoption of and contested relationship to neoliberalism as well as the ways in which national imaginings and the epistemological anxieties invoked by the AIDS pandemic have shaped the early years of the "new dispensation."[23] Postcolonial paradoxes are not only felt by and dealt with at the state level, the poor also contend with their exigencies and place pressure on the state to resolve the crises of liberation they experience. This book will consistently draw connections between the macro- and microlevels—insisting therefore, not only on the reciprocal nature of causality, but also on the often complex and contradictory relationship between global processes, national policies, and local practices. The book traces the history of the biopolitics of AIDS in the post-apartheid era, but it positions this story within the squatter camp, considering HIV/AIDS politics from the perspective of those in whose name these battles are fought but who have been rendered voiceless in the telling. As such, the book details what it is like to live with and die of AIDS in South Africa's urban slums.

Neoliberal Regulation and Governance

In an attempt to deconstruct the teleological myths of Western versions of "modernity," postcolonial scholars have begun to retell the story of colonialism, highlighting the mutually constitutive nature of the "encounter."[24] A similar recasting is required of the era of neoliberalism. Not to downplay the coercive means by which neoliberalism was force-fed to countries in the global periphery through structural adjustment programs and bilateral trade agreements—mostly for the financial benefit of the industrialized North. But the story simply does not end there. Countries in the global South fought back and have thus been major players in the reconstitution of neoliberalism at the global level.

Peck and Tickell (2002) argue that Margaret Thatcher and Ronald Reagan implemented "roll-back" neoliberalization in the 1980s, which was characterized by the active destruction of Keynesian-welfarist interventions and the deregulation of the market. Neoliberal policies were introduced in this period to deal with either perceived crises of Keynesian regulatory regimes (more often in the global North) or with postcolonial national development (in the global South) (Brenner, Peck, and Theodore 2010, 214). This form of neoliberalism led to growing inequality, a series of recessions throughout the world, and widespread public protest—from Seattle, to Chiapas, to Johannesburg. However, instead of imploding, neoliberalism was reconstituted such that market liberalism was accompanied by socially interventionist reforms "epitomized by the Third Way regimes of Clinton and Blair" (Peck and Tickell 2002, 384, 388–89). This "rollout" neoliberalism retains its economic bottom line but buttresses it with attention toward institution building, civil society participation, good governance, social safety nets, and poverty eradication. Here, more government is needed to "mask and contain the deleterious social consequences . . . of the deregulation of wage labor and the deterioration of social protection" (Wacquant 1999, 323).

Porter and Craig, in their analysis of how Third Way regulation has impacted the "Third World" (2004), deploy Karl Polyani's "double movement" thesis to explain how in the first era, "economic liberalization . . . involves the breaking up or disembedding of traditional and local social regulation by market relations, enabling increased, unfettered penetration of market forces," which is then followed by a second embedding movement whereby "'enlightened reactionaries' rally to mitigate the social disruptions of market-led liberalization" (Porter and Craig 2004, 391). The reconstitution and rearticulation of neoliberalism was necessary in the wake of violent and vocal global protests against structural adjustment programs, the privatization of public services, and the contraction of social welfare. "By way of successive, crisis-riven and often profoundly dysfunctional rounds of regulatory restructuring, the ideological creed, regulatory practices, political mechanisms and institutional geographies of neoliberalization have been repeatedly reconstituted and remade" (Brenner, Peck, and Theodore 2010, 210).

The history of South Africa's adoption of neoliberalism differs from other countries in sub-Saharan Africa largely because the apartheid state had already embraced the doctrine and begun to implement its policies long before the ANC took power in 1994—making structural adjustment programs unnecessary. In the mid-1980s, the ANC began negotiations with the South African business elite—the outcome of which was the ANC's reluctant adoption of neoliberalism as a concession to help end apartheid rule.[25] South Africa became a signatory of the General Agreement on Tariffs and Trade (GATT)—the precursor to the World Trade Organization (WTO)—in December 1993. In 1994, the Reconstruction and Development Programme (RDP) was passed. This program was meant to ensure the provision of basic services (housing, land reform, and water and electricity provision) through increases in government subsidies. However, this more progressive development plan was replaced by a neoliberal macroeconomic strategy for development in 1996, when the ANC unilaterally adopted the Growth, Employment, and Redistribution Macroeconomic Strategy (GEAR)—a "home grown version of structural adjustment" (Hart 2008, 681).[26]

"Drawn up by a coterie of mainstream economists, and apparently based on a Reserve Bank model . . . GEAR's prescriptions lit the faces of business, which could not fail to recognise its neoliberal character" (Marais 2001, 163). The plan stipulates measures for liberalizing trade and enhancing export; it advocates fiscal austerity to service national debt, tax incentives for big business, the privatization of "non-essential" state enterprises and state-run utilities, cuts in social spending, and the introduction of wage restraints and "regulated flexibility" in the labor market (ibid., 164–65). There was a subsequent contraction of labor-intensive forms of production, which resulted in sudden increases in unemployment (Hart 2008, 681). Desperate to establish itself as a supporter of the free market, the ANC liberalized trade beyond the rules the WTO demanded (Hunter 2010, 107). The lifting of tariffs left local industry extremely vulnerable, forcing many companies to casualize labor to compete in a newly competitive environment thereby informalizing large swaths of the labor market (ibid.). The ANC's adoption of neoliberalism sparked immediate resistance and drew considerable international attention. Joining forces with activists from Seattle to Chiapas, South Africans forged sustained social movements articulated around antineoliberal themes.

Some have argued that it was in response to these protests that President Thabo Mbeki[27] rather belatedly introduced Third Way politics during his second term of office (a theme I will explore in great detail in chapter 2).[28] I argue against such oversimplifications. In fact, evidence presented throughout this book will highlight the ways in which the economic policies and governmental projects of the post-apartheid state volley back and forth between rollback and rollout neoliberalism fairly consistently in a desperate attempt to keep the paradoxes of postcolonialism at bay. It has been argued that neoliberalism itself facilitates such innovation:

> One of the most striking features of the recent history of neoliberalism is its quite remarkable transformative capacity. To a greater extent than many would have predicted . . . neoliberalism has demonstrated an ability to absorb or displace crisis tendencies, to ride—and capitalize upon—the very economic cycles and localized policy failures that it was complicit in creating, and to erode the foundations upon which generalized or extralocal resistance might be constructed. (Peck and Tickell 2002, 400)

And yet, such an analysis not only yields too much power to an abstract structural system, but it also fails to attend to the forces of resistance that have had and continue to have real effects on the operations of neoliberal power. Further, such an approach tends to afford too great an emphasis on the *economic* aspects of neoliberal regulation and governance. Neoliberalism has become a universal signifier that scholars have yielded tremendous causal force—as such, it has come to stand in for any and all complicated processes associated with the contemporary configuration of global capitalism. Therefore, it is essential to be clear in one's deployment of the term.

Neoliberalism is not simply a particular form of capitalism and therefore should not be understood in economic reductionist terms. It is a global rationality of rule that has enacted massive shifts in the constitution and action of nation-states, in the operation of governance regimes, in the production and circulation of knowledge and expertise, and in the formation and contestation of identities. Capitalism is not always the driving causal force behind these shifts, but is implicated, constituted, and transformed through them. This is not to say, however, that neoliberalism has no outside, that it is everywhere and there are no alternatives. Rather, neoliberalization must be conceptualized as a series of contested processes, which can only be properly analyzed in context-specific ways (Brenner and Theodore 2002). This book and the history of biopolitics it chronicles will reveal the very important ways in which neoliberal governmentality has shifted in response to resistance. In addition, in describing the experiences of those most marginalized by these policies, I will show how the translation of global processes and national policies, at the local level, is replete with contradiction and uncertainty. The failures and fissures involved in population regulation and processes of incorporation leave open important spaces of potential for radical social change.

Fantasies of Independence

In his compelling analysis of economic decline in the Zambian Copperbelt, James Ferguson (1999) shows how deindustrialization shattered the teleological myth of modernization, resulting in a profound sense of betrayal and loss, as people's capacity for making meaning of their situations was compromised (13–14); thus the economic crisis was coupled with an epistemological one. He argues that the processes of globalization have "abjected" Africa from the hope of a modernist future (236). While his careful ethnographic analysis of the effects of deindustrialization is insightful and informative, I would like to suggest that the "myths of modernization" that have captured the hearts and minds of Africans are not the same as Western teleological narratives of progress. Rather, they are postcolonial to the core and involve a radical rejection of Western versions of "modernity."

If nationalisms in the rest of the world have to choose their imagined community from certain "modular" forms already made available to them by Europe and the Americas, what do they have left to imagine? History, it would seem, has decreed that we in the postcolonial world shall only be perpetual consumers of modernity. Europe and the Americas, the only true subjects of history, have thought out on our behalf not only the script of colonial enlightenment and exploitation, but also that of our anticolonial resistance and postcolonial misery. Even our imaginations must remain forever colonized. (Chatterjee 1993, 5)

Taking heed of Chatterjee's warning, I would like to forward a theory of the fantasies[29] of independence that are fueled by but also shape South Africa's postcolonial paradoxes. The primary current undergirding these fantasies is a desire to prosper economically through engagement with the global market while rejecting Western imperialism and dependency, and cultivating some unique, national articulation of Africanness. There is a certain impossible teleology of development implied, wherein all South Africans share equitably in the profits earned from playing the neoliberal market, coupled with a simultaneous recognition that certain portions of the population will have to be forsaken, for the sake of the nation. But in fact this contradiction is a key characteristic of the neoliberal era. The polarization of structural inequality that has led to the conspicuous accumulation of decadence and the simultaneous immiseration of the poor is constitutive of the same neoliberal totality, despite all of the teleological promises of "development" (Žižek 2011).

Jean and John Comaroff (2000) note that one of the prevailing characteristics of what they term "millennial capitalism" is the way in which nation-states have been disarticulated (the nation and the state have been ruptured from each other) by various global forces: nation-states have come under attack by supranational institutions, by civil society organizations, and by their own attempts to trim down to meet the needs of neoliberal capital. This makes constructing narratives of nationalism and fabricating senses of community, based on something more than money, an absolute imperative in the millennial era (327). The fantasies of independence of which I speak attempt to articulate the boundedness of the nation in precisely this way. Mbeki recounted the tale of an African renaissance, while the current president, Jacob Zuma,[30] tells a more populist narrative, a kind of South African version of the American Dream, tinged with Zulu symbolism.

Theorists of nationalism have often discussed the Janus-faced quality (McClintock 1995, 358) of national imagining: "[Nationalism] presents itself both as a modern project that melts and transforms traditional attachments in favour of new identities and as a reflection of authentic cultural values culled from the depths of a presumed communal past" (Kandiyoti 1991, 431).[31] South African national fantasies of independence similarly make use of the tropes of "modernity" and "traditionalism"—which are reconfigured in the post-apartheid era and deployed toward divergent political ends by different actors. Incommensurability is the language used to make political claims about South Africa's position in the global market, relationship to Western states and institutions, and ability to fulfill the promises of liberation. The binary between "traditionalism" and "modernity" sustains and reinforces other dichotomous divisions, which still operate with force in contemporary South Africa: urban/rural, white/Black, healthy/diseased, rich/poor, male/female. Bruno Latour famously warned that "we have never been modern" because the binaries on which modernity relies unconsciously and necessarily produce hybridities that always exceed and defy categorization (1991). Similarly, the deployment of "traditionalism" and "modernity" in South African national imaginings produces a whole series of disavowed hybridities. This is particularly the case with AIDS—as people infected with HIV are asked to "choose" either indigenous or biomedical approaches to healing, but instead defy the state and the biomedical community by using both forms of healing simultaneously.

Because fantasies are constructed to disguise a repressed recognition of their own lacks, they are fragile and take constant and vigilant "ideological work" to maintain (Žižek 1989; 1997). As such, they must be told again and again—especially and most forcibly when they are in peril. The poor undermine the post-apartheid imaginary, but they also expose the disavowed truth at its core: that not everyone will reap the rewards of liberation. Most Black South Africans fought with or alongside the ANC in the violent struggles against apartheid, and many of the poor feel as though they were subsequently abandoned by the ANC once freedom was won. "We trusted the ANC with all our hearts. We helped to put them in power, and they turned around and treated us like shit."[32] The poor have fought back against their symbolic and material marginalization—through their participation in new social movements, through violent uprisings that consistently spring up spontaneously around the country over basic service provision, and through their voting power. The ANC cannot ignore the poor—they are a powerful force in the post-apartheid imaginary. And I argue that it is, in part, through the savvy political manipulations of "traditionalism" and "modernity" that the state attempts to salvage its image as *post*colonial and thus *post*racist, despite the exacerbation of racial, gender, and economic inequalities. The tropes of "modernity" and "traditionalism" become powerful tools in the tricky political maneuvering required of leaders who must represent the interests of the people, while subscribing to the economic policies of global capital—which often requires using the politics of recognition to cover up the lack of material redistribution (Fraser 1997).[33]

The Poors

Everywhere there is evidence of an uneasy fusion of enfranchisement and exclusion.
(COMAROFF AND COMAROFF 2000, 299)

I first went to Johannesburg to conduct exploratory field research in the fall of 2002, which was a watershed moment in the post-apartheid era. When it became clear that the ANC's adoption of neoliberalism as a macroeconomic strategy was going to make it impossible to fulfill its liberation promises and address South Africa's legacy of racial and economic inequality, many South Africans became disenchanted with the ANC. The World Conference Against Racism (WCAR) held in Durban in 2001, and the World Summit on Sustainable Development held in Johannesburg in 2002 provided platforms for launching "new social movements," framed around antineoliberal themes, partially because they allowed for networking with other social movements of their kind throughout the world (Hart 2008, 681). Ashwin Desai (2002) argues that a new collective identity was forged out of these community struggles—"the poors"—who fight on the front lines of a war against neoliberal capital and the postcolonial compromises made by the state and its ruling elite.

I became immediately involved in two of the "new social movements" active in Johannesburg at the time: the Anti-Privatisation Forum (APF), which mobilized against the privatization of water and electricity mostly in African townships, and the Landless People's Movement (LPM), which represented the rights of slum dwellers and fought against the World Bank–sanctioned approach to land redistribution, which has been largely responsible for the fact that only 7 percent of South Africa's land has been redistributed since apartheid fell (Lahiff 2010). In fact, it is through these social movements that I first met Thulani Skhosana and Pheello Limapo, who made this project possible because they welcomed me into their lives and introduced me to their communities of Sol Plaatjie and Lawley.

Hein Marais (2011) has recently suggested that the scope and impact of these "new social movements" have been romantically overexaggerated by leftist intellectuals: "Protests were talked up as proof of growing disgruntlement with the government, of a potential shift in allegiances and the beginnings of a 'counter-hegemonic movement.' . . . The expectancy was overcooked" (450). In addition, despite the development and growth of "new social movements" positioned in opposition to the ANC, election results show increasing support for the party throughout the post-apartheid era. Although voter turnout has decreased from the 86 percent of South Africans who voted in the first democratic elections in 1994, it is still dramatically high compared to the United States, and support for the ANC has only grown in each subsequent election. In the 1999 election, there was 68 percent voter turnout, and 66.36 percent of the votes were for the ANC; in 2004, there was 77 percent voter turnout, and 69.69 percent of the votes were for the ANC; and in 2009, there was 77.3 percent voter turnout, and the ANC earned 65.9 percent of the votes (EISA 2010). In addition, the "new social movements" that once enjoyed diverse and wide-reaching support in South Africa's urban centers in the early 2000s began faltering and losing both local support and political clout in the late 2000s—suffering from brutal assaults and clampdowns from the state but also from their own political fracturing.

Despite all of these complications, one cannot discount the power of the poor to challenge state policy or the seriousness with which the poor have continued to experience a crisis of liberation in the post-apartheid era. Spontaneous uprisings erupt in squatter camps and townships throughout South Africa on a daily basis, but especially in the run-ups to local government elections—often in direct protest against ANC elected officials and policies like the privatization of water and the installation of prepaid meters. Mark Hunter suggests that the "weak form of social citizenship" offered by increases in social grants was used strategically by the state to cover up for the lack of structural redistribution and its overwhelming failure to address rising unemployment and inequality—a strategy essential for maintaining its "continued support at the ballot box" (2010, 107–8). In addition, growing disgruntlement with neoliberal economic policy is often cited as one of the primary causes of Mbeki's ousting from the office of the presidency in 2007 and his eventual replacement by the populist and supposedly "pro-poor" figure of Jacob Zuma in 2009. Zuma's impoverished, self-educated, guerrilla-warrior background made him the first public persona with whom the poor could actually identify.

The double-edged character of official deployments of nationalism in the context of escalating inequality and persistent deprivation is also crucial to grasping popular support for Jacob Zuma . . . part of what Zuma represents is a move to seize the mantle of the liberation struggle, and present himself as its rightful heir. Positioning himself as the hero of national liberation is the key to Zuma's capacity—at least for the time being—to articulate multiple, often contradictory meanings into a complex unity that appeals powerfully to "common sense" across a broad spectrum. (Hart 2008, 692)

The poor continue to support the ANC at the polls, despite their resentment of never having shared in the spoils of the anti-apartheid struggle and their anger over the fact that their daily living conditions are in many ways worse than they were under apartheid. This contradiction is a primary example of how the poor are tied into and informed by the paradoxes of postcolonialism. The poors' experience of an acute crisis of liberation (and jealousy and anger over growing economic inequality *within* the African population) often involves a certain volleying among belief, trust, and hope in the government to resistance against it. Thulani's criticisms of the failures of the ANC have been a major focus of this chapter, and yet when I returned to South Africa in 2009 (after Zuma's election), Thulani had rejoined the

ANC Youth League. He explained that the ANC under Mbeki had, momentarily, forgotten its base—they had gotten tied up with trying to get rich, supporting the interests of the Black bourgeoisie alone. The way in which the poor perceived the shifting configurations of racial inequality, watching as some few African politicians and businessmen got rich, while the rest of the African population was further immiserated, was a major source of resentment and betrayal among the South African masses in the early years of democracy.

Mbeki's ANC . . . represented the rich, you know. And then most of them, they wanted—they benefited from things like BEE [Black Economic Empowerment], but the rest of us . . . we didn't. But Zuma's vision is that everyone benefits from democracy. . . . We see even the ANC calling on all the people of South Africa to come together and protect the democracy. [*Pause*] That's when we revived [*pause*] our struggle with the ANC, that, you know, we need to protect the democracy so that we can also benefit. . . . Zuma is not that much of an intellectual, who will sideline people, poor people, you know, most of the poor people, people who didn't go to school and that. We . . . We identify with him . . . and I believe in him as a true leader of the poor people of our country.[34]

The poor get wrapped up in the promises the nationalist fantasies of independence foretell. This is, for many, because they desperately need something to hope for. And this is precisely what Zuma provided—momentarily, at least. As of August 2012, his popularity is already being replaced by a renewed sense of political betrayal. This cyclical waxing and waning of support for the ANC leadership and the national liberation they continue to both promise and forestall is a sign of the unresolved postcolonial paradox that haunts the political unconscious of the nation.

The Biopolitics of AIDS

AIDS has been rewriting the global geopolitical coordinates within which we think and act. . . . Coming as it did at the time of a radical restructuring of the axes of a bipolar world, of the liberal-democratic nation-state and the workings of capitalism itself, the disease served as both a sign and vector of a global order-in-formation—and with it, a new sense of the nature and possibilities of the political. (COMAROFF 2007, 198)

With the rise of neoliberalism, one can hardly discuss global governance without paying heed to the politics of the pharmaceutical industry, the struggles over intellectual property rights and access to essential medicines, not to mention the important ways in which biomedicine, through the public health industry, seeks to ever expand both its cultural and economic hold over the regulation of population health. There is, therefore, an intimate and complicated relationship between neoliberal macroeconomics and global biopolitics. This is why AIDS politics has consistently been one of the primary terrains for managing and attempting to resolve the paradoxes of postcolonialism.

Thabo Mbeki will be remembered throughout the world for his "AIDS denialism." This is the label most commonly used to refer to the belief held by the former president and several key members of his Department of Health that HIV does not cause AIDS and that antiretroviral treatment[35] is toxic. In a macabre kind of irony, this denialism, which stalled the rollout of antiretrovirals and subsequently contributed to the loss of almost half a million lives,[36] most of them within the African population, was inspired by a strong belief that the international public health approach to AIDS was inherently colonialist and racist. Mbeki was critical of the assumptions about African sexuality underpinning international epidemiological approaches to HIV causality, and he questioned the power of the pharmaceutical industry and the massive profits it stood to gain from the AIDS pandemic in Africa should antiretrovirals be purchased to stem its tide. Further, Mbeki suggested that biomedical science was couched in an imperialist paradigm that ignored the cultural and racial identity of Africans. "The Western way of fighting AIDS will not transfer to Africa" (ANC 2002). Indigenous healing was therefore introduced into public sphere discourses on HIV/AIDS. In this way, the state pitted indigenous healing against biomedical science, thereby maintaining an ideology of incommensurability.

The Treatment Action Campaign (or the TAC)—the primary treatment activist organization in South Africa—fought a long and arduous battle against the denialist state and finally secured the public provision of antiretrovirals, which have been available free of charge in South Africa's public health clinics since 2004. In their battle against denialism, however, the TAC buttressed the idea that biomedical and indigenous forms of healing are mutually exclusive. This quote is from an interview with a prominent treatment activist:

The philosophical division between Western biomedical medicine and traditional medicine is something that you can't overcome . . . either you believe in science or you don't. It's like religion. How it's going to pan out will depend on to what extent . . . the traditional health system is able to give in . . . because it's for their benefit. . . . But you won't be able to get away from the fundamental conflict.[37]

In an effort to distance himself from Mbeki's denialism, Zuma's Department of Health has fully embraced biomedical orthodoxy. In fact, in 2009, Zuma announced a massive expansion of both treatment and prevention efforts in South Africa (Dugger 2009) in which he vowed to cut new infections in half and scale up treatment to 80 percent of those who need it by 2011 (Sidibé 2009). Because the battle over denialism has officially ended, many have suggested that AIDS no longer figures prominently in South Africa's national politics. And yet, I argue throughout the book that AIDS continues to be a terrain upon which postcolonial paradoxes are played out. The biomedicalization of AIDS governance has simply shifted the focus and form of the politicization of the disease.

The provision of antiretrovirals (or ARVs as they are commonly referred to) has restructured welfare rights in the post-apartheid era by biomedicalizing citizenship. This significant shift in policy dovetails other transformations in neoliberal governance at the global scale, but I argue it also serves to reconfigure the contours and technologies of exclusion. As a consequence of these efforts, citizenship rights have become dependent upon the successful adoption of certain health behaviors sanctioned by biomedical practitioners. But people in informal settlements often cannot or will not assume the biomedical technologies of the self required to take ARVs either because of structural obstacles associated with squatter conditions or because the regimen includes a rejection of indigenous healing.

In fact, AIDS has radically shaken the epistemological moorings of both biomedical and indigenous healing paradigms. The fact that the disease is incurable but treatable seriously challenges the ontological foundations of South African indigenous healing. And yet, biomedicine's answer, antiretrovirals, comes with its own complications (a topic I cover in detail in chapter 3). Because of serious underresourcing, public clinics and hospitals have been unequipped to properly manage this epidemic, and so indigenous healers have taken on the huge burden of providing the psychological and social support AIDS sufferers require, in addition to treating symptoms and opportunistic infections.

In many ways, then, living with HIV/AIDS actually *requires* the mixture of biomedical and indigenous approaches to healing. People believe that their illnesses come from multiple different sources (which may be social, spiritual, or physiological); therefore, they require multiple treatment methodologies. Indigenous and biomedical healing are often used for different purposes and cannot always substitute for each other. It is, therefore, unlikely that the increasing availability of biomedical health care (and ARVs in particular) will lead to the demise or disuse of indigenous healing. In people's daily lives and practices, the two forms of healing operate in symbiosis. The perceived incommensurability between the two paradigms of healing, deeply entrenched by the historic struggle between treatment activists and a denialist government, means that there is a profound disjuncture between people's health behaviors and official public health policy.

AIDS also elicits profound epistemological anxiety, as it not only challenges what we know about the world, but also how we live in it, especially in the wake of such tragedy. As Adam Ashforth notes: "The effort to persuade people in this part of the world about the dangers of a retrovirus named HIV also constitutes one of the greatest cultural impositions in the history of these parts. Awareness of AIDS, of the incurable disease brought on by an invisible virus, rarely suffices to make sense of the suffering and death it occasions" (2005, 107). As such, we have much to learn about HIV/AIDS from those who struggle to domesticate it and make sense of the ways it has radically (re)shaped their lives.

Outline of the Book

Overall, the book traces the politics of AIDS from 1994 through 2010 analyzing the political economy of the post-apartheid health system, the shifting symbolic struggles over the signification of HIV/AIDS, and the ways in which communities profoundly affected by the epidemic incorporate culturally hybrid subjectivities, informed by both indigenous and biomedical healing paradigms. The sociological analysis offered in this book is unique in three ways. First, it links together three fields of analysis often atomized in sociological research: the economic, the cultural/discursive, and the subjective/experiential. By showing the multidirectional interrelationship between these different fields, my work addresses core antinomies and rifts within sociology as a whole, but it also highlights the complex interactions among the international, the national, and the local.

Second, the project situates a detailed ethnography within a macro-sociological analysis of global health inequality. In order to provide a context to the experience of suffering,[38] my analysis combines an ethnography situated within communities ravaged by the dual pandemics of poverty and HIV/AIDS,[39] with an analysis of both the *symbolic* and *political* economies of the post-apartheid health system. It locates people's understandings of and experiences with the disease within an analysis of developmental state policy, neoliberal economics, and international policy interventions. In this way, the project links "large-scale events and structures of the world AIDS pandemic" and the "lived experience" of the people in the ethnographic community (Farmer 1992, 262). Ethnographic methods are an essential tool for exploring the way in which disease and health care are experienced and understood by those who are most affected by the disease, but who have been systematically excluded from participation in discussions about how it is addressed at the national and international levels. Each chapter in this book links together the macro and micro, the theoretical and experiential, the structural and the agential. The book interweaves often desperate and disturbing ethnographic details about daily life in South Africa's slums with cultural and politico-economic analysis. To do so, it draws on a rather eclectic toolkit of social theory and in so doing marries abstraction and application.

Finally, my work contributes to a postcolonial critique of sociology by illustrating the ways in which a postcolonial standpoint forces a reconsideration of core tenets of social science research and theory. The three primary theoretical contributions of this book are made possible by this postcolonial orientation. First, I show how "modernity" and "traditionalism" are powerful ideological tools wielded in symbolic struggles for hegemony, but they are also replete with contradictions and inconsistencies. Mbeki and Zuma have recoded the *colonial* tropes of "traditionalism" and "modernity" to deal with the *post*colonial paradox of satisfying the demands of neoliberal capital while simultaneously convincing the masses that their liberation is imminent. Second, I argue that when the shift toward governing health through biomedical citizenship is centered on the squatter camp, it can be understood as a form of exclusionary inclusion. By doling out pills without providing sustainable living conditions, the post-apartheid state has abandoned the poor. Finally, in illustrating how people's health-seeking behavior is informed by *both* Western biomedical healing *and* indigenous healing, I develop a theory of hybrid subjectivity, that contributes to core debates in sociology about agency and identity and their relationship to structural inequality and oppression.

Chapter 1 describes the ethnographic setting for the book as a whole by painting a picture of everyday life in South Africa's squatter camps. It introduces the reader to each of my primary ethnographic sites as well as the central characters in the narrative. It also provides background on people's ontological orientations and vulnerabilities. More than anything, this chapter details the realities of contending with the mutual pandemics of poverty and AIDS.

Each of the next three chapters introduces a main protagonist in the symbolic struggle over AIDS, but also illustrates a shift in the articulation of the postcolonial paradox and in the governance of the poor. Chapter 2 deconstructs Mbeki's "AIDS denialism," and argues it can be understood as both a means of resolving the postcolonial paradox and as a new construction of postcoloniality—one that defies African dependency on Western finance and culture. In the end, I contend that Mbeki's denialism amounted to a form of "necropolitics"—the political decision on whose life is worth living and who must die for the sake of the nation. The chapter ends with a consideration of the effects of political abandonment on the subjectivities of those forced to haunt the margins of the postcolony.

Chapter 3 focuses on the Treatment Action Campaign and its struggle for the public provision of antiretrovirals. The international struggle against patent protection on essential medicines is the backdrop of this movement's success. I argue that the TAC instigated the introduction of biomedical citizenship by linking welfare rights to certain disciplinary biomedical behaviors. The chapter asks: what happens when structural inequality makes the assumption of biomedical technologies of the self impossible?

Whereas Mbeki reconfigured racial politics in his attempt to avoid financing ARV provision while simultaneously promoting African renaissance, Zuma's reign has been characterized by a certain sexualization of politics that I analyze in chapter 4 by comparing the "traditional" sexuality performed by Jacob Zuma with the complex practices of sexuality in the communities where I conducted research. This chapter also illustrates how shifts in the political economy have instigated transformations in gender ideologies and sexual practices in the post-apartheid era.

Chapter 5 analyzes the relationship between indigenous and biomedical healing in South Africa. In so doing, it explores the ways in which people in my ethnographic sites have embodied culturally hybrid identities by amalgamating different African cultures with cultural ideologies derived from international, national, and local influences. This cultural hybridity is made possible by the historical conjuncture of events that marked the transition from apartheid to post-apartheid, and it allows the subjects of post-apartheid to circumnavigate the material strictures erected by both neoliberal economic restructuring and the pandemic itself.

Because AIDS has challenged what we know and how we know it, it has instigated ontological and epistemological crises that have serious ramifications for not only how we understand and respond to the epidemic, but also for how it is lived. The book ends with a coda that reflects on the contribution this book makes to the political battle against the disease in its fourth decade of existence. In so doing, it provides a critique of the ways in which technocratic neoliberal and biomedical solutions have failed to address some of the underlying, fundamental causes of the epidemic. As inequality has become a bemoaned but accepted facet of life in the late neoliberal era, the survival of the poorest of the poor becomes an increasingly political project.

ONE

The Struggle for Life in South Africa's Slums

Pheello Limapo believes he has been HIV-infected since 1994, when he suffered from a serious bout of tuberculosis. "At the time, one of the doctors mentioned HIV, but no one was really familiar with the disease at this point, so this meant nothing to me and I quickly forgot about it."[1] Pheello moved from the Free State to Johannesburg in 2001, where he initially worked in construction, but his constant illnesses made this work difficult at first and eventually impossible. He first lived in central Johannesburg and then moved to a squatter camp about an hour southwest of Soweto, named Lawley, where he still lives today. "My wife and I had a child before we knew we were HIV positive, and the child died. We went to many doctors trying to figure out what was wrong. Another child died before we realized that we were both HIV infected, and that breast-feeding was part of the problem. We had a third child and did *not* breast-feed the child. This child is still fine, healthy and HIV negative."[2] Pheello and Elizabeth had another HIV-negative child (thanks to nevirapine[3] and formula milk) in 2008.

In 1999, Pheello became so ill he was hospitalized, and he was given an HIV antibody test. When he returned for the results, "the doctor called me into a special room where he actually disclosed my status to tell me that I'm positive. . . . Well, I chose not to believe it. . . . When I went home, I decided to keep quiet, not to tell

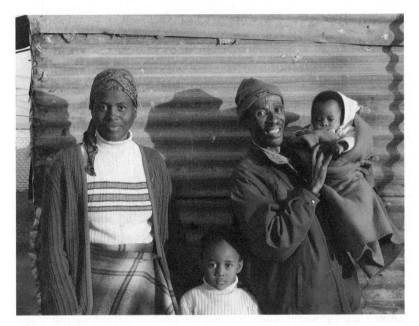

FIGURE 2. The Limapos in front of their home in Lawley. Photo taken by the author in June 2009.

everybody, because I actually saw the kind of circumstances that will come with it, especially if I disclose, because I will be discriminated against at home and by everybody."[4] At another point, he explained: "No one was talking about AIDS. I went to two funerals of comrades I worked closely with in my community . . . and no one mentioned the disease." He paused and took a deep breath, "it was when my brother died that I realized that if I didn't take a chance and talk to people and ask for help, I was going to die just like everyone else . . . with no one knowing."[5]

And so Pheello started talking. He became a strong advocate for himself and the other people in Lawley who were living with or affected by HIV/AIDS. In addition to battling the silences and stigmas that cloak the disease in his community, Pheello has learned there are other more insidious forms of political silence that need to be broken. He became involved in my research, he never ceased to remind me, because he strongly believed that the stories of people living with HIV/AIDS in squatter camps needed to be told as it was all too easy for the government to forget they existed.

It's not that the government has got no capacity or no money to assist people living with HIV. There is a lot of money that is there for AIDS. A lot of this money is
donated from different countries all over the world. . . . And the government is
only the custodian of that money. But instead of the government using that money
where it is supposed to be used—like in the squatter camps, it uses this money
to make millions of condoms and millions of fancy pamphlets. Spending a lot of
money on things that are secondary and not primary. . . . But it's the people in the
squatter camps who are vulnerable. The government does not even try to go to the
squatter camps to find out what is needed. It is the people with the nice lives who
are deciding on the money. People are struggling as we speak—in different squatter camps. But the government does not want to help *us*.[6]

As Mike Davis (2006) points out, the rapid urbanization that has accompanied the global implementation of neoliberal economics has resulted in a "late capitalist triage of humanity" (199) in which millions
of people throughout the world have been converted into surplus populations, abandoned on the peripheries of hypercities, and marginalized
by their inability to participate in the accumulation or consumption of
capital. The plight of informal settlement residents has recently become
a focus of international attention. Indeed, one of the United Nations
Millennium Development Goals is to significantly improve the lives
of slum dwellers globally by 2020 (UN 2010). Despite this increasing
global awareness, there is still much to be learned about the intricate
causal relationships between neoliberalism, urbanization, and disease
epidemiology, as postcolonial countries the world over fight to stem
the tide of increasing informality. In this chapter I provide historical,
ethnographic, qualitative, and quantitative data on two squatter camps
outside of Johannesburg where I have been conducting research since
2004: Sol Plaatjie and Lawley. I begin by providing detailed evidence of
the endogenous relationship between poverty and HIV/AIDS, and then
explain the material and ontological vulnerabilities associated with living in slum conditions.

Informal Settlements

As in other developing countries, the historic "mushrooming" of informal settlements in South Africa began in the 1980s due to rapid
deindustrialization and rising unemployment; however, in the South

African context, the relaxation and eventual eradication of influx controls[7] at the end of the decade accelerated an already escalating rate of urbanization (Hunter 2007; Harrison 1992; Crankshaw 1993). There are different kinds of housing informality in South Africa: "informal settlements" are squatter settlements of the urban poor that develop through the unauthorized occupation of land (Huchzermeyer and Karam 2006, 3). Other informal dwellings include shacks built on serviced sites or in the backyards of formal township houses (Huchzermeyer 1999). From 1996 to 2003 the number of informal dwellings rose by 688,000 in South Africa, despite the existence of house-building projects funded by the state (Hunter 2006, 160–61; *Mail and Guardian* 2006a). By 2009, 14.4 percent of households (1.9 million) in South Africa were informal dwellings or shacks (South African Cities Network 2011, 49).

People move to informal settlements for a number of reasons, which can be attributed to either push or pull factors. Push factors include overcrowding, unaffordable housing, stigma, and eviction, and pull factors are usually associated with job opportunities (or, for HIV-infected South Africans, health care accessibility) (Smit 2006, 108). Often the push factors are more likely with intraurban movement and pull factors with rural-urban migration (ibid.). Intraurban migration is becoming increasingly common. Greenberg notes that the rural-urban migration that marked the apartheid era has simply turned into perpetual migration in the post-apartheid period—as people move from one informal location to another in search of economic security (2004, 31). A community participatory research survey I conducted in Sol Plaatjie and Lawley in 2009 revealed that 75 percent of residents from Lawley and 85 percent of those from Sol Plaatjie most recently lived somewhere else in the Gauteng province[8] before moving to these locations.[9]

Housing is a basic right enshrined in the 1996 South African Constitution (Republic of South Africa 1996b). This right includes not only housing but also secure land tenure, domestic access to basic services (like water, electricity, and sewage), and "socially and economically integrated communities" with "health, educational and social amenities" (Department of Housing 1994). Post-apartheid housing policy is marked by the same antinomy I argue is a result of South Africa's attempt to resolve the postcolonial paradox: the state is committed to and proud of its constitutional goal of providing "adequate housing" to every citizen,[10] and yet it selected a market-based delivery procedure that made this goal practically impossible to achieve.[11] In the early years of democracy, the national government attempted to provide housing through a "one-off product-linked capital subsidy scheme."[12] In other words, people signed on to a queue at the Department of Housing (filling out what is commonly referred to as a C-form), and were slowly allotted small one-room homes, usually on the outskirts of urban centers (where the land is cheaper). But it soon became evident that not only was this an untenable solution but it also exacerbated spatial racial segregation (Huchzermeyer 2001; Greenberg 2004). This venture also sidelined the unemployed or those employed in the informal sector as it assumed access to mortgage finance (Huchzermeyer 2001, 313); it also left completely untouched the tricky political question of informal settlements and squatting (ibid., 323–24). "The challenge," according to Paulos Ntsooa, deputy director of Human Settlements, "is that the residents in these [informal] settlements live in a permanent state of legal and social insecurity. This makes them reluctant to invest in their dwellings to make better living environments" (Social Housing Foundation 2010, 3).

Building low-cost housing has been a key priority of the ANC government in the post-apartheid era. The homes built by the state are referred to as "RDP houses," named for the Reconstruction and Development Programme (the plan adopted in 1994 to deliver services through government subsidies). From 1994 through 2003, the state funded the building of one million RDP houses, which was accelerated in the late 2000s, so that two million had been built by 2007 (Hunter 2010, 110–11; Statistics South Africa 2007a). But during this same period, the number of informal settlements was steadily on the rise. By 2007, two million households still lived in informal dwellings (Statistics South Africa 2007a). Mark Hunter suggests that this is, in part, because unlike the "matchbox" houses built by the apartheid government, which were four rooms and 51.2 square meters, the RDP houses are two-room residences and provide a living space of less than 30 square meters (Hunter 2010, 110).[13] As a result, households have had to break apart, and average household size has decreased dramatically in the post-apartheid era. "Put simply, as the state built RDP houses, thousands of new, overwhelmingly poor, households mushroomed—a reality speaking to the dynamic nature of movements, space and the household. Shacks are not simply a 'legacy' to be overcome through technocratic 'development'" (ibid., 111).

Because of the continued proliferation of squatter camps in the urban areas of South Africa, the national government developed an Informal Settlement Upgrading Programme in 2004 (Huchzermeyer 2006, 41)—intended to move South Africa "towards a shack-free society" (Sisulu 2004; quoted in Huchzermeyer 2006, 44). A further impetus came when South Africa won the bid to host the 2010 World Cup, thus clinching the policy that "visible" informal settlements should be replaced with formal housing,[14] whereas nonvisible informal settlements were to receive in situ upgrading (Huchzermeyer 2006, 45).

The city of Johannesburg established a new approach to "Informal Settlements, Formalisation and Upgrade" in 2008 (Masondo 2008), with the goal of formalizing all informal settlements in the city by 2014. At the time, there were 180 informal settlements in the city, containing 200,000 households (ibid.).[15] "In summary, the policy states that, where possible, informal settlements will be upgraded *in situ*, i.e. where settlements are safely located and their location does not compromise the development objectives of the City," explains Philip Harrison, executive director of development planning and urban management (Davie 2008).

In the late 1990s and early 2000s, many informal settlements were declared un-upgradable, and residents were told this was because of unsafe environmental conditions like undermining and the existence of dolomite.[16] Residents suspected that the government simply used these environmental justifications to warrant eviction in the face of unauthorized land seizure (propelled by a desire to eradicate rather than manage squatter settlements). These suspicions were confirmed when a few years later the formalization of informal settlements was declared the most economical means of providing housing to the urban poor, and many informal settlements previously declared "un-upgradable" were upgraded. Sol Plaatjie is undermined and already suffers from sinkholes, and Lawley residents were told the land was dolomitic. Both were nonetheless upgraded from 2006 to 2008.

Basic service provision was also very politically linked to the issue of housing provision and land tenure. Prepaid water and electricity meters were introduced in the early 2000s in South Africa as a means of combating a perceived "culture of nonpayment," which, it was argued, emerged out of the rent boycotts of the 1980s anti-apartheid struggle.[17] Beginning in August 2003, the South African government created Johannesburg Water, a para-statal organization, to implement the widescale corporatization of water delivery. A neighborhood in Soweto, Phiri, was selected as the site of the flagship project, titled Operation Gcin'amanzi (Operation "Save Water"). The discourse of "water conservation" was used to convince poor people that they were wasting water, and that these systems would allow them to become more responsible consumers. Through the Anti-Privatisation Forum (APF), the residents of Phiri led a major campaign against the prepaid water system and the ideologies used to promote privatization. The APF took Johannesburg Water to court in an attempt to get the prepaid meters declared unconstitutional. After six years and several appeals, the APF lost their case in the constitutional court in the fall of 2009; however, they did manage to increase the basic monthly water allotment. Electricity has also been privatized and is now supplied by another para-statal organization, Eskom. The usage of prepaid technology for a basic service provision has not only been introduced throughout South Africa (over five million households were fitted with prepaid meters in the first ten years of democracy), but the state has also exported both the meters and the necessary technical expertise to countries throughout the continent and the global South (von Schnitzler 2008, 900). Now, informal settlements are only upgraded if the residents agree to the installation of prepaid water and electricity.[18]

Sol Plaatjie

Local residents refer to Sol Plaatjie as DRD. DRD stands for Durban Roodepoort Deep, the mining company whose workers were housed in what has become the squatter camp. The community lives in and around the disused mining compound. The DRD mine, like most of the mines in South Africa, became unprofitable when the technology and labor power required to successfully operate the mine began to cost more than the gold would yield on the market. Mines have become iconic signifiers of the postcolonial world. The former sites of immense wealth and white power now house those who are rendered expendable in a neoliberal world order.

When we first moved here, they told us they would finally bring us water, sanitation, houses . . . and we waited, and there was nothing. And what we saw, this place was . . . more like solitary confinement where we thought we were hidden away from the people, you know, in the disused compound.[19]

Disused land for disposable people. This would be a perfect metaphor if it weren't so painfully literal.

Each of the three primary communities that make up the residents of Sol Plaatjie was forcibly removed from another location in the Johannesburg region. The first community relocated to Sol Plaatjie originally came from Maraisburg and the second from Voeras—the former had been squatting on private land and the latter were living on

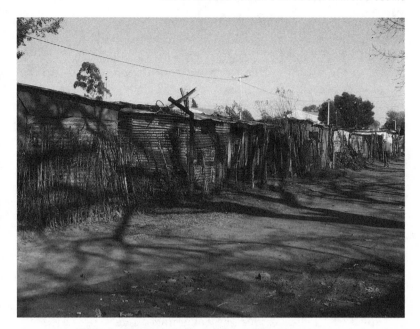

FIGURE 3.   Sol Plaatjie. Photo taken by the author in October 2005.

environmentally unsound land.[20] The residents with whom I worked most closely were evicted from a squatter camp in Soweto, named Mandelaville, in January 2002, which they had occupied since 1976. Mandelaville was a three-block by three-block stretch of land, which was originally the site of a beer hall and police station, both of which were vandalized in the 1976 Soweto uprisings.[21] The community then applied to the local council and received residential permits to occupy the vandalized buildings and turn them into permanent dwellings. The settlement grew throughout the 1980s and 1990s (especially after the influx controls were lifted), and in 2002 there were 1,500 households on the plot.[22]

After the 1994 elections, the residents of Mandelaville (even those who still possessed the original residential permits from the 1970s) were told they were illegally occupying private property. The city had sold the land to a developer to become the site of a new (private) housing development. The community was told they would be relocated to formal housing, but instead they were forcibly removed to Sol Plaatjie. The community fiercely resisted their relocation, but they were finally evicted by court order on January 7, 2002.

In order to justify the forced removal, the Johannesburg Metropolitan Council and the feared eviction company, Wozani Security, told the press that the majority of the residents were "illegal immigrants" or criminals (Human Rights Committee 2002). "[Our] belongings were loaded in the trucks. In fact, the majority of the people had their belongings either willfully damaged or lost . . . [and] most people were not even allowed to take their meager building materials along" (Nimrod Ntsepe, source: Mohlala 2002). Upon their arrival in Sol Plaatjie, the community fought over hostel dwellings that had originally housed migrant mine workers. "It was ugly. Neighbors who had built a community together were fighting each other because if you couldn't get a hostel, you had to build a shack."[23] And many people were forced to sleep outside until they could find materials to build a shack (Human Rights Committee 2002). In the midst of the squatter camp are mine-slag dumps, sinkholes, and the groundwater is heavily polluted from the mining done in the area, making the water provided through community standpipes unpotable. There was no electricity or sanitation service, neither was there a school or clinic. Figures 4, 5, and 6 show Sol Plaatjie prior to its upgrading.

One of the main reasons the community fought relocation was

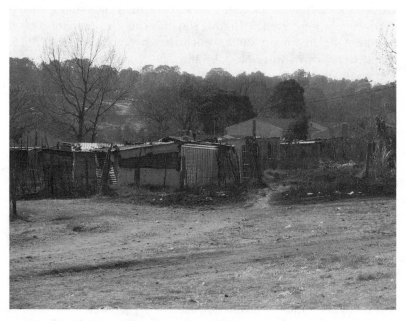

FIGURE 4. Sol Plaatjie shacks. Photo taken by the author in 2005.

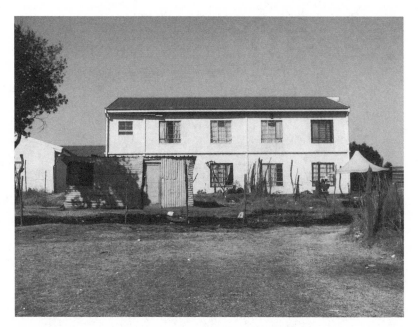

FIGURE 5. Sol Plaatjie hostel. Photo taken by the author in 2005.

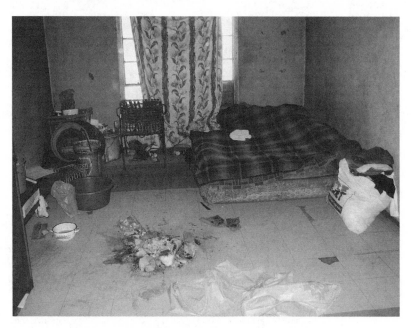

FIGURE 6. Sol Plaatjie hostel—inside. Photo taken by the author in 2005.

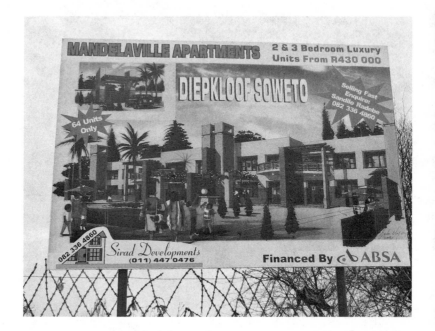

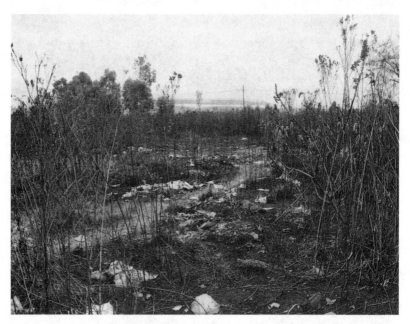

FIGURES 7 and 8.   Mandelaville was still empty four years following the eviction. On the top is an advertisement for the private housing planned for the area. On the bottom is the empty land. Photos taken by the author in 2006.

because although Mandelaville was an informal settlement lacking electricity, water, and proper housing, the residents were close to work opportunities, children could go to school, and there was a clinic that bordered the Mandelaville location. In addition, many of the Mandelaville residents had family in Diepkloof and Orlando, and Soweto had been their home their entire lives. As of June 2006, the land on which the Mandelaville community had lived was still empty (see figs. 7 and 8).

After being relocated, the community fought for proper housing. The court order that led to the relocation stated that the city council had twelve months to provide the residents with *formal* housing. In 2003 the community filed a court case against the city council demanding housing, which was consistently postponed. In late 2005 and early 2006, while I was conducting research in the region, the city developed new plans for the former Mandelaville community. Instead of issuing community members with formal housing in a neighborhood with electricity, water, sewage, education, and health care, the city council had decided to "upgrade" the Sol Plaatjie hostels and build new ones for the shack dwellers in the region. In fact, Sol Plaatjie became the pilot case in Johannesburg for the new Informal Settlement Upgrading Programme. The upgrading process lasted three years, from June 2006 until June 2009. Figures 9 and 10 show the new Sol Plaatjie.

According to the survey I conducted in 2009 (after the upgrades), approximately 51.4 percent of the residents now have formal housing (CPR survey 2009). Of the residents surveyed, 58.3 percent said they lived in a house with running water, but the city is planning to install prepaid water meters, so the residents will be forced to pay 5 to 10 percent of their household income on water. Residents are not sure when they will receive electricity, but the councilor assured me it would also be prepaid.[24] Only 22 percent of residents in Sol Plaatjie are aware that prepaid water and electricity meters will be installed in their communities, but already 65 percent express concerns about how they will be able to pay for these basic services should they be installed (CPR survey 2009).

Despite the so-called upgrading process, people's access to jobs and incomes has changed very little. In 2002 the Centre for Applied Legal Studies at the University of the Witwatersrand conducted a social survey in Sol Plaatjie and found that "households in the lowest quartile received less than R370 [$53] per month. Top quartile households received more than R990 [$141] per month" (Wilson 2003, 5). The survey I conducted in the summer of 2009 revealed that 47.4 percent of the residents surveyed live in a household that has a monthly income

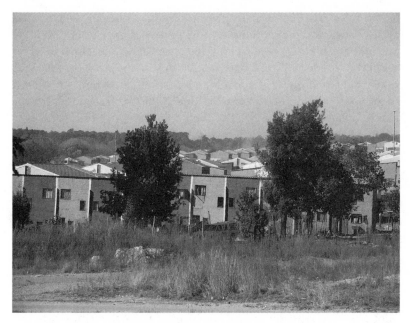

FIGURES 9.   Sol Plaatjie. Photo taken by the author in 2009.

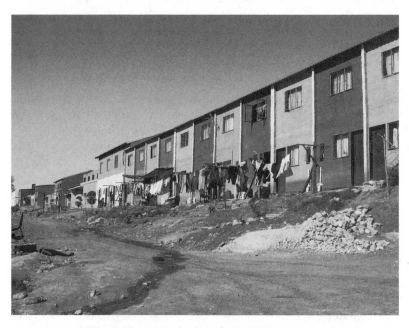

FIGURES 10.   Sol Plaatjie. Photo taken by the author in 2009.

of R500 ($65) or less, and 70.2 percent live in a household that has a monthly income of R1,000 ($129) or less (CPR survey 2009). Obviously, despite the "upgrades," people's capacity to find work and other sustainable forms of survival has not changed.

It is unclear when Sol Plaatjie will be provided a functioning clinic, paved roads, or schools. Most of the houses are two rooms plus a bathroom.[25] Residents insist that this forces the entire household to sleep in the same room, affording very little privacy. In addition, there are no yards for gardens, locations to gather, or places to conduct cultural rituals.

I think sometimes development is a very good thing, but sometimes, I think it comes with challenges. . . . Me, I feel that I'm being taken backwards. I lived in a squatter camp in Soweto, and then they evicted us and sent us here, which was worse. Not only are we still living in shacks, but now we don't have any parks or schools or clinics or anything around us. And we're so far away from everything. But then, they tell us we are finally going to get our houses. And this is what we get? No, it's really not right. We've been fighting for houses our whole lives.[26]

There are three primary problems associated with in situ upgrading. First, local governments struggle to secure land for informal settlement upgrades. In many situations, informal settlements are sites where people are illegally squatting on private land. This land, therefore, has to be purchased by the local government, which often means (as was the case in Sol Plaatjie) people are forced to live on smaller plots of land in overcrowded conditions because of difficulties in securing land tenure.[27] A second serious challenge is that the people must be moved into temporary housing while their settlement is being upgraded. "Transit camps" are thus being constructed, consisting of closely packed prefabricated or zinc structures often without proper water or sanitation. What has also happened in Sol Plaatjie is that after people were moved out of the transit camp and into their permanent residence, they "sold" their shack in the transit camp to a new migrant, so that when the government came to dismantle the transit camps, they found permanent residents who claimed to own their prefabricated shacks. Third, the local government councilor for Region C (where Sol Plaatjie is located) claims one of the most serious challenges for upgrading is the constant influx of new migrants from rural and other urban areas. Development attracts new squatters. Those lucky enough to have received a house out of the court settlement (2,670 units were built)[28] are now surrounded by shack dwellers who still have no access to water, sanitation, or electricity. "We try to stop the growth . . . but when you come tomorrow, you'll find new shacks and stands."[29]

On a recent research trip to Sol Plaatjie in June and July of 2012, I found the community unchanged. There was still no electricity, clinic, or school. Nor were there prepaid water meters. The city was in the process of paving the roads. The shack settlement in the community had grown significantly.

Lawley

People began squatting on the "Lawley Farm" in 1943 after being forcibly removed from Alexandra township in downtown Johannesburg. In the 1960s and 1970s, more people were attracted to the region where they worked for white farmers, engaged in contract construction work in the "Coloured"[30] township of Lenasia, or secured jobs at Corobrick, a brick factory next to the squatter camp. Today, the Corobrick factory is the *only* source of local employment for Lawley residents and still provides the main rationale for living in this extremely isolated, arid flatland. From February 1987 through the beginning of 1988, the local police arrested Lawley squatters on three occasions for contravention of the Illegal Squatting Act.[31] "Coloured" and "Indian" workers for the owner of the land, Mr. Perry, and the local police harassed the Lawley squatters repeatedly for two years until finally a court case was filed in 1988 to evict the squatters. On several occasions the police informed the residents that they were not allowed to settle in this region because "it was reserved for 'coloured' populations." The landowner claimed that he planned to build a company on the plot of land on which the squatters had settled. In November 1989, the ten squatters who were officially charged pled guilty to illegal squatting but asked the court to consider allowing them to remain on the land because it was close to their places of work. The court did not grant permission because the land was privately owned and informed the residents that they had no alternative site for relocation but that they must leave. The residents applied for and were granted permits to relocate to the informal settlement of Orange Farm ten miles away, but the residents resisted relocation. At some point in the ten years between 1989 and 1999, the government seems to have bought the land on which Lawley is situated.

I held a focus group discussion (FGD) with community elders and members of the local ward committee to determine the recent history

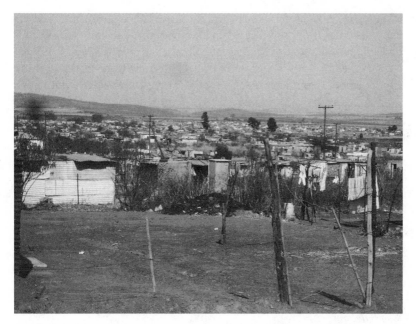

FIGURE 11.   Lawley. Photo taken by the author in 2005 (before the upgrades).

of the Lawley settlement. They claimed that most of the current residents moved to the region in 1999.

Man 1: There were stands here, so people moved here from their locations. They heard from outside that there were open stands. They were R10 [$1.40].

Man 2: From 1999, they wanted to evict us, but we had to fight that—until we started to go to court. We were given the court order that we don't have to move until it is sorted by the High Court in Johannesburg. We were given time. October 11, 1999 was the date we were supposed to move—according to the High Court. The ants came to evict people.

Man 1: The red ants[32] came to evict us, and someone was killed—a small boy, about fifteen to nineteen years. Makhetha was his name. He was shot with one bullet. We had a man by the name of Patrick Kubeka—he was leading the struggle of the people. . . . He came to the eviction, and he talked to the red ants. They stopped the eviction. Then, we were given some time. The community told them to bring the zinc back—the material for the houses, so they can rebuild.[33]

A series of articles run in a local newspaper, the *Sowetan*, in October 1999, corroborates this story. According to the newspaper, the MEC[34] for housing in Gauteng insisted the shacks in Lawley be dismantled despite the court order prohibiting eviction because the area was unfit for development due to the presence of dolomite (Mpye 1999a and 1999b). On October 19, 1999, the state went back to court to resist the prohibition of eviction and won on the appeal (Mpye 1999c and 1999d); however, at a later stage, this appeal was overturned. In 2001, the residents of Lawley were told they could stay.

Man 3: In October 2001, they told us we could stay. Sizakele Nkosi came from the housing department. She called a meeting at the school—this is when they told us we could stay here. . . . They told us we could have the land.

Man 4: Architects came to sample the soil. After the soil was approved, they said we could build. Before, they were saying there was dolomite was here. Then surveyors came. In 2003, they were packing the land—allocating the lands—to make packs, to make the stands. We told them we would register for subsidies, for each and every family. So, we applied for subsidies—everyone. All of us . . . There are about 2,700 subsidies that were approved.

CD: Why did the government change its mind about giving Lawley to the people who lived here?

Man 1: I think because there were already a lot of families. If they had to take us out of here, they had to give us alternative housing because of the Alternative Housing Act. And we were fighting to stay here—it's our land. So, eventually they gave in. The Freedom Charter says we have a right to invade the empty land.

CD: They must have changed their mind about Lawley's upgradability?

Man 1: They were just trying to scare us—with the dolomite. They had already built in this area—they were just lying.[35]

According to the Landless People's Movement's calculations, there were 5,500 shacks in Lawley (with approximately five people per household), when I first began conducting research there in 2005.[36]

At the time, Lawley was quite spread out, so residents built their shacks on rather large stands. There was no electricity or sanitation service, neither was there a school or clinic. The roads were unpaved, so residents usually walked long distances to catch taxis on the main road—this also made ambulance service difficult.

Lawley was also upgraded over the course of my involvement there, though it is not quite clear why it was prioritized for an upgrade over other informal settlements in the region. Some of the residents of the community had been squatting on a piece of prime real estate that the municipality hoped would attract private investors to build middle-class homes.[37] In September of 2007, these residents of Lawley were

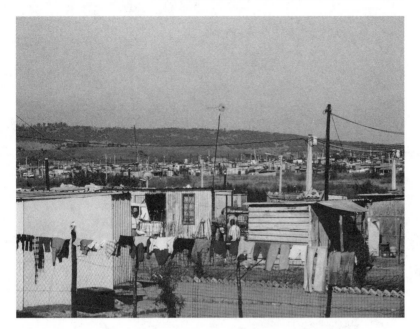

FIGURE 12. Lawley. Photo taken by the author in May 2009 (after the upgrades).

forcibly relocated to a different site within the squatter camp. As either an incentive or in an attempt to squash resistance, the municipality installed electricity, paved the roads, and provided the community with a mobile clinic. Although most of the residents were allocated the plot of land on which they built shacks, other people purchased the stand from someone who sold it rather than building on it. Some residents paid as much as R10,000 ($1,250) to live in Lawley.[38]

As in Sol Plaatjie, the provision of services came with the price of privatization. Residents spend, on average R80 ($11) per month on electricity.[39] In order to help out the poor, the government partially subsidizes residents' electricity purchases. When residents purchase their electricity at the beginning of the month, the government will pay (once per month) 5 percent of their purchase; therefore, if a resident can afford to purchase her entire month's supply of electricity at the beginning of the month, she receives a higher subsidy. However, most residents are forced to purchase their electricity in smaller installments.[40]

The water service was not affected by the upgrades. Johannesburg Water fills plastic, green containers on a daily basis; however, the containers are never cleaned or replaced, so the water is often moldy or contaminated. Residents must purchase additional electricity in order

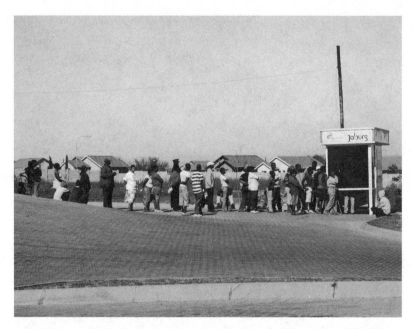

FIGURE 13. Residents queuing to purchase their electricity at the beginning of the month. Photo taken by the author in 2009.

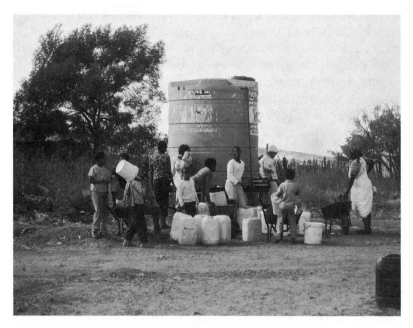

FIGURE 14. Residents gathering water; photo taken by the author in 2005.

to make their water potable. Of those surveyed in Lawley, 37 percent live on R500 or less per month ($62), and 75 percent live on R1,250 or less per month ($156) (CPR survey 2009).

When I returned to Lawley in June and July 2012, the community was largely unchanged; however, the city was in the process of installing pipes to run water to each stand. After this construction, each shack will have an outdoor faucet and outdoor flushing toilet. Other services within the community have since fallen into disrepair—the roads, for example, are practically undrivable. The residents still live in shacks and there is no functional clinic.

The stories of these two communities reveal a strong commitment, on the part of the residents, to develop a tie to the land—for the purposes of security and sustainability, but also in an effort to build a home and community. This desire has been forged through struggle and in response to the state's efforts to eradicate informality by simply displacing it from one location to another. As such, the upgrades in the communities allow the residents to settle. On the other hand, while welcomed, the upgrades have not significantly altered the levels of poverty or increased the quality of living in these squatter conditions because technocratic service delivery does not address the roots of structural inequality. As such, informal settlement dwellers' lives are circumscribed by a host of structural boundaries. In both Sol Plaatjie and Lawley, the lack of social services as well as substandard housing contributes to ill health. Water is often contaminated, informal electricity sources like paraffin cause pollution and congestion, lack of sanitation leads to higher exposure to opportunistic infections, and extreme heat and cold due to lack of proper shelter has a profound effect on people with compromised immune systems.

Environmental Suffering

People living in South Africa's urban slums have by far the worst disease burden and mortality rates in the country[41] because environmental and social conditions increase vulnerability to disease and ill health, and residents are far removed from formal health care.[42] In addition, lack of social cohesion and trust leads to amplified precariousness, as social networks and bonds of reciprocity are constantly threatened, violence and competition are common, and certain forms of informal health care (like indigenous and faith healing, as well as home-based care) rely on strong senses of community solidarity.

The four primary risks associated with living in a shack are: (1) earth floors lead to dampness, which can contribute to rheumatism, arthritis, and respiratory infections; (2) shacks do not offer proper protection against the weather and are thus extremely hot in the summer months and violently cold in winter (Gauteng has some of the coldest winters in South Africa, exacerbated by strong winds in the flatlands, which is a particularly acute problem in Lawley); (3) fires are common, especially when residents utilize alternative energy sources like paraffin or wood; and (4) the poor construction of shacks leaves residents constantly threatened by risks of burglary (Smit 2006, 110–11; see also Murray 2008).

One of the biggest problems in Lawley is the fact that we are living in shacks. They are very cold. Most of the ailments we are facing, because of this disease, our bones—especially in the legs—get very sore, which is worse because of the cold in the shacks. There is also a lot of dust. Sometimes there is not enough space. We keep on having to drink contaminated water. We also don't have electricity or any social services.[43]

One of the biggest problems we are facing is: we stay in shacks. There are all kinds of weather here. If it is windy, then the wind goes straight through the house. This is why so many people in Lawley have TB—our illnesses are reflective of our living conditions. But the treatment is not reflective of our environmental conditions.[44]

Respiratory diseases (including tuberculosis, or TB) are extremely common in informal settlements due to vast temperature fluctuations, the dry high-altitude climate, wind-borne dust, heavy pollution, and indoor tobacco smoking, and their spread is facilitated by taxi transportation where people are crammed into very small spaces for long periods of time (Ashforth 2005, 45). Paraffin (kerosene), the alternative energy source most commonly used in informal settlements, is both expensive and dangerous. It accounts for almost half of hospital admissions for poisoning (Stewart et al. 2000, 417; quoted in Ashforth 2005, 144). During community meetings, the constant rasping and hacking of the people present attests to the effects of both shack living on a windy and dusty plain and the polluting nature of paraffin.

Not having electricity affects people living with AIDS. We normally use paraffin which people suffocate from—it is not healthy for people who are HIV positive.[45]

The paraffin smoke is really bad for you—it destroys people's lungs—even worse for people infected with HIV/AIDS.[46]

The gas stoves are made for poor people, but I'm surprised to see that the prices go up each and every month. . . . People cannot afford them, and the prices still increase.[47]

In 2005, VIP (Ventilated Improved Pit) toilets were installed in Lawley. These are prefabricated outdoor toilets that sit on top of concrete holes dug into the ground; they resemble permanent port-o-potties. A city truck is supposed to come by on a weekly basis to empty the toilets, but residents say they often wait between one to three months for the trucks to arrive, by which point the toilets are overflowing. Some residents purchase acid tablets to manage the volume of their accumulated waste while they wait for respite from the city.[48] "When they don't come to empty the toilets, we are exposed to so many illnesses. They are so full, people are forced to go to the *velds*."[49] Before Sol Plaatjie was upgraded, sewage literally ran through the streets. Environments polluted with human feces increase the likelihood of infection with helminths (worms) (Ambert 2006, 147), hepatitis A, and dysentery. Susceptibility to HIV infection is also higher when people's immune systems are already compromised by other infections.

Prior to the upgrades, Sol Plaatjie's groundwater, and, thus, drinking supply, was contaminated from years of mining in the region. Lawley's drinking water is still unpotable, as the community tanks the city fills are never cleaned out and residents often throw garbage into them.[50]

I think that first of all, if you look at the conditions of the people living in squatter camps. First, look at the issue of water or sanitation. That is where you get germs and other diseases. The kind of water that we drink stays in drums for weeks. It gets contaminated. They never clean the drums of water.[51]

Residents, then, are forced to purchase more energy (in the form of electricity or paraffin) in order to make their water potable. In the community survey I conducted in these communities, I asked respondents whether or not they were satisfied with their basic service provision. In Lawley:

· only 4.4 percent of residents were satisfied with their water provision;
· 45 percent complained the water was dirty;
· 30.6 percent mentioned that collecting water was extremely difficult; and
· 40.6 percent respondents claimed the tanks were not filled regularly (CPR survey 2009).

Table 1. Barriers to healthy living[‡]

	Income	Environment	Nutritious food	Stigma	Sexual practices	Housing
Sol Plaatjie	73.8%	62.7%	73%	49.3%	49.9%	N/A
Lawley	90%	83.7%	82.6%	71.5%	77.1%	95.3%

[‡] Respondents were asked what the primary barriers people in their community faced in trying to sustain a healthy lifestyle (CPR survey 2009).

There is also a serious lack of nutritious food, and in Sol Plaatjie the upgrades have exacerbated this because people no longer have space in their yards to have gardens. In each community there are small stands on virtually every street where residents can buy chips, candy, eggs, and sometimes chicken feet. At the entrance to Sol Plaatjie, men sell cow and sheep heads. Each community also has several *spaza* shops,[52] where more extensive supplies can be purchased, though in Sol Plaatjie, where there is no electricity, nothing is sold that must be refrigerated. In both communities, it is extremely difficult for residents to purchase fresh vegetables and fruits, milk, quality meat, and other perishable items. Travel to the nearest fully operational grocery store takes twenty to thirty minutes via taxi for residents of both communities. Recently, the rising price of food in South Africa has severely intensified this shortage of nutritious food. Between January 2000 and April 2011 in South Africa, white maize increased in price by 75.2 percent and the price of wheat increased 334 percent (Food and Agriculture Organization, United Nations 2011). In 2009, food inflation was 13.7 percent, whereas general inflation in the country was 8.4 percent (*The Star* 2009). Only 27 percent of households in Johannesburg are food secure (De Wet et al. 2008).

Clinics were supposed to be installed in both Lawley and Sol Plaatjie as part of the upgrades, and each community does indeed have a temporary structure that is supposed to house a clinic. However, when I was last there in 2012, neither clinic was fully functional. Both were prone to lengthy and inexplicable closures and when operating provided the most minimal of services.

They don't have ARVs; they don't have medicines.

CD: Then what services do they provide?

They refer you to other clinics . . .

CD: Do you have to have a referral to go to a different clinic?

Yes. So, you start at your local clinic, and you wait there for three or four hours, but I mean, sometimes you have to wake up early because the clinic opens at 7:30, at least, so you have to be there before then, because after it opens, the queues are longer. . . . So then you wait for three hours and get a referral from the nurse, then you have to get transportation to go to Lenasia [the closest fully operational clinic to Lawley]. . . . It's a struggle because sometimes, depending on whether you do have money, because when they refer you at that time, if you've got money and you are lucky, you can immediately go there. But sometimes you resort to coming back and actually going tomorrow to that referral or to come back to the community and loan some monies from people so you can better go to the other clinic.

CD: How long do you have to wait at Lenasia?

. . . four, five, six hours . . . the clinic in Lenasia is a little bit bigger. It opens twenty-four hours. And then it services a bigger area. And also there, it's not just to come in and see the doctor. You have to go through the process of registering, going through the queue, before you see the doctor. And so they need to diagnose you and there is a physical. And then you can get help. But at most, four to five hours . . . even with them, it's not that they provide one-stop service. Sometimes there are things that they cannot help you, where they have to refer you to Bara.[53] And then also they've got a stationary bus which they use to transfer people to Baragwanath. But I mean, you have to get it at certain time. It's actually going there once a day. If it's left, the following day, or if you've got money, you can immediately go to Bara. . . . From Lawley, it's R7 ($1) to go to Lenasia, and R9.50 ($1.35) to go to Bara . . . And then if they write you a script for a medication, then you have to go and queue again at the dispenser.[54]

Pheello also told me that ambulance service is a problem. Before Lawley was upgraded, ambulances were not able to drive on the roads of the settlement, so the ambulance service would ask residents to wait for them down on the main road, and from Pheello's stand, this would take a healthy person at least ten minutes to walk. Now that the roads are paved, the ambulances can come straight to the home, but it often involves waiting up to five hours. The only other option is to pay someone who owns a car in the community for their services.[55] Transportation costs to established clinics and the hospital are often so prohibitive that for many informal settlement dwellers the cost is only worth paying if their condition is immediately life threatening.[56]

Those of us who are infected with HIV or AIDS, when we are sick, we are supposed to take the last money we have, which we should use to purchase nutritious food, and instead use it to take the taxi to the clinic. . . . Sometimes you don't even have the money you need to go get your treatment. Maybe the treatment says you must come in once a month. You don't get enough money so you can't go there, so we can't get our treatment regularly.[57]

Table 2. Barriers to health care[‡]

	Cost	Transport cost	Travel time	Poor treatment at the clinic	Queues	Stigma	Lack of ambulance service	Prefer indigenous or faith healer
Sol Plaatjie	50.1%	88.7%	74.6%	64.8%	83%	52.4%	52.4%	36.1%
Lawley	71.5%	81.3%	76.6%	89.8%	85.8%	70.9%	79%	61.4%

[‡] Respondents were asked what primary barriers people in their community faced in accessing healthcare (CPR survey 2009).

For people who are HIV-infected, bearing children can also lead to difficulties. Nevirapine was provided by the state and reduced the chances of mother-to-child transmission (often referred to as vertical transmission) by 40 percent (McIntyre 2007).[58] However, mothers are then forced to choose between the possibility of vertical transmission through breast-feeding and the alternative likelihood that children will get sick from common infections because they are not breast-fed (Coovadia and Coutsoudis 2001). Formula milk is not only costly, but it also requires purified water, and often bottles and nipples cannot be sterilized (Heimer 2007, 569). Further, not breast-feeding can lead to stigma (as it may reveal the HIV status of the mother to partners and community members), which might affect long-term social and financial support (ibid.). Finally, HIV transmission is often more likely when breast milk is mixed with food, and yet this is often the cultural practice (Coovadia and Coutsoudis 2001; Iliff et al. 2005).

The Mutual Pandemics of Poverty and AIDS

You can't see AIDS, but I saw it in Sol Plaatjie.[59]

In 2005, it was estimated that informal settlements had HIV prevalence rates twice as high as formal urban settlements (Shisana et al. 2005). For some, HIV infection is the rationale for moving to an informal settlement. For example, several women in my study moved to Lawley or Sol Plaatjie in order to escape the stigma they faced from their families and communities of origin. Others move to urban environments in search of better health care opportunities. But informal settlements are also sites of high HIV contraction. Although only 8.7 percent of the South African population lives in informal settlements, they account for 29.1 percent of the total estimated number of *new* HIV infections (Rehle et al. 2007, 198).

When asked to explain this correlation, the residents of informal settlements are generally unanimous in their response: the reason is poverty. They mention various causal factors, including "transactional sex,"[60] alcohol and drug use, lack of social solidarity, and desperation. Poverty and the conditions in which people are forced to live exacerbate disease progression, destroy bonds of solidarity and trust, and can lead to increased risk taking. Again and again in interviews, when I asked people *why* community members do not use condoms or avoid multiple partners, despite the fact that they are well educated on HIV transmission and watch their community members die on a daily basis, the reply was:

Many people think that HIV might kill them in ten years, but poverty or violence will kill them first, so why worry about it?[61]

People are dying all the time in my community, so many people just accept that as . . . you know, their future. So, they aren't careful about HIV 'cause they expect to die anyway. They don't care what kills them.[62]

Lots of people are hopeless. That's why lots of people are getting HIV. This is why it is still spreading. People are just living like it's not there. People are not scared. They should be, but they are not. When you see people are sick, you need to feel something. But people are not feeling anything. They don't care, or they don't think it exists . . . They are hopeless. If you don't have any plans for the future, or hopes or dreams, then you become like this.[63]

People have reached a point where they aren't afraid to die.[64]

The message is quite clear: until abject desperation is no longer the everyday experience of millions of South Africans, the disease will continue to spread.

The epidemic not only feeds off of but also *increases* socioeconomic vulnerability. In a household survey conducted in Soweto, Naidu and Harris (2006) found that households with an HIV-infected member earned less regular income (386). In a survey of 771 AIDS-affected households spread throughout South Africa, Steinberg and colleagues (2002) found that two-thirds of the households reported a fall in the total household income as a direct result of having to cope with HIV/AIDS (16). "The drop in income was exacerbated by the fact that most of the households studied were already very poor" (ibid.). In addition to direct costs of health care, medicines, transportation, and food associated with hospitalization and funerals, there are indirect costs of

Table 3. Income and poverty

	Average household size	Percentage of households with no regular income	Percentage of households that live on less than R500 ($71) per month	Percentage of households that live on less than R1,000 ($143) per month	Average income per person per month	Percentage of households that are grant dependent
Sol Plaatjie	3.8	53.2%	48%	70.2%	R216 ($31)	17.6%
Lawley	4.2	46.1%	38.5%	54.3%	R232 ($33)	22%

CPR survey 2009

HIV/AIDS morbidity and mortality, which include the loss of income from prolonged illness (by those infected as well as their caregivers) and the loss of social grants (Naidu and Harris 2006, 387). Funerals, on average (with prefuneral, day of, and postfuneral costs added together) cost R32,190 ($4,600) (ibid., 391). The average direct cost (associated with health care and transportation) of morbidity to an affected household is R333 ($48) per month per ill person, and the average indirect cost (income lost for care and inability to work) per ill person is R1,011 ($144) per month (Booysen et al. 2004). It is patently clear, therefore, that the epidemics of poverty and HIV are not simply correlated, but symbiotic.

As this survey data reveal, informal settlements are characterized by not only high levels of unemployment, but high levels of abject poverty. In South Africa, a person who lives on less than R431 ($62) per month lives below the poverty line (Statistics South Africa 2007b), but a household is considered indigent if it survives on R1,880 ($269)[65] per

Table 4. Household expenditures

	Average family size	Average household income	Percentage of income spent on food	Percentage spent on energy[‡]	Average cost per year of hospital visits*	Average cost per year of clinic visits*
Sol Plaatjie	3.8	R819 ($117)	49.41%	33.27%	R171 ($24)	R158 ($23)
Lawley	4.2	R976 ($139)	44.87%	11.67%	R869 ($124)	R938 ($134)

‡ Sol Plaatjie does not have electricity and Lawley has prepaid electricity (CPR survey 2009).
* There are a variety of explanations for the discrepancy in hospital/clinic costs between these two regions. Lawley residents reported a higher average number of visits per year (11.22 versus 3.96) and higher average costs per visit (R70.25 versus R44.12). Lawley is geographically farther removed from both clinics and hospitals, so transportation costs may explain part of this differential. In addition, however, many more respondents from Sol Plaatjie answered this question (n = 280 for Sol Plaatjie versus n = 130 for Lawley), so this may have contributed to the reported discrepancy as well.

Table 5. Sources of income

	Average household size	Average household income	Receives salary (average amount)	Receives grant (average amount)	Receives pension (average amount)	Receives money from relative (average amount)	Works in informal sector (average amount)	Self-reported employment rate
Sol Plaatjie	3.8	R819 ($117)	35.2% (R1,448 or $207)	35.8% (R761 or $109)	3.1% (R1,113 or $159)	9% (R443 or $63)	28.3% (R816 or $117)	46.8%
Lawley	4.2	R976 ($139)	54.4% (R1,339 or $191)	54.3% (R1,059 or $151)	7.4% (R1,289 or $184)	9.6% (R606 or $87)	9.6% (R1,006 or $144)	53.9%

CPR survey 2009

month (Statistics South Africa 2008b). Informal settlements are often characterized by quite high levels of economic differentiation between households (Smit 2006, 113).

As table 5 shows, people rely on a variety of sources of financial support. When people reported that they received a salary (or were employed), the CPR survey did not ask residents to define whether this was in the formal or informal sector—rather, it asked residents to self-report whether they received a salary or were employed. People who earn the highest incomes most likely are employed in working-class jobs (for example, in Lawley, at the Corobrick factory). Both Lawley and Sol Plaatjie are too far removed from Johannesburg for most people to commute to regular jobs in the city, though some residents work in smaller bordering towns (like Roodepoort for Sol Plaatjie residents and Ennerdale for Lawley residents). Other higher income earners would include owners and operators of spaza shops and *shebeens*.[66] Some women are employed as home-based care workers (earning R500–R1,000 per month from the government). Informal, irregular income-generating activities include collecting wood, selling meat or offal, selling paraffin, or selling sweets or other foodstuffs.

The formalization of informal settlements can threaten certain income opportunities. For example, location is important for spaza shop owners and others who sell food and supplies within the settlement; therefore, relocation can threaten their livelihood. Meat traders have been displaced with formalization as residents are no longer allowed to slaughter and cook meet on open fires because of health regulations in formal areas (Smit 2006, 117). In addition, many people earn money by renting out space on their stand for others to build shacks, or by renting out rooms in shacks—formalization also threatens this livelihood strategy (ibid.).

One of the most important forms of financial support for the poor is social grants; however, there are no grants available simply based on indigence. Pensions are available to South African citizens over the age of sixty who do not earn more than R31,296 ($3,912) per year; this grant is currently R1,080 per month ($135) (South African Social Security Association 2011). Child support grants are available for South African parents who are primary caregivers to a child under fifteen years of age (and who do not earn more than R30,000, or $3,750 per year) (ibid.). These grants equal R250 per month ($31.25), but parents can earn multiple grants for multiple children (ibid.). As of 2008, 7.2 million children benefited from the grant (UNICEF 2008). Disability grants are given to South African citizens (between the ages of eighteen and

Table 6. Quality of life

	% of households living in shacks	% of female-headed households	% of grant-dependent households	% of immigrant households	% of households with running water	% of households with electricity	% of respondents who completed high school
Sol Plaatjie	40%	15.5%	17.6%	10.4%	58.3%	2.2%	30.1%
Lawley	98.5%	20.8%	22%	10.9%	N/A	99.2%	37.8%

CPR survey 2009

fifty-nine) who are medically certified with a physical or mental disability that makes the person unfit to work (South African Social Security Association 2011). Again, the person must not earn more than $3,912 in income, and the grant is $135 per month. There are about fourteen million South Africans who receive social grants (Republic of South Africa 2010, 103). In Sol Plaatjie, 39 percent of those surveyed received grants and 17.6 percent of households were grant dependent (CPR survey 2009). In Lawley, 62 percent of those surveyed received grants and 22 percent of households were grant dependent (ibid.). Generally, entire households use the grants, so each grant supports approximately 4.5 household members (Altman and Boyce 2008, 12). "The result is an arbitrary divide between the poorest households, which have no state support at all, and the otherwise very similar households that receive comparatively generous support simply because they are 'lucky' enough to include grant-eligible children, elderly, or disabled persons" (Ferguson 2007, 78). The grant provision system has been criticized for being overly complex: it requires detailed and updated paperwork and documentation, people often get stuck in window periods when grants have expired but their renewal has not yet been processed, there is no real mechanism for detecting fraud, and a byzantine bureaucracy is needed to sort out the qualified from the nonqualified but equally needy.

In 2009, Pheello was receiving R250 ($36) each month from a child support grant, which was his family's only source of income, and yet he said that his costs (many of which are associated with health care since both he and his wife are HIV-infected) range from between R3,000 to R4,000 each month. When asked how he manages, he quietly responds: "It becomes a serious challenge. There is nothing that you can do. . . . Mostly, I live on hand-outs."[67]

Loss of "Ubuntu"

The African ethic of *ubuntu*, usually defined by the adage "A person is a person through other people," became a feature of the post-apartheid state's African renaissance movement, ironically at the same time this philosophy was crumbling due to the strain of unemployment and increasing inequality. The philosophy attempts to epitomize the African ethos of reciprocity and the strength of kinship ties. One of the most horrifying testaments to the destruction wrought by HIV/AIDS is the emergence of orphanages. Children of deceased parents were always cared for by extended family networks of care and support; therefore, orphanages signify the loss of whole kinship structures (see, for example, Guest 2001; Foster, Levi, and Williamson 2005). Africans' definition of family in no way resembles the Western nuclear ideal. Most of my African friends were raised by a group of adults (including grandparents, parents, aunts, and uncles) and shared their home with cousins, nieces, and nephews. In fact, the person referred to as "mother" or "brother" does not necessarily reflect a biological relationship. The bonds of kinship are defined, in part, by a system of reciprocity. If one is financially successful, s/he is expected to share that wealth across the kinship structure, and in times of need, one could also rely on that structure for support.

However, in the context of extremely minimal resources, continually asking others for help can strain and even destroy social networks of support and care.

Long-term structural unemployment and the virtually permanent state of dependency it entails have corrosive effects in families and communities. Although there are deeply rooted norms of sharing and reciprocity within families and communities, these function best when capacities for giving are relatively evenly distributed. . . . But when some people's needs are permanent and their capacities for reciprocity limited, habits and ethics of sharing come under strain. (Ashforth 2005, 28)

I started to notice, in 2009, a certain slippage of signification between poverty and HIV. People started mentioning that if you borrowed money, people in the community would begin to gossip about your HIV status.

Gossiping is ripe. You can't borrow R100 because people will talk about your status. Eventually that person will gossip about your financial status. Even though you are sick, or someone is sick at home, but they will always gossip. You can't find any help anywhere.[68]

If one is HIV positive, and he sometimes feels weak in his body, he's not also strong to go and get means to try to make ends meet because he is sick and he is hungry and he is not able—then he is forced now to go and ask. And you can't always ask because once you ask, sometimes people get tired . . . they even say remarks that, you know, this thing of HIV is becoming a burden to me because people are coming to me and asking things.[69]

Not only are poverty and HIV/AIDS deeply causally related, they also have come to substitute for each other, as stigmata of shame.

When I was conducting research in Lawley in 2005 and 2006, Pheello ran a small support group for people affected by HIV/AIDS in his community. With the permission of the members, I often attended the support group, and I even conducted interviews with many of the members. One day, after a support group meeting, I drove a few of the members home. As we dropped one particularly ill woman off at her door, Pheello mentioned that she was really suffering and he wished he could help her. I had brought groceries for Pheello's family with me that day, so I said we could offer her some groceries to help out. Pheello looked at me, and sadly shook his head, "no." Pheello has always done everything he can to help members of his community, but if it comes down to saving his family and himself over others, he knows where his priorities have to be.[70] This is perhaps the greatest testament to the way in which scarcity destroys the bonds of reciprocity and solidarity.

When asked to discuss symptoms of the social discord that have come to characterize daily life in informal settlements, people very often give examples of residents willfully infecting each other. For example:

People don't use condoms because they want to deliberately spread the virus because they know if they are already infected they are going to die. They want to make sure they are not going to die alone, they will take others with them.[71]

In those water tanks, there is tendency to put used nappies, used condoms, dead cats, etc. There are some people who take this idea that "I don't want to die alone." They want the disease to spread, so they put their used condoms in the water. So, that everyone will get what they have. We are killing each other here. . . . Some deny to use condoms. . . . People want to spread this HIV—if I've got this thing, then so should everyone else. We don't love each other.[72]

While I doubt that the prevalence of such vindictive behavior is as high as people seem to *think* it is, these expressions reveal an underlying fear of widespread malevolence and a definite distrust of one's neighbors (both of which are reverberated in conversations about the prevalence of witchcraft, which I discuss below). This manifests itself in a general sense of people's destructive sentiments and in suspicion that some might be willing to act on them to the point of murder.

Profound stigma is another indication of the breakdown of community solidarity and trust. One day when I arrived in Sol Plaatjie, Thulani said he had been waiting impatiently for me and that he needed my help. He took me into one of the hostels, down the dark and narrow hallway, and then into one of its tiny rooms, where a family of four lived on top of one another. In a bed (the only one in the room) lay a young woman who was very clearly dying of AIDS. Her body was emaciated and she was completely despondent to words or touch. It was also very obvious that in addition to suffering from the illness, this young woman was suffering from neglect. She was lying in her own bodily waste, she had oozing bedsores, and the whole room smelled of death. The woman's mother was busy preparing dinner and barely looked at us as she spoke quickly with Thulani. I asked (through Thulani) if she wanted us to take her daughter to the hospital. The mother responded abrasively and irritably, "I don't care where you take her— just get her out of here."[73]

In a survey conducted in the early years of the pandemic in Soweto, 38 percent of adults believed that people living with HIV should be separated from society, 6 percent believed that they should be killed, and only 34 percent said that they should be cared for by their families (cited in Webb 1992, chapter 3).[74] In December 1998, after openly declaring her HIV-positive status on a local Zulu television program, Gugu Dlamini was stoned to death by her neighbors in her hometown, KwaMancinza, in the KwaZulu-Natal province (Bareng-Batho and S'Thembiso 1998; McNeil 1998; Nicodemus 1999). Although the level of violence Gugu Dlamini experienced is rare and is perhaps indicative of a particular moment in the history of AIDS in South Africa, it does reveal the level of fear this pandemic inspires. As the story I told about the young woman in Sol Plaatjie reveals, stigma often leads to neglect and isolation, both of which can contribute to the earlier onset of death from AIDS.

Many of the participants in this study went to great lengths to maintain silence about their status due to fears of stigmatization. In the support groups in which I conducted ten months of participant observation in Soweto,[75] most of the participants traveled vast distances to attend a support group in a neighborhood where no one knew them.

The treatment in the hospital is much nicer than the treatment at the clinic. But the . . . the nicest thing about it is that it's far away from . . . from where I stay. Because I thought I'm all alone from DRD, but, wow, I saw two people, you know, from my area, seeing *me* now, and we're all in the HIV ward [*laughs*]. . . . But really, that's a horrible feeling. This is why I hate going to the clinics and hospitals.[76]

One young community member in Lawley explained that one of the reasons there is so little community solidarity has to do with the fact that people do not have anything to do since there is no work, and the only places where residents can gather together are shebeens.[77] Rates of alcoholism are extremely high, which can lead to both heightened violence and unsafe sexual practices. In 2000, alcohol accounted for 7 percent of all deaths, and men suffered from four times as many alcohol-related deaths as women (Schneider et al. 2007). Alcohol use is also a contributing factor to the astronomical rates of violence and crime in South Africa.

In 2000, the "age-standardized homicide rate (65 per 100,000) was more than seven times the global average, placing South Africa among the most violent countries in the world" (Norman et al. 2007, 653). South Africa has the highest incidence of *reported* rape in the world (Ashforth 2005, 36), and rape is the crime perhaps least likely to *be* reported in South Africa. It is estimated that every six hours a woman is murdered by an intimate partner (Coovadia et al. 2009, 825). In Johannesburg in 2010, there were 38.5 murders (per 100,000), 618.5 aggravated robberies (per 100,000), and 193.2 sexual offenses (per 100,000)—each much higher than the national average (SAIRR 2010a). In fact, Johannesburg is widely considered one of the most dangerous cities in the world.

The absence of law in informal settlements seems to lead to an increase in violence. Under apartheid, Black South Africans grew to distrust the police, and there is still a pervasive disdain for the institution of policing, which is widely believed to be corrupt, inept, and under-resourced (Ashforth 2005, 37). Reporting violence, especially for rape, is seen as pointless.

Women don't feel comfortable reporting rape. There are so many cases of rape that go unreported. Children especially are scared to report.[78]

The issue of rape is very serious. Children and women are being raped. And the thugs get arrested, but only for one day. You see them back in the community the next day.[79]

Rape is normal. It's very, very normal. But, there are no official *charges* of rape. You can go to the local police station. No one is getting a rape charge.[80]

One woman who was the victim of HIV-related stigma in Lawley asked other residents, in a focus group discussion, what she should do. Residents informed her that reporting the crime to the police was futile.

The closest police station is forty kilometers away, and costs R90 ($13) in transportation, round trip. "The magistrate will write down your story, but it won't assist you. Also the court order is useless."[81]

There used to be a strong sense that communities should solve their own problems—this is particularly true in more formal townships like Soweto (Ashforth 2005, 39). In informal settlements, though there are community policing units, these can sometimes turn into vigilante groups. This was especially the case when xenophobic violence erupted throughout South Africa in May 2008, leaving sixty-two dead. On May 11 and 12, brutal riots broke out in Alexandra township (in northeastern Johannesburg), where locals brutally beat African immigrants (and three were killed). These events spawned weeks of xenophobic attacks against African immigrants in urban areas throughout South Africa (*Mail and Guardian* 2008). African immigrants increasingly make up a large percentage of the population in urban informal settlements (they make up 10 percent of the community in both Lawley and Sol Plaatjie [CPR survey 2009]). In addition to facing potential violence and stigmatization from neighbors (due, in many ways, to what has been labeled "relative deprivation" [HSRC 2008a]), immigrants face difficulties in finding work, securing social welfare or health care, and their vulnerability to arrest and deportation means they are hesitant to signal their presence to police or government officials.

Political differences can also spark rather brutal violence among community members. Sol Plaatjie was originally made up of people from three different regions in the Gauteng province. These three communities kept to themselves, but there were often points of contention between them, based on different political affiliations or presumed rural, ethnic identities.[82] When asked to comment on community solidarity in Lawley, one resident explained that differences were usually expressed through allegiances to different political parties, based, in part, on which parts of South Africa people hailed from:

We are quite mixed here. You see, so the conflict, it comes through the political parties. Because at first, there was no ANC . . . only IFP.[83] Now, we're divided by blocks. This block is ANC, that block is IFP. So, during the upgrades, when people were being moved around onto new stands, there was a lot of accusations about whose stand was better or bigger and why.[84]

These kinds of political differences, as well as violence aimed at immigrant populations, arise from acute vulnerability associated with shared social exclusion and deprivation.

Conducting research (or simply living) in and around Johannesburg requires an adjustment in one's habitus.[85] As Ashforth puts it: "considerations of security infuse every aspect of everyday life" (2005, 36). It requires not only a spatial and temporal accommodation (I was cautioned against being in the informal settlements at night—a serious obstacle to ethnographic research), but also certain physical adjustments—being consciously aware of one's surroundings, having escape routes in mind, and making sure to have no phone, money, or other valuables visible in the cab of the car. But being able to avoid crime and violence is also an incredible privilege—yet another privilege withheld from the residents of informal settlements, especially female residents. On my last visit to Lawley in 2009, as I said good-bye to community members, one quiet and studious young man who enjoyed discussing sociology with me said, "Well, I'll see you in the next life." I responded, "no, don't worry, I'll be back in two or three years." And he smiled ruefully, "chances are, I won't live that long." Growing old is also a privilege, it seems, in South Africa's slums.

In many ways, the historic, cultural practice of *ubuntu*, of reciprocally supporting one another, has been privatized under neoliberalism. The rise of competition over scarce resources contributes to heightened forms of individualism. Many people blame "development" itself for destroying community solidarity and eroding bonds of reciprocity. Usually, people are simply referring to the lack of employment and resources for the poor, which seems, to many, to have accompanied the fall of apartheid. But it goes beyond this. Here is a conversation from a focus group discussion in Lawley:

CD: *Is Lawley a tight-knit community, with a lot of solidarity, or rather, is there a lot of disagreement and competition?*
Female 1: Before development, it was a tight-knit community.
CD: *What has changed?*
Female 1: Before development, we would rally around each other on one issue, or we fight not to be evicted. And that thing would bring us together. Now, because everyone is allocated a stand and everyone is free, now there is not so much community. And also, there are new people who have come to stay here.
Female 2: The community is no longer the same. Before, we would come together and do things together and fight for each other. One example is "Mary," she has been victimized where she stays, and she has to face that. But before development, other people would go and reprimand the culprits, but now she is alone in trying to solve that problem.[86]

And so, many experience the arrival of "development" with a tremendous sense of loss—of tradition, of solidarity, of a shared sense of culture and identity.

Thus far in this chapter, I have tried to paint a vivid picture of the precarious nature of surviving squatter conditions. However, precariousness is caused by not only material deprivation but also by spiritual anxiety and ontological vulnerability, both of which are exacerbated by a strong sense that certain cultural norms and traditions have been forsaken over the years. Before I can properly address these feelings of loss, it is important to elaborate a bit on what constitutes an indigenous ontological orientation in South Africa.

An Indigenous Ontological Orientation

In Adam Ashforth's masterful book on witchcraft in Soweto (2005), he insists that the people with whom he works "live in a world of witches." As opposed to a belief, medical, or cultural *system*, he insists that witchcraft entails a certain ontological orientation, which suggests that witches (as well as ancestors) have agency on and in the social world, and that this agency is often occult in nature (129–30). While I find this a compelling approach, Ashforth's "world of witches" implies fundamental difference—as if the inhabitants of Soweto occupy an alien world altogether in addition to occupying "the same world as people like me" (121). Rather, I would like to insist on the perspectival nature of different ontological positionings. Whereas a sociologist explains social phenomena, events, and actions, by uncovering (often invisible) causal mechanisms like structures, institutions, networks, and discursive formations, an indigenous healer would explain those same phenomena and events as interventions by certain spiritual causal forces and mechanisms. According to an indigenous ontological perspective, *muthi* (a generic Zulu word used to describe any herbal medicinal substance fabricated by an herbalist), a person's deceased ancestors (*amakhosi* or *amadlozi*), and a syncretized interpretation of the Christian God, all have causal power over the social world and people's personal relationships. Healers, prophets, and witches can also mobilize these forces to intervene in people's lives in either protective or destructive ways.

Like any paradigm or episteme, the South African indigenous ontology is historically and socially contingent—reflecting radical structural transformations within the social world. In addition, there are certain epistemological and practical differences associated with the various ethnic cultures in South Africa. Most importantly, and in contradistinction to Ashforth, throughout this book, I will show how indigenous ontology is constitutively hybrid—there is nothing pure, delimited, or radically other about it. This ontological orientation allows those who subscribe to it to navigate a social world interwoven by a wide array of cultural systems, influenced by international, national, and local sources. Despite these caveats, it is possible to characterize an ideal type of indigenous ontology (by reading fragments articulated by different healers and scholars against the grain).

I was first introduced into the world of indigenous healing by my interpreter, Torong Ramela,[87] who had spent many years working with and advocating on behalf of healers in the Gauteng province. Torong had personal connections with the leaders of all of the major indigenous healing organizations and the Department of Health officials who were working closest with the indigenous health sector. I developed a very close relationship with two indigenous healers working in Soweto, Drs. Martha Mongoya and Robert Tshabalala. Much of what I explain below (though corroborated with academic scholarship) was learned over hours and hours of interview time spent sitting in Martha's living room with the two of them.[88] Dr. Tshabalala has been practicing as a *sangoma* (diviner) in Soweto since 1968, and Dr. Mongoya is both a faith healer and *sangoma* and has been practicing since 1993. The differences in their genders and generations had implications for their experiences with the world of indigenous healing (and its confrontation with HIV/AIDS). They often respectfully disagreed with each other, which provided me insight into different epistemological perspectives and methodological approaches to healing.

The first essential component of an indigenous ontology is that the self is not "well-bounded" (Niehaus 2002, 189). It is contiguous with both the spiritual world (from which it comes and toward which it is heading) and the social world (the self is built, sustained, and enriched through interaction with others). In other words, the self is made up of ancestors who came before, is added to throughout the life through various social interactions, and then in death will continue to contribute to and shape the lives of the next generation. Thornton describes this as being a nodal point in a network of relations that extend both vertically (across the generations and over time) and horizontally (across social networks and through space) (2008, 205). People's bodies and selves are constantly being incremented by various different gifts (material, social, and spiritual) and flows (bodily and ancestral), making them "compound sites of [the] relations that define them" (Niehaus 2002, 190). The body is, therefore, not the sole property of the individual but is linked to a whole host of ancestral spirits who use it to communicate with other ancestors and who bestow the individual with a unique cultural and familial identity and guide his/her life choices. It is also due to this contiguous notion of the self that certain stages of the life course, in which a person is in a liminal state between birth and death (during pregnancy, widowhood, when suffering from disease) are considered moments imbued with both power and danger. Indeed, healers are considered to be in a rather constant state of liminality due to their ability to be possessed by the ancestors.

According to indigenous cosmology, the body is the site of four synchronized components. These are: the spirit (*umoya*), the body or flesh (*umzimba*), the blood (*igazi*), and what is directly translated as "charisma," which can be understood as a person's "aura," "shadow," or "presence" (*isithunzi*).

Healing the body involves a careful balancing of all of these components, "with excesses of blood or spirit being purged . . . and with deficits being made up through ritual treatments involving the 'calling' of the spirits (*pahla*). . . . Health results from a balance of substances both within the body and between others involved in the person's social and sexual network" (Thornton 2008, 214). Practices of amplifying the body (because of a bodily or spiritual insufficiency) might be done through the inhalation of herbal fumes, being washed with herbal remedies, or the rubbing of medicines into small incisions made on the body (Henderson 2005; Thornton 2008). Cleansing or purging unwanted toxins or infections would call for drinking medicines that will induce vomiting or diarrhea, or steaming the body with herbal infusions to sweat out the infection (Henderson 2005; Thornton 2008).

Illnesses can also be caused by the ancestors or by witchcraft. Ancestors may intervene in daily life, wreaking havoc or demanding attention in some way.[89] Usually, this type of intervention can be accom-

Table 7. The body's four synchronized components (in bold)

	Enduring	Transient
Substance	**Blood**	**Body**
Nonsubstance	**Spirit**	**Shadow**
	Fluid	Immanent[‡]

‡ Thornton 2008, 213.

modated by a ritual or gift. For example, an ancestor may be angry because his/her grave is not being paid proper respect, and thus the illness the ancestor caused can be cured by cleaning and honoring the gravesite. In fact, the "calling" by the ancestors to become a *sangoma* (or diviner) manifests itself through illness. Witchcraft can cause illnesses of a more maniacal and serious sort. Before explaining this type of illness, it is necessary to categorize the different types of indigenous healers in South Africa.

"Indigenous healing" refers to many different practices and trades. It includes diviners (*sangomas*), herbalists (*inyangas*), *muthi* traders, spiritual healers (of various faiths), "traditional" birth attendants, "traditional" bonesetters, and "traditional" surgeons. These different practices are characterized as "indigenous" or "traditional" because they all rely on and invoke "African conceptions of cosmology and cosmogony" (Devenish 2005, 243; Xaba 2002, 24). It is most common to distinguish between three types of healers: (1) the *sangoma*, or diviner, who has graduated from a long period of training and self-healing; (2) the *inyanga*, or herbalist; and (3) the faith healer, usually a member of a syncretic African Christian church (Thornton 2009, 20). These categories are not discrete (i.e., people often engage in one or more of these professions), and they are often complicated by different levels of expertise in various "disciplines" of healing.[90]

Usually, diviners and herbalists are distinguished by their relationship to the *amakhosi* or *amadlozi* (ancestors).[91] The *sangoma* communicates directly with the ancestors and is in a fairly constant state of spiritual possession. "Each sangoma belongs to a 'school' or 'family' of fellow healers that have been trained by a senior sangoma-trainer, the *gobela*. This is called the *mpande* or 'root,' and signifies the closely bound group of healers that come from a common 'core' of understanding, treatment, and training" (Thornton 2002).[92]

The *inyanga* does not have a relationship with the ancestors and simply acts as an indigenous pharmacist. S/he does not diagnose patients. They are either referred to the herbalist by a *sangoma*, or with less serious conditions, the patient self-diagnoses. The *inyanga* is often a hereditary profession. Meaning, the knowledge of herbs was often passed down from one generation to the next. *Inyangas* generally learn their trade through apprenticeship with a master. However, anyone can become an *inyanga*, which makes it very different from the process for becoming *sangoma* (Abdool-Karim, Ziqubu-Page, and Arendse 1994).

In order to become a *sangoma*, one must first be "called" (*ukubiza*) by the ancestors. "This generally manifests itself as an illness, anxiety or pain in the body, and is due to the desire of the ancestors to communicate with this person, or due to the failure of the person to recognise and respect their ancestors" (Thornton 2002). When an individual is "called," s/he must at the very least conduct a ritual to honor the ancestors. However, if this does not cure the illness, then it is necessary for the person to undergo training (*ukuthwasa*) to become a *sangoma*.

The *sangoma* initiate must select a *gobela* (trainer) under whom s/he apprentices. The *gobela* "both heals and trains their *umthwasa* [trainee] in the arts of spirit possession . . . and therefore initiates the trainee into the secret knowledge of the traditional healer" (Thornton 2002). This training can take anywhere from several months to several years. During the apprenticeship, the *thwasa* lives in the home of the *gobela* and is "expected to serve and respect his/her teacher in all ways" (ibid.). Once the *gobela* decides the *thwasa* has completed his/her training, it is necessary for the trainee to go through a "graduation" ritual, which serves to publicly test the *thwasa*'s skill and to show off the new *sangoma* to his/her community.

The graduation ceremony begins when the *thwasa* goes into a trance and channels his/her particular spirit guide, who then greets the guests. The guests are invited to hide objects for the *thwasa* to find through communication with the ancestors and also to ask the *thwasa* questions about their own ancestors. Finally, a goat is slaughtered, and the trainee drinks the blood of the goat as it is dying. The *gobela* then hides the gall bladder of the goat. If the *thwasa* can find the gall bladder, with the help of the spirits that possess him/her, then the final test has been passed and the trainee becomes a *sangoma*. This process can fail, and the trainee will either continue his/her apprenticeship or leave the profession. The graduation is held publicly and actively involves the community, so that the community can judge for itself the strength or weakness of the *sangoma*'s powers. And community members take it seriously. If the *thwasa* cannot find the items hidden by the audience or the *gobela*, and then tries to practice in the community, s/he will be shunned and considered a charlatan.[93]

In order to diagnose an illness, a *sangoma* will "throw the bones." Unlike in Western medicine, patients do not report symptoms to the *sangoma*. It is the *sangoma*'s duty to determine what ails the patient, through ancestral mediation. "The bones" are a set of divinatory objects, which are unique to the *sangoma*. They include bones from the animals slaughtered at the *sangoma*'s graduation ceremony, objects that represent the *sangoma*'s particular spiritual guides (e.g., if the *sangoma* is linked to a water spirit, there might be a rock from the river that the spirit inhabits), or objects from deceased relatives who now possess the *sangoma*. In addition, there are a series of objects that help the *sangoma* narrate a story of illness. These include pieces to represent family members (e.g., brother, sister, mother, father, child, and grandfather) and pieces to represent sex. There may also be pieces that represent good and evil. In addition, there are objects that serve as "adjectives" indicating degrees of importance, size, seriousness, and distance (Thornton 2002). When one asks the *sangoma* to "throw the bones," one must place money on the mat in order to "open the mouths of the spirits" or to "make the spirits talk." The *sangoma* will give the patient his/her "bones." The *sangoma* will breathe on the set of bones and then ask the patient to also breathe on the bones. Because the *umoya* (spirit) is connected to breath, this invites the ancestors of both the *sangoma* and the patient to guide the bones. Then the patient throws the bones onto the mat for the *sangoma* to interpret.[94]

Another means of consulting with a *sangoma* entails direct communication with the ancestors, without the use of "the bones." The *sangoma* will burn *impepo* (an indigenous herb) in order to facilitate a trancelike state the *sangoma* requires to communicate with the ancestors. This takes quite a bit of time and saps great energy from the *sangoma*. The *sangoma* will call forth the patient's ancestors and talk directly to them. Often, one or more of the patient's ancestors will actually appear before the *sangoma*. The *sangoma* will describe the person to the patient, so the patient can identify the ancestor. The patient can also ask questions and is invited to tell the *sangoma* when s/he is incorrect.[95]

Faith healing is generally associated with Zionist and Apostolic churches, which are without a doubt the "most significant expression of Christianity in Southern Africa" (Ashforth 2005, 185). Although the growth of these churches is usually attributed to missionary and apartheid racism (thus promulgating the creation of African churches, with syncretized religious practices), their popularity also arises from the "spiritual security they offer their congregations" against the evils of demons and witches (ibid.). Most of these churches offer their congregations some form of spiritual healing. In fact, "most healers of all kinds in South Africa have a formal religious background in Christianity, even if they do not practice" (Thornton 2002). Faith healers share a common theory of health and disease with other indigenous healers, but they synthesize Christian and indigenous healing practices. I held an FGD with a group of women who were trained as both faith and indigenous healers. I asked them to explain the relationship:

You talk to your ancestors, but you pray to God.

The ancestors are closer to God than you are.

The ancestors are between us and God. So, the ancestors take the message to God. And when the answers come, God replies to the ancestors, and the ancestors will tell the traditional healer.[96]

Faith healers utilize prayer, the laying on of hands, and the application of holy water, ashes, and herbs (Abdool-Karim, Ziqubu-Page, and Arendse 1994). They also use candles and the Bible to channel the spirit of God (Staugard 1985, 74). The Zion Christian Church (ZCC) uses water, coffee, and tea to cleanse the body of pollutants and evil spirits. Faith healers do not need to diagnose patients with a particular illness. Prophets simply pray with the patient and conduct private rituals that "cleanse them spiritually 'from inside' so that the illness might heal itself through the intercession of the holy spirit" (Thornton 2002).

The practice of witchcraft (*ubuthakathi* [Zulu] and *bomoloi* [Sotho]) is cloaked in silence. "Since the arts of witchcraft are secret, the practices and procedures of witches are generally inferred through analogy with their antitheses: the healers" (Ashforth 2005, 137). And yet, due to historic confusion between the two professions, healers are very insistent on the differences between the professions. Indigenous healers can detect and sometimes heal witchcraft, but do not engage in the "dark" arts. The most common forms of witchcraft entail the usage of *muthi* to entrance people (or cause them to fall in love); instigate misfortune, illness, or death; or elicit wealth and power for the witch (ibid., 133). However, witches can also act on a person through his/her dreams, use his/her personal effects (especially clothing, which carries the person's aura) or picture to cast spells, or turn him/her into a zombie— which occurs when a witch makes a double of a person and leaves it at home as a corpse in order to use the original as a slave (ibid., 225–35). Ashforth notes that the young people he studied in Soweto often use the analogy of technology to explain how people are able to mobilize the agency of *muthi* toward nefarious ends: "spiritual powers and technological powers are equally mysterious—but the capacity is the same" (ibid., 142). If a healer believes a particular illness or condition is caused by witchcraft, she can cleanse the substance from the person's body (through bathing, steaming, purgatives, or enemas); counter the "intentionality and direction of the poisonous agent"; or "protect and strengthen the victim against further assault" (ibid., 140). I will return to the significance and prevalence of witchcraft in the next section.

Overall, then, the spiritual world is, according to Ashforth, a very "tumultuous place":

> Relationships with invisible beings can be either hostile or friendly, supportive or antagonistic. What they cannot be is neutral. . . . [T]he image of a well-ordered cosmos ruled by a single almighty deity . . . has incomplete purchase on the imaginations of people struggling to manage relations with hosts of invisible beings wielding forces that are experienced as shaping the lives of the living in every detail. Managing relations with these beings is the central part of life." (Ashforth 2005, 170–71)

These multitudinous spiritual forces must be managed along with and in relation to other material, structural, or interactional social forces (like disease, the market, the state, civil society organizations, or kin). Inequality, economic deprivation, and a loss of community and tradition, which have all accompanied urbanization, deindustrialization, and postcolonialization, make many South Africans feel that they are the target of forces unknown and ungraspable, which can lead to profound feelings of vulnerability and anxiety.

Ontological Vulnerability

Along with forms of physical, social, and economic insecurity, Ashforth (2005) argues that in the post-apartheid era, South Africans are increasingly suffering from "spiritual insecurity." The fall of apartheid initiated important changes in the constitution of the bourgeoisie—some of the African population became exceedingly wealthy, but others faced growing unemployment and poverty. AIDS, crime, new forms of socioeconomic inequality, and the "erosion of community spirit" (101) have left South Africans with a profound sense of anxiety as well as feelings of resentment and jealousy. Without discourses or sites of social authority to make sense of (or redress) these rapid changes, Ashforth argues people have turned increasingly to religion and have sought explanations in the malicious theories of witchcraft. Witchcraft entails a presumption of malice on the part of community members. Ashforth argues that this is the negative corollary of *ubuntu*—where "a person is a person through other people . . . [with witchcraft] . . . because they can destroy you" (86).

In the ancient times, people were scared to engage in witchcraft, because during those times, people took care of each other. People would come together to denounce such practices. Now they are free to do such things.[97]

The reason most often cited for the increasing prevalence of witchcraft is jealousy:

Yes, there are witchcraft acts in Lawley. It is very prevalent. Because if one progresses, maybe I buy myself new furniture or something of value, people will start to get jealous and start to bewitch. And if there was no witchcraft, we would not be having a lot of work as traditional healers to heal those who have been bewitched.[98]

Witchcraft, it is so common.
CD: Why?
Because people are jealous. Sometimes you've got a car, or something of value, and someone sabotages you to stop you from progressing. It's to try to jeopardize other people's lives.[99]

In this context, any fortuity, economic success, or even moral pride that might offer a moment of respite from the daily destitution of abject poverty can actually lead to additional misfortune in the form of witchcraft. People, then, hide their economic triumphs because it may require reciprocal payback to those who previously offered a lending hand, *or* it may invite the scornful gaze and wrath of jealous neighbors.

In addition, Ashforth notes that to presume people living in your community have the capacity for "extraordinary action in the form of witchcraft creates an epistemological double bind" (2005, 13). This is because one can never be certain who may have malicious intent, but one can also never really know who has the capacity to practice witchcraft; thus, one has to simply be suspicious of everyone. This creates epistemic anxiety, according to Ashforth: "a sense of unease arising from the condition of knowing that invisible forces are acting upon one's life but not knowing what they are or how to relate to them" (127).

I believe there is witchcraft because of what is happening amongst and between the Black people. It's true that you cannot point to somebody to know if they are a witch because that person is invisible. . . . He knows what he is doing and he knows what is the end result . . . sometimes there are different ways of identifying or exposing a witch. Those who are believing in traditional or spiritual healing, they are likely able to see who is a witch—through their own powers. They can see who is causing troubles in your life. And there is a general notion that someone who is likely to be successful in bewitching you is someone who is in your extended family or someone who knows you well. But sometimes it's someone from outside. Witchcraft is there, they are everywhere.[100]

People who don't regularly use the services of indigenous healers will use them if they believe they have been bewitched. Everyone believes at least in the possibility of witchcraft—it would be impractical and dangerous not to. "There are witches even in our own midst. They are everywhere."[101]

This pervasive fear of something absolutely ubiquitous but unidentifiable is a primary source of ontological vulnerability for people living in informal settlements. Accompanying this fear, however, is a general unease about the loss of certain cultural practices and traditions, and the knowledge of them. In fact, the two are directly related. If one's ancestors are unknown, or one has lost the knowledge of how to properly thank them or ask them for their protection, then one is left defenseless against onslaughts from not only witches but also from an unknowable number of sources, be they material, social, or spiritual. One indigenous healer once discussed with me the ancestral impact of the changing family structure. She explained that male children's names were usually chosen from the father's side of the family as a way of identifying an ancestor who could protect the child. Since many children grow up never knowing their fathers, they also live without the knowledge of or protection from their father's ancestors.[102]

Some informal settlement residents have discussed the ways in which "development" has made it difficult to continue to practice certain rituals and traditions. One resident explains the restrictions associated with the small C-form structures built in Sol Plaatjie, which resemble row houses:

If you look at these new structures which they build here, they are not so convenient for us, especially Black people, because sometimes, we make traditional feasts where a lot of people are coming. Imagine if you are not getting along very well with your neighbor, then your neighbor doesn't want anything on her space. So the people cannot overflow to sit even, you know, in that space. And then worst part is that when there's a funeral, you can't get the coffin through the doors. You can't put it in the house, so how would you have a night vigil? We are pretty much inconvenienced. So I think this space, it could have been built, these structures, the way they are, for migrant workers who come in here and work knowing that they can go back home, you know. It's not a family—it's not a place to raise—to have a family.[103]

One healer explained that the reason witchcraft is so prevalent is because traditions are no longer followed, and so people feel they can take spiritual matters into their own hands.

It's because we left our original places where we grew up and where we used to stay. We came to the urban areas, where there is competition. We see that Pheello is being visited by a white person, and others get jealous, so that's where it starts from. One of the contributing factors is that here we are so mixed . . . there are those who go to the Faraday market[104] to buy the *muthi*. People will go to find *muthi* to hurt someone, and the seller will give it to you. This thing may cause problems when they get it home. That's why we were sitting with witchcraft. Sometimes there is a *muthi* that actually allows you to interact with the ancestors. Normally people buy it at Faraday. But traditionally you are not supposed to do that. You are supposed to dig it from the *veld* yourself. And most of the people who are selling the *muthi* at Faraday market are not initiated, they are not *inyangas*. They will see someone digging something in the field, so they will dig it, but they don't know the qualities of the *muthi*—or what it does. That is why we've got so much spread of HIV because other people they go there and buy an *imbiza*[105] for R10 and think it will assist you. But that *imbiza* is making more complications for a patient. After that, the patient will consult an *inyanga* to ask for assistance. By the time you attempt to assist that person, it will be too late, and that person dies. Then, others will think you are just killing people.[106]

Apartheid destroyed many African traditions and practices, with its forced migrations, urbanization, and legislation restricting African healing, but the "development" associated with the post-apartheid era, as well as catastrophic unemployment and AIDS, have led to further losses, which contribute to not only economic and social insecurities but also to ontological and spiritual ones. "Since ancestors are by definition guardians of tradition . . . the forgetting of rules and prohibitions in urban life has undermined the sense of ancestral efficacy" (Ashforth 2005, 176).

A final factor contributing to ontological vulnerability is that the social discord prevalent in informal settlements leads to a profound distrust of indigenous healers, despite their prevalence in the regions.

We do have a lot of them. Lawley is their kingdom, but I, for one, don't trust them and never use their services.[107]

Sangomas cannot tell you how long you have been sick or what your status is. . . . Sangomas mostly they lie, they say you have been poisoned, and others will say your ancestors are punishing you. So, they don't have a straight answer when it comes to HIV/AIDS.[108]

In a survey I helped to conduct in 2006 in Sol Plaatjie, only 12.5 percent of the respondents ranked indigenous health care an "effective strategy for fighting HIV/AIDS" (APF 2006, 28).[109] In 2009, 33.1 percent of residents of Sol Plaatjie listed indigenous healing as a form of health care used when someone is sick in the household. In Lawley, only 10.2 percent of residents indicated a usage of indigenous healing (CPR survey 2009).[110] There are four primary reasons why residents of informal settlements might be less likely to trust indigenous healers (than residents of formal townships or rural areas). First, charlatans of all shades have a tendency to feed off the most desperate—this makes shantytowns a primary target.

These impostors . . . they target the people who are really, really vulnerable. You won't find these signs advertising "cures" in the wealthier areas of town. The people who use this kind of "treatment," I think are low class, or who are, you know . . . desperate.[111]

You cannot find charlatans everywhere—they target the places where they see people need health care, and where they see people who are desperate. They target those people—mostly the poor.[112]

But in fact, some shantytown residents were more likely to try the random remedies packaged and sold by charlatans than use indigenous healers. These various tonics and mixtures (which are perhaps the form of "healing" *most* available to informal settlement residents) include "immune boosters," miracle vitamins, and hundreds of mysterious powders and liquid remedies that claim they can treat everything from asthma and low blood pressure to impotency and, always, HIV. At one of the support group meetings I attended in Lawley, a representative from a random organization touting a powder formula as an effective treatment for HIV/AIDS was given space to sell her product.[113] In addition to the sales representative, there were two women who served as witnesses, testifying to the formula's potency and miracle qualities: "Before I took this treatment, I was wasting away, and now look at me! I've gained twenty pounds, I have so much energy, and I've never felt better!" On the bottle, it claims to be an "herbal cure for AIDS." But then it also suggests it can cure the following:

Diabetes

TB

Kidneys

Arthritis

Back Pain

Boosts Erection

Flu

Joints and Inflammation

Period Pains

High Blood

Ulcers

Digestion

Dizziness

Purifies Blood

Sore Bones

Eyes

Ears

Kills Worms

Gives Appetite

Rheumatic

Diarrhea

Sweating

I expected Pheello to tell these people to stop exploiting the support group members, but instead, he tried the treatment and then forked over the R80 ($11) for the "first bottle." The remedy is usually packaged as one of a series of treatments that get progressively stronger. In order to buy the whole package, one would need R240 ($34)—an incredible amount of money for people whose entire household subsists on an average R976 per month ($139). When I asked Pheello why he tried this product, when he was such an adamant believer in biomedical treatment, he shrugged and said with a bit of embarrassment, "well, it couldn't hurt."

The second reason indigenous healers are not trusted in informal settlements is that they are often confused with witches.

People have norms that traditional healers are associated with wrongdoings. That's why there might be stigmas of traditional healers. But also, some people don't want to use them because they will then be accused of bewitching their neighbor.[114]

Sangomas will tell you that you are sick because your neighbor is using some *muthi* to bewitch you, so they are misleading people.[115]

And yet, indigenous healers are also recognized as the only source for remedying witchcraft. Healers in both Lawley and Sol Plaatjie told me that the primary demand for their services is associated with the prevalence of witchcraft in the region.

Most importantly, there are no regulatory mechanisms for ensuring the quality and legitimacy of indigenous healers who work in informal settlements. In formal townships, organizations of indigenous healers have developed to protect the profession against charlatans. Further, in formal townships, people *know* one another. They know family histories, they know their local *inyanga*, they know when a particular *sangoma* received his/her calling and probably attended his/her graduation. In informal settlements, people cannot rely on history or reputation. And because there are no regulatory institutions, impostors, fronting as indigenous healers, would fare far better in an informal settlement than in a formal township.

I think that there are some *sangomas* who are only doing business. Those who will judge you according to the way you dress. If you wear expensive shoes, then you will pay R1,500 to get cured.[116]

We respect the fact that in other communities, they are standing up and helping the community as best they can. In Lawley, they don't do that. They still haven't come out to the community to let us know what they know about HIV and how they might be able to help. They also don't seem to have any training on the disease at all—and traditional healers in other communities maybe do. . . . In their own respective practice, we believe they are not taught in a right way. I say this because when a new *sangoma* graduates, sometimes we go to that graduation. During the ceremony, we are supposed to hide something that they will find through their communication with the ancestors. But they battle to find that hidden object, and sometimes they fail completely. This is why we say they are undertrained.[117]

Table 8. Average cost per visit for health care

	Hospital	Local clinic	Regional clinic	Home-based care	Indigenous healer	Faith healer	NGO	Social worker or counseling
Sol Plaatjie	R44.12 ($6.30)	R17.78 ($2.54)	R23.52 ($3.36)	R72.50 ($10.36)	R302.86 ($43.27)	R35.85 ($5.12)	R13.00 ($1.86)	R32.50 ($4.64)
Lawley	R40.00 ($5.71)	R60.14 ($8.59)	R32.87 ($4.70)	N/A	R106.63 ($15.23)	R60.00 ($8.57)	N/A	N/A

CPR survey 2009

Finally, indigenous healers may be trusted, but simply not afford-able. Indigenous health care is more expensive than biomedical care, which the state subsidizes. As one healer in Sol Plaatjie explained: "Yes we are expensive . . . it is because of the hassles associated with organiz-ing all the things you need as a traditional healer. Because sometimes we are expected to . . . go and dig the medications. Or we need to stage a ritual or ceremony. Those things cost money, so we have to charge our patients more, and the people here are poor."[118]

Indigenous healers always have a primary role to play in funerals. As people who are able to straddle the multiple worlds of the living and dead, they help guide the dead on their journey to the spiritual world, but a healer's presence is also necessary to protect the living. When someone dies, his/her relatives enter a liminal zone, from having been close to death (especially those who shared sexual intimacy with the deceased). A series of important taboos serve to help protect the liv-ing from the pollution associated with bestriding the ancestral and material worlds (Douglas 2000; Hammond-Tooke 1981). Because people have lost knowledge of the various funereal rites and rituals, they can be major sites of danger and vulnerability. Therefore, although funerals are expensive (which are exacerbated by the need to hire indigenous healers to conduct purification rituals), people are willing to pay the cost.[119] In fact, an entire industry has developed around the production of death.[120]

The Production of Death

Due to the overwhelming toll AIDS has had on African communities in South Africa, Avalon, the cemetery on the outskirts of Soweto, has become a primary focal point of community activity. On any given

Saturday,[121] the entire geography of Soweto is reconfigured to accommodate the "production" of funerals. Torong and I drove to Soweto on August 13, 2005, where we waited at a corner and joined a convoy of twenty cars, buses, and bakkies[122] heading toward Avalon. On our way, our convoy was mixed up with several others. There seemed to be no other traffic on the roads. Police officers were directing traffic. I was struck by the efficiency of the operation—both on the streets of Soweto and at the gates of the cemetery—a rare occurrence in post-apartheid South Africa with its byzantine bureaucratic regulations. The "production" of funerals has in fact become a kind of industry of death due to the AIDS pandemic. And Avalon, generally a horrific, austere, and sinister site of mass-scale death, with its tombstones that stretch silently and disquietingly for miles on end[123]—was transformed into a bustling site of community participation. But with all of this obvious attention paid to the genocidal level of deaths the epidemic has produced, the words HIV or AIDS are never mentioned at funerals. The bodies are piling up, but their significance is cloaked in silence.

Accompanying the pervasive proliferation of discourses *about* AIDS and the various cacophonous symbolic struggles in which the post-

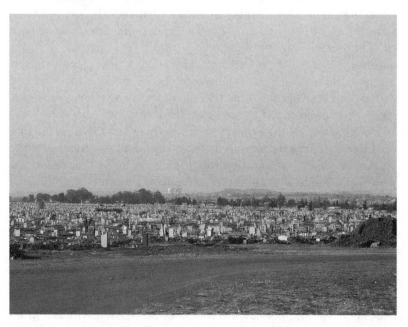

FIGURE 15.   Avalon cemetery. Photo taken by the author in 2005.

apartheid state is embroiled, is an eerie silence that circulates with deadly force within communities stricken by the dual pandemics of poverty and AIDS. The lack of words is a response to the answerlessness of thanatopolitics—the incomprehensibility of being abandoned by the state, civil society, and the community—left with a terrifying and debilitating disease as one's only company.

But the unaudibility of talk about AIDS is often less a matter of brute repression or secrecy than of complicated practices in the context of *radical uncertainty*. Nuanced registers and indirect forms of speech flourish in a field haunted by the ubiquitous presence of the disease. For death is the unspoken referent around which much everyday signification has been reoriented. (Comaroff 2007, 202; my emphasis)

The "epidemic of signification" (Treichler 1999) that marks the social landscape of AIDS in South Africa does not succeed in abating the lingering sense of unease and anxiety about a disease that has such an incomprehensible capacity to kill and destroy. As discourses abound, communities' own sense of meaning is destabilized. They are unable to make symbolic sense of the genocidal destruction they are suffering.

TWO

A State in Denial

There is this kind of illogical contrariness which celebrates so-called questioning of accepted truths when it comes to HIV and medicine, but doesn't see
any contradiction in . . . [embracing] the orthodox when it comes to economic policies. MARK HEYWOOD

As this quote from Mark Heywood[1] implies, Thabo Mbeki's
political leanings were often considered contradictory because while he rejected conventional health norms by suggesting that biomedical science had an imperialist agenda
(and even supported indigenous notions of healing over
biomedical ones), he embraced "modern," rights-based
gender initiatives and was a staunch promoter of neoliberal economic restructuring. I argue that Mbeki's logic is
only contradictory from a particular Western perspective.
In fact, his denialism operated as a rather coherent narrative that attempted to resolve the paradoxes created by colonialism and globalization. The perceived contradiction
is fully synthesized (even sublated) in Mbeki's dreams of a
postcolonial Africa reborn out of the ashes of colonial rule
and Western domination; his denialism was an indispensable feature of his postcolonial fantasy of independence
and autonomy. Before providing evidence for this analysis, a bit of historical contextualization is necessary.

The History of Denialism

The history of Mbeki's presidency and AIDS denialism
have been scrupulously documented by several scholars

(Nattrass 2007; Fassin 2007b; Gumede 2005; Johnson 2004 and 2005; Mbali 2002, 2003, and 2004; Jacobs and Calland 2002). Here I will only foray briefly into this history in order to provide background for my own analysis. The first manifestation of Mbeki's unorthodox views on HIV/AIDS emerged in 1997 when he threw his weight, as then deputy president, behind clinical trials on a new experimental drug, virodene. Two scientists at the University of Pretoria (Ziggy and Olga Visser) presented evidence to the cabinet from their unofficial trial with AIDS patients indicating that this antifreeze solution was an effective antiviral medication (Nattrass 2007, 42). They received a standing ovation. One cabinet member explained, "The thing I will always remember is the pride in South African scientists" (ibid.). Another cabinet member noted: "Virodene's champion was Mbeki himself. He couldn't wait to prove Africa's potential in the field of science and technology" (Myburgh 2012). Despite the eventual scandal and subsequent abandonment of the drug, it was originally touted as a possible "cure," and the ANC government (under the leadership of Mbeki) went to extraordinary lengths to promote the drug and to support the possibility of extensive human trials (Myburgh 2007).[2] Eventually, the Medicines Control Council (MCC) blocked clinical trials in South Africa.[3]

In 1999, as part of a mother-to-child-transmission-prevention (MTCTP) campaign, the Treatment Action Campaign (TAC) promoted the provision of AZT and nevirapine to pregnant women attending antenatal clinics (Heywood 2004b). In direct response to this campaign, Mbeki reported to the National Council of Provinces[4] that AZT was "toxic" and then asked the health minister to find out "where the truth lies" (Mbeki 1999a; quoted in Nattrass 2008a, 161).[5] One month later, he questioned the safety of AZT in a speech to Parliament (Mbeki 1999b). Then, in 2000, Mbeki convened a Presidential Advisory Panel on AIDS that included well-known AIDS denialists, including Peter Duesberg, the originator of the international AIDS dissident movement (Mbali 2003 and 2004; Specter 2007).

Peter Duesberg was one of the first scientists to discover key properties of retroviruses in the 1970s, for which he received international acclaim and recognition from the scientific community. Then, in 1987, he wrote a paper arguing that HIV is a mere "passenger" virus that causes no harm to the body (Specter 2007). Duesberg and his colleague, David Rasnick, noted that HIV "did not conform to the expected epidemiological patterns for viral pathogens. Instead, it looked more like the linear progression of illnesses caused by environmental factors" such as toxins, pollution, and lifestyles (Thornton 2008, 38). They concluded that HIV did not cause AIDS. Their inherently incongruous logic still managed to convince Mbeki that: (1) the drugs that were used to treat AIDS were actually the cause of it; and (2) because parasites and bacterial and viral infections are carried at a higher disease load by people living in poverty, many Africans were probably already infected with AIDS by the time they contracted HIV (ibid., 39). Mbeki wrote in 2000: "By resort to the use of the modern magic wand at the disposal of modern propaganda machines, an entire regiment of eminent 'dissident' scientists is wiped out from public view, leaving a solitary Peter Duesberg alone on the battlefield, insanely tilting at the windmills" (Specter 2007).

It was not until the International AIDS Conference held in Durban in late 2000 that Mbeki was publicly identified as a denialist for the following statements, which have been construed as a clear indication of his belief that poverty rather than HIV is the cause of AIDS:

The world's biggest killer and the greatest cause of ill-health and suffering across the globe is listed almost at the end of the International Classification of Diseases. It is given the code Z59.5—extreme poverty. . . . As I listened and heard the whole story told about our own country [as presented by the WHO], it seemed to me that we could not blame everything on a single virus . . . what is to be done, particularly about HIV-AIDS? One of the questions I have asked is are safe sex, condoms and antiretroviral drugs a sufficient response to the health catastrophe we face! . . . We remain convinced of the need for us better to understand the essence of what would constitute a comprehensive response in a context such as ours which is characterised by the high levels of poverty and disease to which I have referred. . . . The world's biggest killer and the greatest cause of ill health and suffering across the globe, including South Africa, is extreme poverty. (Mbeki 2000)

Mbeki never exactly claimed poverty *caused* AIDS.[6] Rather, he pointed out the structural vulnerabilities the poor face and suggested that attention paid to poverty might go a longer way toward curbing transmission than "safe sex, condoms and antiretroviral drugs." While public health professionals were focused on epidemiological solutions, Mbeki was debating structural causes.

In April 2002, an article titled "Castro Hlongwane, Caravans, Cats, Geese, Foot & Mouth and Statistics: HIV/AIDS and the Struggle for the Humanisation of the African" was posted to the ANC website anonymously. It is generally interpreted as a kind of denialist manifesto, and there has been widespread speculation that Mbeki penned it himself.[7] It is a fascinating read, especially since the article clearly draws on a history of science critique of biomedicine as well as historical evidence about the unethical treatment of Africans in pharmaceutical testing.[8] It suggests a conspiracy between scientists, doctors, and the pharmaceutical industry by branding biomedicine the "omnipotent apparatus"[9] and lambastes the international pharmaceutical industry for its corporate logic and greediness in the face of a humanitarian crisis.

Stridently and openly, the omnipotent apparatus disapproves of our effort to deal with the serious challenge in our country of health, poverty and underdevelopment. It is determined that it will stop at nothing until its objectives are achieved. What it seeks is that we should do its bidding, in its interests. In this respect, all of us are obliged to chant that HIV=AIDS=Death! We are obliged to abide by the faith, and no other, that our immune systems are being destroyed solely and exclusively by the HI Virus. We must repeat the catechism that sickness and death among us are primarily caused by a heterosexually transmitted HI Virus. Then our government must ensure that it makes antiretroviral drugs available throughout our public health system. (ANC 2002)

By 2002, Mbeki had stopped voicing denialist rhetoric publicly. In fact, he stopped talking about the epidemic altogether (*Mail and Guardian* 2002; Mbali 2004). Instead, Mbeki's minister of health, the controversial Manto Tshabalala-Msimang[10] became the public face of denialism.[11] Tshabalala-Msimang promoted a health paradigm that highlighted the importance of micronutrients and a healthy diet and lifestyle. Perhaps the most striking illustration of her position occurred in early 2005, when she stated publicly that garlic, olive oil, beetroot, and lemon could delay the onset of AIDS (Cullinan 2005).

Mbeki's denialist position on HIV/AIDS served to stall the public provision of antiretrovirals. From 2002 to 2004, the TAC had pursued action against industry abuse of patents through the Competition Commission, essentially suing GlaxoSmithKline and Boehringher Ingelheim and eventually securing seven voluntary licenses for antiretroviral drugs (Heywood 2009).[12] This radically transformed the landscape of AIDS health care in South Africa. By drastically reducing the cost of ARV treatment and thereby obliterating the last logical rationale the Department of Health had presented to providing ARVs through the public health system, a reluctant government was forced to finally adopt a National Treatment Plan that included the large-scale rollout of ARV medication (Department of Health 2003). As of 2004, ARVs were slowly becoming available in the public health sector free of charge. However, Tshabalala-Msimang (presumably at Mbeki's bidding) attempted to stymie the provision of ARVs in multiple ways. Although the rollout began in 2004, within two years "fewer than one third of the originally planned number of people were on HAART" [13] (Nattrass 2008a, 167). Tshabalala-Msimang's promotion of beetroot and garlic was part of a governmental critique of its own health policy on antiretrovirals. In addition, Tshabalala-Msimang was always ready to highlight the "toxic" side effects of the drugs, which she claimed were killing people (Nattrass 2008a, 166). For example, she declared: "When we were being pressured to use ARVs, we did warn about the side-effects, and when I get reports about the people on ARVs, nobody presents to me how many have fallen off the programme or died because of the side effects. . . . We need this information" (Adams 2005).

In early 2007 there was widespread speculation that the government's position on HIV/AIDS was changing. The minister of health received a lot of negative international attention because during the International AIDS Conference, held in Toronto in August 2006, the South African government's stall, which Tshabalala-Msimang designed, featured beetroot, lemons, and garlic, but not antiretrovirals. The United Nation's top official on HIV/AIDS, Stephen Lewis, denounced the South African government's position on ARVs as "wrong, immoral and indefensible" (*Mail and Guardian* 2006c). After this debacle, Tshabalala-Msimang was less visible in the public sphere. Rumors circulated that "Manto [had been] muscled out in a palace coup" (Cullinan 2006), but her absence was actually due to a prolonged illness and hospitalization. The press seemed to imply that Tshabalala-Msimang's illness was allowing the "real work" on HIV/AIDS to progress unchallenged.

On May 2, 2007, the cabinet approved the National Strategic Plan for HIV/AIDS and STDs "as a strategic framework that will guide the national response to HIV and AIDS over the next five years" (Cabinet 2007). Civil society organizations that had worked against the denialist government in support of the ARV rollout (like the TAC, the AIDS Law Project, and the AIDS Consortium) were thrilled at the work Deputy President Phumzile Mlambo-Ngcuka, Deputy Health Minister Nozizwe Madlala-Routledge, and acting Health Minister Jeff Radebe were able to accomplish in Tshabalala-Msimang's absence. Many thought AIDS denialism was dead (Cullinan 2007). But it kept on kicking for a few more months. Mbeki fired the deputy health minister and reinstalled Tshabalala-Msimang in August 2007. Mbeki himself was then ousted from the ANC leadership (replaced by his former deputy president, Jacob Zuma) in December 2007—though he remained president of South Africa until he resigned in September 2008. At that time,

Barbara Hogan replaced Tshabalala-Msimang as minister of health. Hogan immediately distinguished herself from her predecessor in her first public speech as minister by acknowledging the causal link between HIV and AIDS, commending the efforts of "the scientific, medical and activist communities," and committing the government to achieving the targets indicated in the National Strategic Plan—all moves that were considered historical turning points in South Africa's AIDS politics and that were publicly celebrated by the TAC (TAC 2008). Tshabalala-Msimang passed away in 2009 from complications from a liver transplant.

There was never any consensus on denialism within the internal structures of the ANC, though the sharpest criticisms emerged from members of ANC's tripartite alliance partners, the SACP (South African Communist Party) and COSATU (Congress of South African Trade Unions) (Heywood 2004b, 14; Robins 2008a, 107n10). In addition, despite denialism, a pilot HAART project was rolled out in the Western Province in 2000 through collaboration between the provincial leadership (which was controlled by parties oppositional to the ANC) and Médecins sans Frontières (MSF) (Nattrass 2008a, 174).[14] Despite these complicating factors, denialism "did nevertheless become de facto state policy" (Heywood 2004b, 14). One of the main reasons denialism was able to have such a profound and long-term effect on South Africa's AIDS politics was because health policy was fully centralized in the early years of democracy, as opposed to incorporating civil society participation (Thornton 2008, 161). This was in part due to Mbeki's rather autocratic style of governing, which entailed ousting ANC members who disagreed with his policies (Gumede 2008, 264). This approach changed once Zuma took power in 2009.

In the end, denialism shaped South African AIDS policy from at least 1999 through 2007. It has been estimated that 365,000 people died as a direct result of denialism. This number represents the people whose lives would have been saved if the rollout of ARVs had been implemented in 2000 instead of 2004 (Chigwedere et al. 2008; Dugger 2008). The TAC routinely issued WANTED posters plastered with Manto Tshabalala-Msimang's visage, suggesting she was responsible for "not stopping 600 HIV/AIDS deaths every day." Denialism was not only the scandal of the Mbeki presidency; it was also his most enduring legacy. Mbeki's denialism was often represented as simply "the ravings of a madman." However, such an interpretation underestimates his political acumen, the postcolonial dilemma he faced, and the depths to which he was willing to go to resolve it.

Complicating Denialism

When once more the saying is recalled, *Ex Africa semper aliquid novi!* (Something new always comes out of Africa!), this must be so, because out of Africa reborn must come modern products of human economic activity, significant contributions to the world of knowledge, in the arts, science and technology, new images of an Africa of peace and prosperity. Thus shall we, together and at last, by bringing about the African Renaissance depart from a centuries-old past which sought to perpetuate the notion of an Africa condemned to remain a curiosity slowly grinding to a halt on the periphery of the world. (MBEKI 1998B)

The discourse of "African renaissance" was a primary feature of Thabo Mbeki's presidency, and I argue that it is through this fantasy of independence that we can make sense of his AIDS denialism and its deadly effects. Mbeki initiated the call for Africa's renewal during a very evocative and memorable speech titled "I Am an African," which he made to Parliament in 1996 (as then deputy president) on the occasion of the adoption of South Africa's constitution:

I am an African. I am born of the peoples of the continent of Africa. . . . The dismal shame of poverty, suffering and human degradation of my continent is a blight that we share. The blight on our happiness that derives from this and from our drift to the periphery of the ordering of human affairs leaves us in a persistent shadow of despair. This is a savage road to which nobody should be condemned. This thing that we have done today, in this small corner of a great continent that has contributed so decisively to the evolution of humanity says that Africa reaffirms that she is continuing her rise from the ashes. Whatever the setbacks of the moment, nothing can stop us now! (Mbeki 1996)

Mbeki's renaissance is reminiscent of the various strands of Pan-Africanism that marked African struggles for independence throughout the continent—from Ghana's Nkrumah, to the Congo's Lumumba, to Tanzania's Nyerere (Ajulu 2001). And like these previous discourses, two primary goals are implied: (1) to construct and reassert a renewed culture and identity of Africanness, and (2) to emphasize Africa's economic regeneration within a globalized world order (Vale and Maseko 1998).

Because the struggle against apartheid ended so much later than other African countries' struggles against colonialism, Mbeki watched neighboring countries go through various crises of independence. He was aware of the problems associated with corruption and the rise of an elite postcolonial class manipulating power at the cost of the masses:

When its upper echelons are a mere parasite on the rest of society, enjoying a self-endowed mandate to use their political power and define the use of such power such that its exercise ensures that our continent reproduces itself as the periphery of the world economy, poor, undeveloped and incapable of development. (Mbeki 1998a; quoted in Ajulu 2001, 34)

He was equally aware of the devastation wrought by structural adjustment programs and the uneven distribution of the benefits of economic globalization:

The message that comes across is that the market is a cannibal that feeds on its own children . . . it feeds on the emerging adolescent it has spawned, taking advantage of the fact that this fattened being, described as being in transition, is fat enough to be an attractive meal and not yet fat enough to defend himself or herself from attack by the cannibal progenitor. . . . So does it come about that the market feeds on its most robust children, seemingly as an expression of a necessary condition of its existence (Mbeki 1998c; quoted on Ajulu 2001, 36).

This did not disenchant Mbeki from the promises of global capitalism, it only made him wary of its imperialist tendencies and made him ever more committed to pursuing economic development, but without the aid of the West (see also Johnson 2005). Ajulu (2001) explains that Mbeki's belief in Africa's renaissance is predicated on two related processes: "first, economic development is based on fostering the productive forces of capitalism; the second, political stability and accountability, [which] draws authority and legitimacy from the will of the people" (34). And thus Mbeki was committed to a version of global capitalism that required active participation on the part of Africa's citizens, in the words of his political advisor Vusi Mavimbela, "*to deliver themselves* from the legacy of colonialism and neo-colonialism and to situate themselves on the global stage as beneficiaries of all the achievements of human civilization" (Mavimbela 1997; quoted in Ajulu 2001, 34; emphasis added). As I explain later in this chapter, Mbeki's adoption of "rollout" neoliberal capitalism required the poor to become entrepreneurs of their own development and deliverance.

"An African solution to Africa's problems"—this mantra of the Mbeki era expresses the particularities of his nationalist fantasy for independence. Mbeki sought to secure South Africa's position as an economic and political leader on the continent (a goal he actively pursued through the New Partnership for Africa's Development, NEPAD), but he was extraordinarily antagonistic toward Western imperialism and expansionism. He promoted the active development of the poor through their self-responsibilization, which required the implementation of certain pedagogical forms of citizenship. Thus his vision combined economic neoliberalism with strong anti-imperialist sentiments.

Mbeki's denialism fits precisely within this framework. His views on antiretrovirals can be summarized as such: (1) he claimed that ARVs were not only toxic, but also their promotion at the global scale served the greedy interests of the Western pharmaceutical industry; (2) the notion that HIV was caused by "unsafe" sexual behavior seemed to provide support for age-old, racist, colonial assumptions about African sexuality and ignored more fundamental, structural causes like poverty; (3) he believed Africans should learn to develop their own solutions to the problems plaguing the continent and stop depending on the Western world—both financially and epistemologically; so, (4) he promoted indigenous forms of healing as an "African" approach to health, and he endorsed neoliberal economics as a means by which South Africa could secure a position as an economic leader on the continent.

Like all nation-building projects, Mbeki's postcolonial national imagining required the deployment of the tropes of "traditionalism" and "modernity," which served to (re)signify race, gender, and sexuality in the post-apartheid era. For example, his critique of the racist representations of African sexuality that characterize Western approaches to solving the "African AIDS crisis" as well as his dreams of an African renaissance led him to embrace modern, liberal, gender rights.

The women of our country carry the burden of poverty and continue to be exposed to unacceptable violence and abuse. It will never be possible for us to claim that we are making significant progress to create a new South Africa if we do not make significant progress towards gender equality and the emancipation of women. (Mbeki 2002)

Mbeki supported a woman to succeed him and introduced quotas for women's representation in political office and ANC structures. But it was in his attempts to delegitimize biomedical healing that he invoked "traditionalist" notions of race, which required the promotion of indigenous healing as the only true "African" solution to the epidemic. As such, in what follows, I show how Mbeki mobilized a certain cultural capital (Bourdieu 1986, 247) of indigeneity and authenticity. He sought to racialize biomedicine as anti-African and imperialist in nature; he attempted to delegitimize the Treatment Action Campaign by painting them as a group of white liberals who were only out for economic gain. Not only did Mbeki use race as a weapon in the symbolic struggle against treatment activists, but also in so doing, he redefined racial politics in the post-apartheid era *in direct response to* the AIDS pandemic.

The poor were important to Mbeki's vision of national development and progress. Their successful integration into the national and global economy represented postcolonial victory, and they still made up the majority of the ANC's voting base. However, Mbeki was not a populist leader (unlike his successor), and the poor did not identify with him. He was highly educated, had grown up in exile in England, and he was aloof and autocratic. His plan was to earn the trust of the poor through a series of technocratic service delivery projects, which were linked to disciplinary measures. These provisions to the poor replaced more profound structural redistribution. But he also used indigenous healing to cultivate his "authenticity" capital—in part because of his lack of popular support. It was through indigenous healing that he attempted to claim his position as a rightful heir of the liberation struggle.

For Mbeki, however, the poor could only be incorporated into the post-apartheid body politic if they were willing to "develop themselves." He therefore introduced a series of rollout neoliberal measures, with disciplinary strings attached. In this way, the state provided a series of social safety nets for the poor in an attempt to change their behavior. Those who could not adapt would be left behind on the road to development. And thus one begins to glimpse the more insidious features of Mbeki's denialism. The rebirth of Africa required letting a certain portion of the population die, for the perceived interest of the national good. Foucault labels this sovereign decision "thanatopolitics" (1990; 1997).

In this chapter, I address four important features of Mbeki's denialism: the way in which he utilized and thus resignified racial identity, his promotion of indigenous healing as an alternative to biomedical care, his undermining of the antiretroviral rollout program, and his attempt to entrepreneurialize the poor. I then explore the deadly costs of his vision for a renewed Africa and illustrate how HIV-infected South Africans have responded to their own social abandonment.

Resignifying Race

AIDS lays bare schisms of inequality long in the making, but it has also instituted new exclusionary practices. Contemporary analyses of inequality in South African have suggested that the political transition and the adoption of neoliberalism have served to supplant race for class as the leading structural force in post-apartheid politics (Bond 2000 and 2002). In these analyses, structural racism is simply an unfortunate leftover from apartheid. Against this trend, I argue that racial politics have instead been complicated and newly rearticulated in the post-apartheid era.

The history of colonial and apartheid racism undergirds Mbeki's denialism. In his detailed account of Mbeki's views on HIV/AIDS, Fassin (2007b) argues that South Africa has been rendered amnesiac. Only through a reading of the present in light of the colonialist past (ibid., 169–70) can we begin to make sense of Mbeki's "ghosts" (Mbali 2002).

I speak of courage because there are many in our country [who] would urge constantly that we should not speak of the past. . . . The story of Sarah Bartmann is the story of the African people of our country in all their echelons. . . . It is an account of how it came about that we ended up being defined as a people without a past, except a past of barbarism, who had no capacity to think, who had no culture, no value system to speak of, and nothing to contribute to human civilization—people with no names and no identity. . . . The legacy of those centuries remains with us, both in the way in which our society is structured and in the ideas that many in our country continue to carry in their heads. (Mbeki 2002)

Mbeki's denialism incorporates an analysis of the role colonization played in creating the conditions for the AIDS epidemic, and he urges South Africans to remember the scientific racism inherent in the eugenics movement and the apartheid government's various health violations. In a report prepared for the Truth and Reconciliation Commission, the American Association for the Advancement of Science and Physicians for Human Rights provide evidence of the various health violations the apartheid government exercised, including: the inequitable allocation of resources (that is, failing to provide funding for the prevention of diseases common among the African population, like tuberculosis or asbestos poisoning); evading the punishment of doctors who covered up torture; refusing emergency medical care to activists; or breaching patient confidentiality to provide information to security forces (American Association for the Advancement of Science [with Physicians for Human Rights] 1998). Women were often injected with Depo-Provera (a controversial contraceptive) without their consent or knowledge (ibid.). In addition, Dr. Wouter Basson (or "Dr. Death" as he is commonly referred to), a key member of the chemical and biological warfare program of the apartheid government, was accused (though never convicted) of poisoning anti-apartheid activists, manufacturing cholera and anthrax, and injecting salmonella and botulism into chocolates (Selva 2005; see also Fassin 2007b, 161–68). This history provides some of the context for Mbeki's skepticism of biomedical science.

Mbeki used the controversy surrounding the drug nevirapine (an ARV given to mothers during childbirth to prevent vertical transmission[15]) to lambaste the pharmaceutical industry's historical usage of Africans for clinical and drug trials. In September 1999, a report from a clinical trial in Uganda found that a single dose of nevirapine given to a mother and her infant during labor would halve the chances of vertical transmission. This became the basis for the drug's usage throughout the continent. In 2004, the Associated Press ran a story that unveiled the fact that this Ugandan clinical trial downplayed problems with the drug and failed to communicate them to the US Food and Drug Administration (FDA) (Cohen 2004). The South African government had been hesitant to fully license the usage of nevirapine, and when this story broke, Mbeki clearly felt vindicated in his reservations. Nevirapine had never been approved by the FDA, according to Mbeki, because its application for review was furtively withdrawn. He thus insinuated a conspiracy on the part of the United States and the pharmaceutical industry to simply use Africans as "guinea pigs":

This tells the deeply disturbing and frightening story that "top" U.S. government officials were ready to hide from "African countries looking for U.S. guidance on the drug," the adverse effects of Nevirapine they knew very well, and which they were certain would oblige the FDA to reject the license application of the drug maker. In other words they entered into a conspiracy with a pharmaceutical company to tell lies to promote the sales of Nevirapine in Africa, with absolutely no consideration of the health impact of those lies on the lives of millions of Africans. (Mbeki 2004a)

Mbeki's concerns are not unfounded. Medical research sponsored by wealthy countries is still conducted in poor countries. Paul Farmer notes an ongoing "global Tuskegee experiment" whereby "afflictions of the poor," when consistently ignored become, in essence, a "control group of unfortunates [who] exhibit the natural history of untreated disease" (1999, 35). Unfortunately, however, because Mbeki's critiques were used to stall the rollout of life-saving medications, his entire argument was discredited.[16]

Similarly, Mbeki was concerned that Western representations of the "AIDS crisis" were derived from racist assumptions about the voracity of Africans' sexual appetites. In fact, Mbembe and Nuttall claim that

Western representations of AIDS in Africa are "fraught in ways that go beyond even the paradigm of orientalism first introduced by Edward Said" (2004, 348).[17]

[History] . . . created an image of our Continent as one that is naturally prone to an AIDS epidemic caused by rampant promiscuity and endemic amorality. (Mbeki 2001, 7)

We [Africans] are germ carriers, and human beings of a lower order that cannot subject its [sic] passion to reason. We must perforce adopt strange opinions . . . convinced that we are but natural-born promiscuous carriers of germs. . . . They proclaim that our continent is doomed to an inevitable mortal end because of our devotion to the sin of lust. (Mbeki, from Forrest and Streek 2001)

Mbeki rejected the epidemiological and public health response to HIV/AIDS that focused on individual sexual behavior as the causal factor for transmission. To him, this response implies that Africans have far more (unprotected) sex than Westerners. In other words, the international epidemiological approach decontextualizes behavior and ignores the structural factors that create conditions of vulnerability to disease. Obviously his concerns and his focus on structural causal factors are not only relevant but also provide an important critique of the global health industry. But they also provided fuel for his denialism.

In addition to highlighting the racism inherent in historical and contemporary biomedical health campaigns, Mbeki used race to delegitimize the TAC and to thus portray antiretrovirals as an imperialist imposition. The TAC was founded and initially operated by a group of anti-apartheid activists who were mostly intellectuals (lawyers, academics, and other professionals). This original leadership used its class position to mobilize tremendous economic and symbolic capital in the fight against denialism and for the public provision of treatment. However, the racial and class makeup of the TAC's leadership invited scorn and accusations of racism for maintaining a largely white leadership,[18] while its volunteer and activist base was made up of poor, African, HIV-positive community members. Accusations were made that the TAC paid its African members to attend rallies in order to boost its public image.[19] In April 2003, Mark Heywood (whose quote began this chapter) was attacked in a public speech by Health Minister Tshabalala-Msimang, who accused him of being a "white man misleading black people in TAC to demonstrate against the government" (Heywood 2004a). Similarly, the National Association of People with AIDS (NAPWA) criticized the

TAC in an AIDS Consortium general meeting held in March 2004: "we are sick of white people sitting at the front of the meeting; it causes us pain" (Heywood 2004a). Recognizing the validity of the critique,[20] the TAC eventually changed its leadership by replacing the national chairperson and incorporating community activists into its leadership at all levels (Heywood 2004b; Jacobs and Johnson 2007). In addition, the organization became much more involved in grassroots initiatives after winning the battle against denialism.[21]

In the end, much of Mbeki's denialism attempted to portray biomedicine as a racialized science masquerading as an objective epistemology. He not only suggested that international (or national) programs based on biomedical treatment neglected the fundamental causes of disease (poverty and underdevelopment) in order to serve the greedy interests of the pharmaceutical industry, but also that biomedical public health is itself an imperialist project that ignores the cultural and racial identity of Africans. Thus the denialist state *wielded* race as an ideological weapon in its battle with the TAC, *and* it promoted indigenous healing *in the place of* antiretrovirals, which were represented as "foreign" and "toxic" (*Sunday Independent* 2004).

Indigenous Healing

The denialist government invoked indigenous healing in the symbolic struggle over the management of HIV/AIDS for two reasons: first, to delegitimize biomedical healing as incapable of addressing an *African* disease, and second, to attempt to garner support from the masses who rely so heavily on "traditional" health practices. And so indigenous healing became one of the primary ways in which Mbeki invoked "tradition" and thus attempted to resignify Africanness. In fact, Mbeki went the furthest of any South African public official to institutionalize indigenous healing not because he was a strong proponent of the profession himself, but rather in an effort to position it as a viable alternative to antiretrovirals, thereby providing a nonbiomedical health care option for the poor.

The Traditional Health Practitioners Act was first signed into law in early 2005 (Republic of South Africa 2005),[22] was subsequently challenged, and then was reenacted as of January 2008.[23] Overall, the act provides guidelines for the definition of indigenous healing and the registration and certification of practitioners. It establishes a Traditional Health Practitioners' Council, the members of which are appointed by the minister of health. An indigenous healer is chosen as chairperson, and each province and each indigenous health profession is represented by an indigenous healer sitting on the council. In addition, a biomedical doctor and pharmacist sit on the council, though no indigenous healer sits on the South African Medical Association or the Health Professions Council.

The healers the act defines include: herbalists (*inyangas*), diviners (*sangomas*), "traditional" birth attendants, and "traditional" surgeons. This categorization was first suggested by the Select Committee on Social Services in 1998 (Select Committee on Social Services 1998; Ashforth 2005, 291). Ashforth notes that "traditional" birth attendants and surgeons can be easily integrated into a biomedical system because such a step would only require healers to be trained on hygienic practices; however, incorporating *inyangas* and *sangomas* is much more complicated because the premise of their work is radically different from biomedical principles (2005, 292). "Implicit in the description of healing categories presented in the Committee's report is a model of functional differentiation of professions and modes of training that is thoroughly Western and modernist in conception and that ignores the possibility of unseen evil forces acting in both the etiology and the treatment of disease" (ibid.). Faith healers are ignored altogether.

Despite these challenges, most indigenous healers welcome the legislation because they believe it will salvage the reputation of the profession from being associated with charlatanry and witchcraft. However, the act mostly subjects the profession to scrutiny and does little to actually provide institutional support for indigenous healing or provide healers with remuneration for their services—two moves that would be essential if the profession were ever to be considered a health care option on equal footing with biomedical healing. The legislation further bifurcates the two approaches by providing them each with separate legislation.[24] This means that the mixing of health approaches is literally outside of the law. There is no policy or legislation that contends with the relationship *between* biomedical and indigenous approaches to healing. Finally, even though the act was first passed in 2005, there has been virtually no movement, on the part of the state, to actually implement the policies detailed within it. In fact, "a significant critique of this Act is that it does not propose concrete measures through which to implement its objectives" (Mills 2005, 146). In an interview held in 2009, an indigenous healer explained, "we have the Act, but we don't have the Council, which is quite frustrating . . . you do have the Act, but we don't have any policy on how are you going to, you know, to . . . implement the Act."[25]

On the subject of the legislation, Dr. Robert Tshabalala told me: "I appreciate the fact that Mbeki supports traditional healing, but I don't see any major changes. If there were changes, then people wouldn't come to traditional healers with already made solutions . . . with briefcase solutions to our problems."[26] At the request of some of the indigenous healers with whom I worked, I sat on a task team formed by the Gauteng Department of Health to strategize around the role indigenous healers should play in the AIDS pandemic.[27] While the indigenous healers engaged in this process in order to directly participate in the professionalization and institutionalization of their vocation, the Department of Health was only concerned with providing workshops to indigenous healers to explain to them the biomedical definitions of HIV, sexually transmitted infections (STIs), and tuberculosis (TB). In terms of their service to the state, the Department of Health wanted healers to be part of the home-based care (HBC) initiative—which provides funding to lay volunteers to provide palliative home care. In other words, indigenous healers' knowledge and expertise on healing was only considered valuable as HBC volunteers who could help ease the financial and human resource burden on the public health sector.

There is no real budget for traditional healing, apart from moneys allocated for AIDS. . . . So it means if we didn't have this pandemic, there would be no money given to traditional healers at all.[28]

Some members of the Department of Health did try to act on the government's mandate to incorporate indigenous healing, but they were not given any directives or a budget. In fact, the Gauteng Department of Health was quite proactive;[29] however, without any national government support or direction, and with so many complications involved in the process, even those with the best of intentions were forced to resort to "briefcase solutions." From what I can tell, most of these initiatives have slowly disintegrated.[30]

Both my ethnographic and textual data suggest that the government was content to use indigenous healing as an ideological weapon in the symbolic struggle over HIV/AIDS without making any significant efforts to change the current state of affairs in which indigenous healing subsists as a peripheral and informal health care option for poor, African communities. In promoting an ideology of "indigeneity" and using race politics to undermine the legitimacy of the TAC and other biomedical proponents, Mbeki constructed a false dichotomy between African "authenticity" and biomedical care—thus contributing to a myth of incommensurability and insinuating that the usage of antiretrovirals was un-African or imperialist in nature. He therefore attempted to convince those who most needed antiretrovirals to eschew them and use only "natural" or indigenous forms of healing.

Undermining the Rollout

Prior to the passing of the National Treatment Plan in 2003 and the subsequent (but slow) rollout of antiretrovirals in 2004, the state had simply tried to avoid financing the public provision of antiretrovirals, but once this became impossible, the state resorted to a number of tactics to undermine its own ARV program. As Nicoli Nattrass (2008b) explains, the voluntary licenses (won in the Constitutional Court case from Boehringher Ingelheim and GlaxoSmithKlein)[31] were delayed, and the Medicine Control Council (MCC) then had to approve the medicines. The state awarded tenders to producers of branded products instead of generic producers and interfered with provincial governments' attempts to gain grants from The Global Fund to Fight AIDS, Tuberculosis, and Malaria to facilitate the ARV rollout. Further, the state failed to invest in laboratory capacity or the training and retention of health professionals. In addition (as already mentioned), the minister of health called the safety of ARVs into question and promoted indigenous remedies and vitamin supplements in the place of ARVs. "In so doing, both the supply of HAART services and the demand for them was artificially constrained by government" (Nattrass 2008b, 576). But beyond these more direct means of sabotaging the rollout, the denialist state used a series of governmental strategies to discourage people from using antiretrovirals—by suggesting they were unsustainable in squatter conditions, that their side effects were dangerous, and that due to severe nutritional lacks, citizens should utilize vitamins and indigenous forms of healing instead

There is this notion that if you haven't treated patients with ARVs (antiretrovirals) then you have not done anything. . . . With a population which has high levels of micronutrient deficiencies caused by food insecurity, as well as health system challenges means adopting a model which focuses exclusively on ARV therapy would not solve the problem. (Tshabalala-Msimang, South African Press Association 2006)

You can't say the response to an unhealthy human body is drugs. Your first response is proper feeding. The Minister of Health repeats this thing every day and what do they do, they mock her. It's like she's some crazy person from the moon! (Mbeki 2004b)

This approach is typified by the Rath Foundation—behind whom the state hid once Mbeki decided to damper his own public denialist exhortations. Key members of the Treatment Action Campaign and AIDS Law Project argue that the Rath debacle was a "shocking demonstration of where our government stands in relation to HIV and AIDS . . . because it reveals that denialism, which everybody thought was over when the operational plan was passed, is actually not over."[32] The Rath Foundation,[33] run and operated by the internationally controversial figure of Dr. Matthias Rath, announced its presence in South Africa by running a series of advertisements in national and local newspapers throughout the country. These advertisements not only promoted his own vitamin products—as an "answer" to the ravages of the South African AIDS pandemic—but also defamed antiretrovirals, the pharmaceutical corporations that sell them, and the TAC itself, which, according to Rath, acted as "the running dogs of the drug cartel in South Africa" (Rath 2005a). The Rath Foundation was operational in South Africa from 2004 through June 2008 when the Cape High Court found Rath's clinical trials and vitamin distribution unlawful (TAC 2009a).

The South African government did not overtly or publicly support the Rath Foundation and its propaganda, its rollout of vitamins in townships throughout South Africa, or its controversial "clinical trials" on human subjects; however, its relationship to the organization was suspicious.

The Rath Foundation is just another manifestation of AIDS denial, which is a slight arm's length from the President and the Minister of Health, and the current people who control the apparatus in the ANC, but is nonetheless connected to them, and traceable to them. And the fact that Rath hasn't been closed down is indicative of the fact that it reveals that that thinking has not gone away at that level of government.[34]

One of Mbeki's previous AIDS advisors, well-known denialist Anthony Brink, worked for the Rath Foundation,[35] and investigations into Rath's vitamin supplements and clinical trials were furtively called off and delayed.[36] In addition, the Rath Foundation employed a discourse similar to that of Mbeki's, which highlighted poverty, the social construction of science, and the greed of the pharmaceutical industry.

We focus on health care, which is monopolized by the pharmaceutical industry. When people are sick, in a capitalist system, then the market works only when people stay sick. Some illnesses (like high blood pressure, etc.), which are really part of the natural life course, are created by the pharmaceutical industry in order to create new markets for their drugs. The more people who are sick, the more they make a profit. . . . Disease is therefore in their interest, and they fight against anything that actually prevents or cures the diseases on which they make their profit. . . . We are here to reform primary health care, to promote affordable therapies and cost-effective natural products.[37]

The Rath Foundation promoted its own vitamins as the most natural, cost-effective approach to HIV (which they claimed to be distributing in South Africa free of charge but which were never approved by the national regulatory institution, the MCC). "Denialism is not the issue. The real issues are the toxicity of drugs and the fact that nutrients are the cost effective means of dealing with the disease. . . . Poverty does cause AIDS. We are bringing the science to support the power of the nutrient."[38] Given that the minister of health utilized this exact same discourse in defense of her promotion of vitamins over antiretrovirals (Adams 2005), the South African media often suggested that the denialists and Rath were in cahoots. When asked "why South Africa?," the spokesperson for the Rath organization responded: "Because of the progressive approach of the South African government. They recognize the importance of nutrients."[39]

In addition to sharing a common AIDS denialism and ideology that promoted "natural" health options over "toxic" pharmaceuticals, the Rath Foundation deployed a racial critique that was uncannily similar to Mbeki's. In the words of Anthony Brink:

Why did HIV/AIDS, as an item, seize the public imagination and particularly the white imagination (liberal and conservative) . . . after 1994? AIDS was nothing, in the public consciousness, until the revolution—when the old order had been displaced. So, I have explored AIDS as a manifestation of mass epidemic hysteria. This notion that, let's be frank about this, the thinking is: African people are rife with AIDS. . . . There is a phenomenon of "othering" in play. I find that very interesting. I have set about flushing out, quite brutally—by that I mean, uncompromisingly—the inarticulate, enduring racist preconceptions that fuel this kind of thinking.[40]

But Brink did not stop with a critique of the racist and colonialist assumptions that have historically underwritten medical discourses. He suggested that AIDS in South Africa was constructed and turned into a "mass epidemic hysteria" by "white liberals" who needed to find a sense of belonging after the fall of apartheid.

White liberals lost their voice with the revolution in '94 . . . Now that they're suddenly bereft of a function, they need something, they need a cause. You know, so AIDS has become a cause. . . . But it's driven by a tremendous residual racism . . . It's based on a deeply engrained cultural chauvinism. . . . They need HIV and AIDS to have a cause. But also, HIV and AIDS ideology gives them a continuing sense of superiority. A continuing reason to regard the other as a diseased lot.[41]

In addition to offering an "alternative" to antiretrovirals (supposedly backed up by "science"), in the Rath Foundation, the denialist government found ideological support for its political agenda. In fact, most of the critiques the Rath Foundation put forward were already made by Mbeki in the early years of the transition (Heywood 2004b), so when he withdrew from public debate on HIV/AIDS, the Rath Foundation was there to continue his legacy. The attempt, epitomized so thoroughly by the Rath agenda, was to encourage distrust of ARVs so that people who finally had access to ARV medications that could extend and improve their lives would eschew biomedical treatment and rely instead on immune boosters, vitamins, and nutritious food.

As neoliberal economic restructuring requires the state to cut social services, one cannot ignore the convenience of Mbeki's attempt to avoid financing the public provision of antiretrovirals. Daniel Herwitz has argued that a "smokescreen" becomes essential when a state is faced with a "stark" "Malthusian" choice: "either one denies antiretrovirals to pregnant mothers, guaranteeing an early death to their children, or one floods the society with motherless children for whom nobody can care" (Herwitz 2006, 2). In fact, Parks Mankahlana, the late presidential spokesperson, made this argument in no uncertain terms during the national debates about funding MTCTP. He insinuated, publicly, that it cost less state resources to let HIV-infected children die than to have them become dependent upon the state as orphans (Nattrass 2007, 63–64; Mbali 2004, 110). From such a point of view, denialism was quite simply a convenient excuse for the failure to provide adequate health care to an undesirable population. Although made often enough (Mbali 2004; Bond 2004), I will now show how this is far too simplistic an explanation. Other scholars have also addressed this line of argumentation, suggesting that the provision of ARVs to the country's poor is actually more cost effective than letting them die from AIDS illnesses, especially once the prices of the drugs were reduced (Nattrass 2008a, 163). As such, purely economic rationalization cannot explain denialism.

From Two Nations to Two Economies

As deputy president, Mbeki once labeled South Africa a country of two nations—one white and one Black, one rich and one poor (Mbeki 1998d). But by his second term of office, he had shifted to describing South Africa as being possessed of a first and second economy:

Now, this is, as it were, the modern part of South Africa, with your aeroplanes and your computers and the people sitting around this room who read and write and so on. We, all of us, we are this modern sector. . . . So you have this large part of South Africa, which is relatively uneducated. It is unskilled. It is not required in terms of modern society. I am saying "required" in the sense of employability. So, we have recognised this from the beginning, that large numbers of our people are poor and are in this condition. You can make the interventions we make about modernisation of the economy and so on, but it wouldn't necessarily have an impact on them, because of that degree of marginalisation. Therefore, you needed to make different sorts of intervention. (Mbeki 2003; quoted in Hart 2006, 24)

At this juncture, Mbeki adopted a governmental approach that paternalistically targeted those he deemed superfluous to the modern economy: those bemired in "tradition" could be saved and brought into the modern economy if they were willing to be disciplined so that they could become self-sufficient entrepreneurs. As a means of incentive, citizenship rights would be circumscribed by behavioral norms.

Discourses of self-responsibility were particularly prevalent in the promotion of prepaid water and electricity meters, as well as indigence programs. Von Schnitzler (2008) explains that paying for basic services was framed, from the outset, as a means of promoting "active" citizenship. She quotes from a 1994 White Paper on Water Supply and Sanitation Policy:

An insistence that disadvantaged people should pay for improved water services may seem harsh but the evidence indicates that the worst possible approach is to regard poor people as having no resources. This leads to people being treated as the objects rather than as the subjects of development. . . . A key element influencing a household's willingness to pay for an improved water supply is the households' sense of entitlement . . . and their attitude toward Government policy regarding water supply and sanitation. In general, communities are reluctant to involve themselves in countries where the perception prevails that it is the Government's responsibility to provide services. (Quoted in von Schnitzler 2008, 906)

Von Schnitzler goes on to explain that new economic rationalities were introduced, through the corporatization of water and electricity delivery, to "equip citizens with the ability to calculate and engage in cost/benefit analysis" (2008, 902).

The usage of prepaid technology (which, as explained in the previous chapter, was first introduced in 2003 as part of the government's water delivery restructuring) has become one of the primary instigators for public unrest. In the 2004/2005 year, there were 881 illegal and 5,085 legal social service protests on record (Hart 2008, 682). These subsided during the 2006 local government elections and reemerged with more violence and fury in 2007 (ibid.). In the face of these protests, the government utilized several strategies to attempt to garner South Africans' acceptance of prepaid technology. For example, informal settlement upgrades are provided on the condition that prepaid services will be installed.[42] In addition, new indigence policies allowed for the complete erasure of accumulated debt[43] in exchange for an acceptance of prepaid meters and an agreement to be identified and registered as indigent (Naidoo 2010; Hart 2006).

Some have argued that the shift in Mbeki's second term constituted a belated turn toward Third Way politics—which was meant to quell, at least in part, widespread discontent expressed through a surprising number of spontaneous uprisings of the poor throughout the country (Hart 2006, 26). Mbeki was very clear: only those who could prove their disciplinability, who were capable of self-regulation, were worthy of incorporation into the modern economy. This process ultimately drew a dividing line around the outskirts of the body politic. Those capable of self-regulation were included within the body politic and became objects of regulatory and disciplinary regimes of power. The state deployed a series of governmental tactics, including the privatization of basic services, the outsourcing of health care to community volunteers, and the appropriation of "do-it-yourself" logic, in order to encourage pedagogical citizenship (Von Schnitzler 2009) and shift its welfare responsibilities onto the shoulders of the poor themselves. But those who were incapable of assuming entrepreneurial technologies of the self or who were untrainable in civic lessons of self-regulation were forsaken. This simultaneous process of incorporation and abandonment was buttressed by Mbeki's denialism.

As a means of promoting both Third Way politics and a denialist agenda, the state invoked the "community" as a vector through which citizens were to garner self-control and construct entrepreneurial identities (Rose 1999, 175–76). Toward this end the state encouraged citizens to "do it themselves"—a common move in neoliberal governmentality since it helps cloak the state's abdication of the provision of social welfare and support while simultaneously promoting self-reliance and responsibility. President Mbeki declared 2002 the Year of the Volunteer for reconstruction and development, an eerie reminiscence of the "Volunteer Week" instigated in 1987 by one of the primary leaders of neoliberal ideology, Ronald Reagan. In 2003, the Department of Health launched a media campaign asking citizens to "take responsibility for their own health care": "We need to start owning our programmes and move towards self-reliance. . . . We need to strengthen the spirit of volunteerism amongst our communities" (Tshabalala-Msimang 2003).

The state's home-based care strategy, which provides extremely minimal resources to women who essentially "volunteer" to provide basic palliative care to victims of the HIV pandemic, helps alleviate the financial burden on the state and allows the government to avoid provisioning public health care. The government sells this as an "investment in social cohesion" (Cullinan 2000). Through home-based care, the government insists, "disease may become normalized within society, expensive institutionalized care is avoided, and social networks are maintained and even strengthened" (ibid.). Indigenous healers are also part of this social response to the disease (Gauteng Department of Health 2010, 56).

Community-based care is the care that the consumer can access nearest to home, which encourages participation by people, responds to the needs of people, encourages traditional community life and creates responsibilities. . . . Care in the community must become care by the community . . . it is undesirable, patronizing and promotes dependence if the state does it for them. (A National Guideline on Home-Based Care and Community-Based Care: ANC 2001)

Home and community based care is a very important component of our response to HIV and AIDS, TB and other debilitating conditions . . . it is geared towards community empowerment. It takes a holistic approach to the challenge of diseases related to poverty that is affecting our people and takes into account the cultural beliefs and values of individuals. . . . HIV and AIDS as well as TB . . . [have placed] a heavy burden on our formal health care and social security system. Hospitals are seeing increased bed occupancy rate and average length of stay putting additional pressure on our human and other resources. Partly as a result of all these factors, Cabinet prioritised home and community based care and support as a key intervention to mitigate the impact of HIV, AIDS and TB. (Tshabalala-Msimang 2003)

This ideology of self-reliance resonates well in South African communities, guided by the age-old philosophy of *ubuntu*—"a person is a person through other people." This classic adage stressing communal respect and solidarity is put to neoliberal use, in the post-apartheid era, as a means of promoting community self-reliance as an alternative to government dependence. Every other small, community-based group in South Africa is called "Iketsetseng" or "Vukuzenzele," both of which mean "do-it-yourself."[44]

Iketsetseng means "do-it-yourself," it means self-reliance—not begging and not depending on anyone else to do it for you. People in South Africa suffer from a dependency syndrome, all the time thinking that other people should do things for them. . . . It started under apartheid, this syndrome, but even in post-apartheid, people are finding it hard to change their mentality.[45]

Vukuzenzele means "wake up and do-it-yourself." People waited for the government to deliver, and the government did not. Now, it's a wake-up call. Now, stand up and do-it-yourself because no one will ever do it for you.[46]

As the state cut-back on social support and the rising unemployment rate threw the poor into desperate competition over scarce resources, thus effectively destroying community solidarity, this cooptation of community-based values of care became sardonic.

In addition to the outsourcing of care, Mbeki used the provision of social welfare grants as a technocratic means of avoiding more profound economic redistribution (Hunter 2010, 107–8),[47] which further implicated the poor in their own social abandonment. South Africa's welfare system is set up to provide only to those who cannot work to support themselves (Seekings and Nattrass 2006)—though, as was shown in the previous chapter, the poor often rely on grants as their only means of subsistence.[48] HIV was added to the list of disabilities eligible for welfare compensation, and there was a dramatic uptake in the use of the grant from 2001 through 2004 (Hardy and Richter 2006; Nattrass 2006). Different assessment criteria are used in different provinces, but "a general rule that applies in most hospitals and clinics throughout the country is that an individual with a CD4 count of ≤ 200, which is roughly associated with clinical Stage 4 AIDS, meets the clinical criteria for receiving a disability grant" (De Paoli, Grønningsæter, and Mills 2010, 7).[49] It is also a CD4 count of ≤ 200 that is required for people to begin taking ARVs.[50] People have criticized this policy because often people are very sick by the time they become eligible for ARV provision or social welfare.

The government wants to give the grant to someone who is already dying, and then how are you going to eat that money when you are dead? [The policy] is killing us in disguise.[51]

It seems like what the government is doing is waiting until we are on the brink of death before offering any help. *Or maybe the government is just waiting for us to drop dead.*[52]

When I first met Pheello in 2005, he was receiving a disability grant, which at the time equaled R750 ($107) and had to support his entire family for the month. Pheello was a strong advocate for the provision of ARVs and worked with TAC activists in the Johannesburg region. He and his wife wallpapered their first home in Lawley with TAC posters demanding the right to universal access to ARVs (see fig. 16).

Pheello was hospitalized a number of times with severe illnesses in 2005, and he was finally put onto the state ARV rollout program in October of that year. He began to feel better and get stronger. Six months later, his CD4 count had risen over 200—this often happens when people begin antiretroviral treatment (ART) because their immune system is strengthened. The government threatened to cancel his disability grant, and Pheello was forced to choose between social subsistence for his entire family and life-saving medications. It has become de facto policy that poor, HIV-infected South Africans must "choose" *either* social subsistence *or* life-saving medication (Hardy and Richter, 2006; Nattrass 2006). In this way, the state coerces people into making maniacal choices about the instrument of their own death.

There's this one person I know who is HIV positive, and who was supposed to go and collect his medication. Because his disability grant was cancelled, he cannot

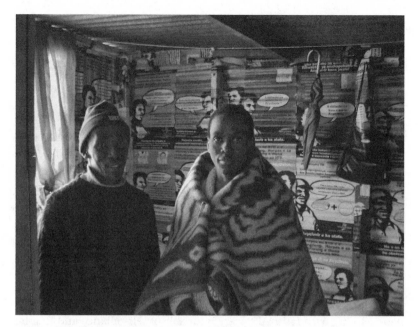

FIGURE 16.   Pheello and Elizabeth Limapo. Photo taken by the author in 2005 in Lawley.

afford the transport money to go and get the medication. I don't see the difference between low and high CD4 count. The government is just tricking people. They give the grant to people who are just 5 minutes from dying. They only give you a grant if you are about to die. This is [the government's] plan to kill people instead of supporting them.[53]

The individualization of blame for the spread of HIV (popularized and hegemonized by the international AIDS industry) parallels an individualization that underpins neoliberal market logic, which serves to shift the obligation of economic welfare from the shoulders of the state to its citizens whose very survival, then, rests solely on their capacity to embody entrepreneurial tactics and engage in aggressive competition over scarce, commodified resources.

It's true, the Department of Health is shifting its responsibility to . . . to the community itself, you know [laughs], yeah. And how . . . how can we have clinics, hospitals in our own homes. Yeah, I think that they are, you know, they're just trying to get rid of these HIV/AIDS patients, you know, because of maybe . . . they don't want to improve the health care sector.[54]

Thanatopolitics

Mbeki's dreams of an African renaissance, where South Africa plays a leading financial and symbolic role in Africa's movement toward self-reliance, oddly never included generic production. Even though Mbeki supported South Africa's development of an AIDS vaccine (Mbeki 2000), he never saw the benefit of investing in the generic production of ARVs, even though South Africa could stand to benefit financially from exporting generic medicines to the rest of the developing world. Since the crux of Mbeki's ideology of renaissance rested on finding "African solutions to African problems," promoting South Africa's economic prowess, and not leaving the poor behind, then why wouldn't he invest in the generic production of ARVs? Such a move would allow him to challenge the pharmaceutical industry, profit from the disease, and build the poor up, so they could take part in the economy. But he only ever discussed South Africa's development of a *cure*, not life-extending medications. The only logical conclusion is that Mbeki decided that people living with HIV/AIDS were incapable of self-reliance and that he was not convinced of the long-term yield on his investment in them. If providing poor people with ARVs simply prolonged their reliance on the state and still ended in their eventual illness and drain on hospital resources (even if these were delayed until the person became resistant to first-line treatment), then why not simply let them die? In the end the withholding of ARVs was a "socially authorized death" (Biehl 2001, 134). Too sick to produce, too poor to consume, too needy to accommodate—impoverished, HIV-infected Africans became the target of what Foucault calls "thanatopolitical" power (Foucault 1990 and 1997; Agamben 1998; Mbembe 2003). "Sometimes what he has to do for the state is to live, to work, to produce, to consume; and *sometimes what he has to do is to die*" (Foucault 2000, 409; my emphasis). I argue that the denialist state engaged in a regime of "thanatopolitics" (or "necropolitics") by denying poor, African, HIV-infected populations access to antiretroviral medication.

For Foucault, modernity ushered in a novel form of power, *biopower* (1990). As knowledge about biological processes advanced and so did techniques for controlling famine and disease, new techniques of control and discipline over the body's functioning were brought into the sphere of political techniques (Foucault 1990, 141–42). Biopower is the productive power to discipline and regulate both individuals and populations in order to cultivate a strong, healthy society.[55] Death is the limit of biopower that is exercised against "those who represent . . . a kind of biological danger to others" (Foucault 1990, 138). The dividing line between thanatopolitics and biopolitics is the decision on the exception—the decision between those whose lives are still worthy of state incorporation and those who can be abandoned to social exclusion and subsequent death.

Carl Schmitt defines the sovereign as "he who decides on the exception" (2005). Vinh-Kim Nguyen points out that because AIDS is an exceptional disease (which has instigated exceptional epidemiological and public health responses), decisions over AIDS have become sovereign decisions insofar as they throw into question who has the power to decide on life and death (2010, 7, 13). Because AIDS has also emerged on the global stage at precisely the moment when state sovereignty is being destabilized and decentralized, this question is particularly acute (ibid.). Whereas for Foucault the ancient sovereign power of *taking* life or *letting* live was replaced in the modern era with the power to *foster* life or *"disallow"* it to the point of death" (1990, 138), Giorgio Agamben (1998) argues that "taking life'" and "letting die" have become indistinguishable under late modernity. Because sovereignty has become decentralized in the contemporary neoliberal era, the sovereign "exception" becomes the rule, enabling more and more people to make decisions about the value of human life.

The clearest example here is the way in which contemporary biomedical practices employ various forms of expertise (risk assessment, prenatal screening, counselling, criteria on the futility of further treatment, notions of brain death, bioethics, etc.) to constitute family members, prospective mothers and fathers, carers, doctors, etc., as loci of decision concerning the termination of life or the attempt to preserve and foster it. (Dean 2002, 133–34)

Mbeki disallowed a certain part of the population the right to life-saving medications. This population was rendered disposable, in part, by the adoption of neoliberal macroeconomic policies that led to deindustrialization and a reduction of the size of the productive labor market, which also made their social welfare too heavy a burden for the newly trimmed neoliberal state to bear. Given the need/desire to reduce social spending, this surplus population was an obstacle to economic development. But further, this surplus population symbolically represented the failure of post-apartheid liberation. By exposing South Africa's schisms of *contemporary* inequality, AIDS undermines the state's claims to a successful liberation, a narrative upon which its postcolo-

nial national identity depends. With the legacy and current manifesta-
tions of structural inequality so clearly emblazoned on their bodies,
AIDS sufferers became the target of a thanatopolitical regime under the
presidency of Thabo Mbeki.

Mbeki couched these "letting die" policies in a discourse that attempted to make people complicit in their own sociopolitical exclusion.
I explained the ways in which he utilized indigenous healing to do this
and also detailed the ways in which he claimed to have the poor's interests at heart in questioning the viability of ARVs in resource-poor
settings.

Thabo Mbeki—our leaders, our politicians, whenever they want to eat at their tables and get fat, they talk about us people who are HIV positive. They like to make
like they are with us—they love us, but they do not love us. HIV is a problem in the
communities. Because HIV affects us, and not them.[56]

"Poverty" was used as an important rhetorical device in the symbolic
struggle over AIDS, but the actual needs and interests of the people
so interpellated were largely marginalized and ignored. The discursive
attention obscures an inability or refusal to attend to the material realities of poverty and disease.

And although Mbeki attempted to bring a certain portion of the
"second economy" into his African modernity through pedagogical
forms of citizenship, this entailed the desertion of those unable or
unwilling to become responsible, self-sufficient citizen-consumers. It
would be a mistake to interpret this abandonment as an accident of
history. Despite Mbeki's attempts to rearticulate race as indigeneity and
to therefore offer a new image of the post-apartheid nation, his policies
very clearly drew a line around the body politic—and race and health,
as much as class, determined the contours of that exclusion.

Abandonment

Several scholars have argued that Foucault's theories of biopower describe the era defined by Fordist regulation (Fraser 2003) and therefore require revision in the age of neoliberalism. Others have argued
that neoliberal societies have suffered from a deinstitutionalization of
discipline, giving way to the rise of a "control society" (Deleuze 1997,
177–82). In disciplinary societies, one moves from "one closed site to
another, each with its own laws" (177)—first the family, then school,

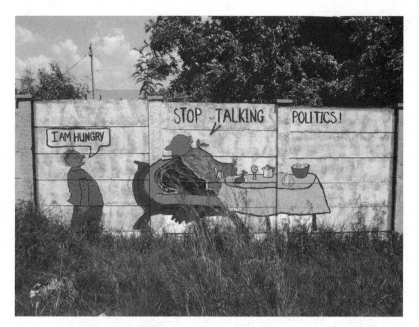

FIGURE 17.   This photo was taken by Emily Squires in Orange Farm, a settlement on the outskirts of Johannesburg, in late 2005.

then the factory or barracks or hospital. But under neoliberalism, control is dispersed as opposed to centralized: "it flows through a network of open circuits," and "one is always in continuous training, lifelong learning, perpetual assessment, continual incitement to buy, to improve oneself, constant monitoring of health and never-ending risk management" (Rose 1999, 234).

Foucault is not given enough credit in these accounts. First of all, Foucault theorized that while disciplinary forms of power are at first linked to particular institutions, they become generalizable, pervasive, and permanent as they are diffused throughout civil society and are incorporated into the bodies of docile subjects—such that in the end discipline functions "in a diffused, multiple, polyvalent way throughout the whole social body" (Foucault 1995, 208–9). In addition, Foucault *did* theorize a shift that accompanied the rise of "advanced liberalism" in the latter part of the twentieth century, which entailed a conversion of normalization to normation (2007). Whereas disciplinary regimes indicate where the norm *should be* and mobilize punitive sanctions against those who are *ab*normal, apparatuses of security, under advanced forms of liberalism, calculate what the norm *is*. As such, probability assessments and risk management supplement surveillance and docility as the order of the day.

There are a number of important implications for this shift to a society of control and of normation. We are no longer dealing with disciplinary tactics of individualization, but rather, with the construction of "dividuals"—not subjects with innate qualities but rather capacities and potentialities (Deleuze 1997, 180; Rose 1999, 234). Castel (1991) argues that this also has an impact on our construction of danger and risk, and thus, our programs for exclusion. "A risk does not arise from the presence of a particular precise danger embodied in a concrete individual or group. It is the effect of a combination of abstract *factors* which render more or less probable the occurrence of undesirable modes of behavior" (287). Different social destinies are therefore assigned to different people depending on their willingness and capacity to live up to the requirements of competition and self-regulation (294), which ultimately yields a "dual society": "the coexistence of hyper-competitive sectors obedient to the harshest requirements of economic rationality, and marginal activities that provide a refuge (or a dump) for those unable to take part in the circuits of intensive exchange" (ibid.).

Nikolas Rose takes this one step further by suggesting that those who fail to live up to the requirements of a control society are either the target of strategies of incorporation aimed at reattaching them to the circuits of civility through pedagogical citizenship *or* they are deemed uneducable and become the target of inexorable exclusion because of the danger they pose (1999, 240)—hence, a "new archipelago of confinement without reformation is taking shape" (270). Although the excluded are fragmented and divided, constituting simply a group of people who resemble one another only insofar as they are unable to "manage themselves and capitalize their own existence" (259), they are also unified both ethically and spatially. Ethically because they have either "refused the bonds of civility and self responsibility" or they aspire to them but are not given the means (ibid.), and spatially "in that the territory of the social is reconfigured, and the abjected are relocated, in both imagination and strategy, in 'marginalized' spaces" (ibid.).

I am suggesting that the squatter camp has become a new means of circumscribing and thus extinguishing the risk posed by a group of people who are imagined as threatening to the post-apartheid nation and to the safety of the species-body because of their HIV status and their unwillingness and inability to assume self-regulatory, self-responsible, and self-entrepreneurial technologies of the self. While the theories reviewed above move us toward an understanding of neoliberal exclusion, they do not go far enough. In developing an analysis of the squatter camp as a prototypical archipelago of exclusion in the neoliberal era, I make two primary interventions into this set of theories. First, I argue that the shift from discipline to control, from surveillance to risk management, and from normalization to normation actually serves to redefine the contours of exclusion. Foucault argued that on the basis of calculating the normal curve, one could conform instances outside of the norm into an acceptable bandwidth of variability (2007, 63). As such, when natural disasters, epidemics, and/or crises of capital occur, they only affect the outliers. Thanatopolitics thus operates at the *limit* of processes of normation. Effectively, I argue, this constitutes a *shift* in the configuration of exclusion—from one of self/other to one of inside/outside.[57]

People are excluded on the basis of *both* their *capacity* (and desire) to adopt disciplined and entrepreneurial technologies of the self and their *externality*. People's abandonment to the threshold of the body politic (a spatial externalization and political marginalization) is compounded by and affects their subjective ability (or desire) to self-discipline. Therefore, this exclusion is spatial, biopolitical, *and* corporeal. Through technologies of responsibilization and entrepreneurialism, the burden of blame for thanatopolitics has been shifted onto the shoulders of those whose bodies cannot be disciplined, who cannot govern themselves. In the classical neoliberal logic of privatizing blame, the victims of HIV/AIDS become responsible for their own abandonment. In the next chapter, I show that the line between incorporation and exclusion has shifted with the provision of antiretrovirals, as tenuous lifelines are thrown to AIDS sufferers. But this extension of social citizenship is weak, precarious, and reliant on the embodiment of *biomedical* technologies of the self. I will argue that this constitutes a new form of exclusionary inclusion.

My final intervention into the literature on neoliberal governmentality attempts to make sense of the effect of abandonment on subjects' habitus—a topic that is never covered by the above theories. What effect does inexorable exclusion have on the subjectivities, habits, and actions of those abandoned at the margins of the social? People abandoned at the social periphery see themselves living in the midst of garbage and shit—the detritus of a postindustrial, postcolonial age. Over time, this abandonment and the precariousness and insecurity of their daily living infiltrates people's bodies and identities. Thulani once told me: "We are not good business according to the government. The poor in this new South Africa, they don't have a space. . . . Not giving

HIV-positive people health care is one strategy that the government uses to get rid of the poor. We are a stress to the government, and they don't want to deal with us."[58]

It is important to show that most available theories of contemporary social exclusion either do not explore the effects of abandonment on subjects' actions and identities or suggest that those so abandoned are bereft of agency and resistance. Giorgio Agamben (1998) argues that the sovereign decision to invoke a state of exception (where the sovereign can deploy the death function against the nation's enemies) has actually come to define the neoliberal era—such that the exception has become the rule. As such, he argues, the concentration camp becomes the political paradigm of modernity because it represents the materialization of the state of exception (174). *Homo sacer* is the name Agamben gives to the inhabitants of these exceptional spaces that mark the boundaries of sovereignty in advanced modernity. *Homo sacer* (he who cannot be sacrificed but who can be killed with impunity) "does not sit outside of law, nor is he indifferent to it, but he is *abandoned by it*" (Agamben 1998, 28). Agamben does not explore the effect such complete abandonment has on people's subjectivities and movements; rather, one gets the sense that the *homines sacri* are devoid of all agency. But as my case will show, without agency, the marginalized cannot be blamed—neoliberalism is a form of government premised on *freedom* (Rose 1999). It is essential, therefore, that the poor retain their ability to "choose" to embody certain technologies of the self in exchange for the rights of citizenship.

Foucault labels the subject of the control society *Homo economicus*—a rationally calculating subject. Because probability is the science of this new regime of governmentality, calculating what is known and being comfortable with risk becomes part of subjects' habitus. But those living outside the norm *cannot* calculate risks because they are immeasurable. Their lives are subsumed by constant risk and unmooring contingency, so they have not only incorporated their own disposability but also face overwhelming uncertainty.

CD: Why don't people talk about HIV/AIDS in your community if so many people are dying?
TS: Because talking isn't going to change the situation. It is not going to change the living conditions. And so, it's not going to change the fact that people are spreading this disease and dying from it. . . . You know, I thought if there could be access to health, access to jobs, access to, you know, basic services, that would enable communities to decide to live. But no one could take a different path, no one could

choose from various types of lives . . . like you could. We don't have an option but to live in the dark . . . we have to live there.[59]

And yet, no one's abandonment is absolute. Certain people are able to assume different subjectivities and social destinies at different times. This provides people a tenuous hold on the rights and privileges of the body politic and also an ability to calculate their own survival. The next chapter explores the ways in which antiretrovirals have afforded subjects a particular biomedical selfhood, which allows them to refuse their position as "leftovers" and charter new trajectories of action (Biehl 2006b, 472). In chapter 4 I show how women in squatter camps are able to *ukuphanda* (to "get by") by using "transactional sex" to assume certain kinds of self-entrepreneurialism. And in chapter 5 I show how hybrid health itineraries allow HIV-infected squatter residents to navigate the material obstacles erected by apartheid and sustained by neoliberal economics and the pandemic itself. The subjectivities people assume are always partial, fleeting, and in constant peril. Meaning, subjects cannot *rely on* the subjectivities only made available to them with certain disciplinary and regulatory strings attached. Therefore, people's life strategies often involve prioritizing different possibilities of action and inclusion. This means that, for the most part, people living on the margins of the social have become savvy *bricoleurs*.

The "bricoleur" is adept at performing a large number of diverse tasks; but, unlike the engineer, he does not subordinate each of them to the availability of raw materials and tools conceived and procured for the purpose of the project. His universe of instruments is closed and the rules of his game are always to make do with "whatever is at hand," that is to say with a set of tools and materials which is always finite and is also heterogeneous because what it contains bears no relation to the current project, or indeed to any particular project, but is the contingent result of all the occasions there have been to renew or enrich the stock or to maintain it with the remains of previous constructions or deconstructions. (Lévi-Strauss 1966, 17)

Countering the theories above, the residents of South Africa's zones of social abandonment are not without agency or possibilities for resistance. In fact, quite the opposite. Most refuse to sit back and wait for deliverance. Earlier in this chapter I mentioned the spontaneous uprisings that spread like wildfire throughout the country, at first in 2004/2005 and then with renewed vigor in 2007 (Hart 2008).[60] These are largely staged in response to the backlog in basic service provision and the installation of prepaid technology. One of the most iconic and symbolic protests used, which is a strategy still being deployed throughout the country today, involves dumping the fecal matter collected in either overflowing VIP toilets or buckets (for those unfortunate enough to be forced to use the so-called bucket system for their waste "management")[61] onto the streets, onto police cars, or in the front yard of local councilors. One cannot help but think of Kristeva's theory of abjection (1982).[62] These residents throw their own abject waste in the face of the postcolonial regime—thereby repudiating their expulsion from the body politic. Their acts render not only their abandonment but also the boundaries of the social visible and legible for all. They refuse to be held responsible for their own abandonment.

THREE

Biomedical Citizenship

When we started TAC, we didn't think there was going to be this battle of denialism. There were two things in our mind. One was about community mobilization and de-stigmatization and the other was a campaign against profiteering by pharmaceutical companies. We didn't think we were going to have to fight the government every step of the way. And it's been a big waste in many respects, because it takes us away from the real issues. . . . We shouldn't be having to establish that ARVs are safe and effective. That shouldn't be the national debate. The national debate should be how do we manage the bad parts of ARVs, like the side effects? How do we deal with adherence issues? What do we do to monitor ARVs better? . . . But instead, we were drug into debates about toxicity and stuff. And so, there hasn't been space for nuance. We've had to take a hard line, and that has its disadvantages. MARK HEYWOOD

As Mark Heywood, who is currently the deputy chairperson of the South African National AIDS Council (SANAC) and the executive director of the AIDS Law Project (ALP) and formerly served as national treasurer of the Treatment Action Campaign (TAC), explains in this quote taken from a 2005 interview, he and the other treatment activists who formed the TAC never expected their primary struggle would be aimed at defeating a denialist government. In addition to battling the international pharmaceutical industry and working to repair an unequal and sorely inadequate health infrastructure, the TAC and its legislative ally, the ALP,[1] were dragged into a *national* battle against the ANC itself. The state's denialism not only presented the TAC with an extreme obstacle but also served to frame their struggle in several important ways.

First, in an effort to combat the denialists' antagonism

to biomedical hegemony, the TAC was forced to adopt a "stridently secular and scientific cosmology" (Robins 2004, 669n34) and to thus sideline (and in some cases disavow) the important role indigenous healing plays in a large majority of South Africans' healing beliefs and practices. As mentioned in the previous chapter, the state wielded indigenous healing as a symbolic weapon in its battle against the TAC. This caused irreparable damage to the already controversial public image of indigenous healing and also served to further exacerbate the myth of incommensurability, thus driving an ideological (in addition to infrastructural) divide between biomedical and indigenous forms of healing. In this chapter, I present evidence to illustrate the ways in which the treatment activists from TAC, ALP, and other AIDS-related civil society organizations contributed to this bifurcation.

The second way in which the battle against denialism had unintended but important consequences for the struggle for treatment in South Africa revolved around the question of poverty. One of the rationales the international public health community, Western states, and the pharmaceutical industry used to avoid funding antiretroviral rollout in the global South was to cast doubt on the viability and safety of introducing antiretrovirals into "resource-poor settings." Often these arguments were decidedly racist and imperialist in tone. The most extreme example of this occurred when George W. Bush's director of USAID, Andrew Natsios, claimed, without any sense of irony, that Africans could not take antiretrovirals because they "don't know what Western time is."[2] More engaged public health officials raised concerns about cost effectiveness, monitoring and evaluation, and drug resistance, but as Paul Farmer noted, most of these concerns were discussed without any evidentiary support or research (2002, 8). When the Brazilian government adopted an official policy of universalizing access to antiretrovirals in 1996, public health officials were skeptical and pharmaceutical companies nervous. But its success proved to the world that ARVs could be successfully rolled out in resource-poor settings and that it would actually save money in the long run by reducing costs associated with hospitalization and the treatment of opportunistic infections and would simultaneously yield a return on labor productivity (Biehl 2006a, 216). "The government doesn't often think about the fact that spending more money up front, actually saves money in the long run. The more a pandemic is left to its own devices, the more people suffer from opportunistic infections, etcetera, which in the end, provides more and difficult work for the health sector to accommodate."[3]

Countries in the global South were therefore burdened with convincing the international public health community and potential donors that ARVs were a viable solution for poor countries, and this often meant sidelining really difficult questions around sustainability, informality, and the challenges associated with poverty. And such was the case with TAC, which waited to discuss the practicalities of rolling out (and monitoring) antiretrovirals in very poor communities until after the battle against denialism was won. In fact, the denialists dominated the conversation about poverty by claiming to defend the poor against toxicity, side effects, and other problems associated with the lack of health infrastructure in impoverished communities. The TAC did not develop an effective strategy for responding to the government on these matters except to insist they were a cover-up for denialism. As such the TAC avoided discussing or preparing for the real complications associated with poverty, and in so doing alienated itself and the fight for treatment from communities hardest hit by the pandemic.

Throughout the book, I argue that the symbolic struggle over HIV/AIDS was about much more than treatment and was therefore deeply implicated in questions about the national imaginary, South Africa's relationship to and position within a globalized world, and the constitution and configuration of race and gender relations and practices. Treatment struggles, therefore, became primary sites for deliberations over the postcolonial paradox. The framing issues TAC faced are reflective of treatment activists' standpoint on key issues associated with "development," modernity, and postcoloniality.

In many ways, TAC's commitment to and faith in science to transform deeply entrenched health inequalities and save millions of suffering victims reveals treatment activists' subscription to a certain myth of modernization (Ferguson 1999). From its stance on gender politics, to its use of legal mechanisms and constitutionality, to its active patient advocacy, TAC showed its deep commitment to a liberal political ideology and "modern" teleology of development. I do not deploy the metaphors of scientific salvation with irony or derision. Rather, throughout the chapter, I will illustrate the role that biomedical soteriology[4] plays in TAC's struggle for treatment and for political power.

TAC has restructured and reoriented its mission and priorities over time in response to its critics and to the needs of impoverished communities suffering from HIV/AIDS. In so doing, I argue in this chapter, treatment activists helped to biomedicalize citizenship rights, which conditioned (and in some cases contractualized) social citizenship on the basis of biomedical behavioral norms, which has profoundly shifted the contours of inclusion and exclusion in South Africa's body politic. I explore the empirical and theoretical implications of these newly emergent forms of "exclusionary inclusion" (Agamben 1998). Further, I argue that this biomedicalization of citizenship is a major feature of the strategies of neoliberalization that came to dominate in the "post-Washington consensus" era—thus forging a collusion between the expansion and realization of biomedical and neoliberal hegemonies.

However, one cannot overstate the tremendous victories TAC was able to achieve in health care access, in addressing health inequalities, or in helping to radically transform international policy on essential medicines. By the end of 2009, 919,923 people were accessing ARV treatment in the public health sector in South Africa, and 56 percent of adults and children needing ARV treatment were receiving it (UNGASS 2010). Because South Africa is the country with the highest percentage of its population infected with HIV, its ARV rollout program is one of the world's largest. New research has recently emerged indicating that treatment is also an important tool for curbing transmission. A study published in the *New England Journal of Medicine* in August 2011 found that people who are treated earlier (when their CD4 count was between 350 and 550) were 96 percent less likely to pass the HIV on to an uninfected sexual partner (Cohen et al. 2011; Brown 2011). This means that though the fight for treatment is far from over, the worldwide expansion of treatment programs could bring about the end of the epidemic (Tutu 2011).

In this chapter, I begin by providing a brief history of the TAC and then provide details on the ways in which TAC fully embraced an orthodox scientific position, which both disavowed indigenous healing and contributed to the reification of the myth of modernization. Next, through an exploration of the international struggle to secure access to essential medicines, I explain the position TAC took in relation to neoliberalism and the state, which subsequently established therapeutic governance and biomedical citizenship in post-apartheid South Africa, once the battle against denialism was won. The chapter then moves to the squatter camp to show how structural obstacles often impede impoverished South Africans from successfully embodying the biomedical technologies of the self required of them to access citizenship rights. I end with a discussion of "exclusionary inclusion" and its broader implications regarding neoliberal governance and public health.

A Brief History of TAC

Since its inception on International Human Rights Day, December 10, 1998,[5] the Treatment Action Campaign has fought and won tremendous victories in the field of HIV/AIDS prevention and treatment and has successfully mobilized tens of thousands of community activists to fight for access to health care and treatment for HIV/AIDS.[6] In 1999, TAC launched a mother-to-child-transmission-prevention (MTCTP) campaign encouraging the government to provide zidovudine (AZT) and nevirapine to pregnant women. After a long and vigorous struggle on the part of the TAC, in 2001, parliament's Joint Monitoring Committee on the Improvement of the Quality of Life and Status of Women ruled that "under South African law, women had a right to treatment and to antiretroviral drugs to reduce the risk of MTCT and HIV infection after rape" (Heywood 2004b). In July 2002, the Constitutional Court ruled that failure to provide treatment violated women and children's constitutional rights—eventually leading to South Africa's first ARV program, targeted at preventing HIV transmission to newborn infants and providing postexposure prophylaxis (PEP) to victims of sexual assault (Heywood 2009).

In 2000, TAC engaged in a Defiance Campaign, led by Zackie Achmat, the founder and longtime national chairperson of the TAC, who was nominated for a Noble Peace Prize because of his decision to wait until all South Africans had access to ARVs before beginning to take them himself. During this campaign, Achmat and other TAC leaders went to Brazil to purchase and then illegally import three ARVs: zidovudine (AZT), lamivudine (3TC), and nevirapine (TAC 2000). In the same year, TAC threatened Pfizer with a legal battle over patent abuses for its antifungal treatment fluconazole, used to treat thrush, a common opportunistic infection.[7] After TAC held an international press conference drawing negative media attention to Pfizer's drug pricing on essential medicines, the company donated the drug, and it was offered free of charge in the public sector as of March 2001 (Robins 2008a, 118).

But perhaps the single greatest victory of the TAC occurred from 2002 to 2004 in the Competition Commission court case against GlaxoSmithKline (GSK) and Boehringher Ingelheim (BI), which, as I explained in the previous chapter, resulted in the issuance of seven voluntary licenses and the eventual passing of a National Treatment Plan

(Department of Health 2003), which included the large-scale rollout of ARVs. As part of this mobilization, TAC launched another civil disobedience campaign, this time aimed directly at the ANC government.

In addition to these triumphs, the TAC has also worked extensively to transform the body politic, so that it envelops and represents the needs and interests of people living with HIV/AIDS. It has utilized a variety of strategies to do so: from encouraging public disclosure, through the use of mass mobilization of people living with the virus, to their renowned t-shirts, which declare in large purple letters, "HIV positive." They have thus waged not only legislative battles, but symbolic ones.

TAC is perhaps best known for engaging in legislative and national media battles, but TAC activists have consistently argued that this image obscures its more community-level engagement and mobilization.[8] Because of its focus on treatment, it brought a largely poor, African (and often female) HIV-positive population group into activism for the first time (Heywood 2004b and 2009). Through its treatment literacy programs and clinical partnerships with Médecins sans Frontières (MSF, Doctors without Borders), it developed community bases in townships, squatter camps, and rural regions throughout the country—a presence that began in Khayelitsha, a township on the outskirts of Cape Town, and has slowly spread to other locations nationally. Heywood suggests that its legal battles would never have been successful without this large capacity for social mobilization (2009).

However, its reach on the ground, in poor and working-class neighborhoods, has always been rather uneven. In Gauteng, for example, its presence was mostly administrative, and TAC activists in the region struggled to build a community presence in and around Johannesburg. Xolani Kunene, the longtime provincial organizer for Gauteng, explained to me that this was partially because of an overrepresentation of HIV/AIDS organizations in the region, but he also notes that politics in the Western Cape, where TAC's national office is located, were always different from other regions of South Africa. For one thing, the Western Cape was able to provide treatment in clinics before the National Treatment Plan was passed due to a partnership with MSF.[9] In addition, however, Kunene explained that people were much more willing to be openly infected and more politically demanding in the Western Cape because of the strong presence of TAC on the ground in Khayelitsha, whereas "Gauteng has more concentrated on books, research, boardrooms and all that."[10] Many of the people with whom I worked echoed this sentiment:

I don't know where the TAC is situated. But I think it is situated somewhere near the courts . . . because you'll see TAC whenever there's a court case. . . . I think TAC's management . . . they are professional. They are intellectuals . . . And their struggle is somewhere . . . up above. . . . It's not within the communities . . . it doesn't have an impact in and it doesn't represent communities. I don't know how it operates, but it's never in this region. I've never heard of TAC in Soweto . . . in this region. No, it is somewhere next to the courts.[11]

In fact, the TAC shifted its focus at two critical junctures in its history, to focus more on community concerns and initiatives. The first shift occurred directly following the rollout of antiretrovirals in 2004. First, TAC needed to address the accusations of racism emerging from the state denialists who quite easily pointed to the fact that TAC maintained a largely white, middle-class leadership, while its volunteer base was predominantly poor and African. Heywood admitted to this perceived "tension between the profile of the leadership and the base" (Friedman and Mottiar 2004, 11), and so Zackie Achmat was replaced by Nonkosi Khumalo as the national chairperson, and the organization attempted to incorporate community activists into its leadership at all levels—from the national to the provincial (Heywood 2004b; Jacobs and Johnson 2007). But after the rollout of ARVs began in earnest, there was also a need to be closer to the ground to monitor the successful implementation of the new national policy, which required the strengthening and capacitating of district structures throughout the country.

The first five years of TAC a lot of the focus was on grassroots mobilization around national and international issues . . . the target was to get the policy change . . . the turning point came after the government approved the comprehensive so-called HIV care and management plan in November 2003. And then I think there was a decision at . . . the executive level in TAC that if TAC were to continue . . . then the real challenge would be to insure that implementation took place at the local community level . . . in terms of . . . use of service delivery, the quality of clinics, the availability of medicines and so on. So it really meant getting the TAC branches to develop programs of action that were community oriented and community based. . . . But I think that the challenge . . . it's TAC's greatest challenge, because it's a helluva lot easier to mobilize people for marches, for demonstrations around a fairly narrow focus. It's much more difficult to sustain [a] grassroots organization of people who are predominantly unemployed, generally very poor, many of them people who have HIV around much more difficult issues that exist that's at community level. . . . Because the resources are just not there, and there's not an ideology that's holding people together . . . we've had patchy success."[12]

In response to the difficulties TAC faced in maintaining a more community-based approach, it went through another organizational restructuring in 2009, when it was decided that "TAC's financial and management capacity would be better applied through the focusing of resources in one 'model district' in each of the provinces in which TAC operates" (TAC 2009c, 14). This was, in part, a scaling back based on fiduciary constraints that also entailed the retrenchment of certain staff and the termination of stipends for hundreds of community treatment literacy practitioners, trainers, and peer educators (ibid.). The TAC lost key funding (especially when the Global Fund to Fight AIDS, TB, and Malaria withdrew its grant), and commitments to universal access to treatment began to decline on a global scale. These were consequences of the economic recession and a subsequent shift in international support for funding HIV treatment. For example, the United States has steadily been reducing its donor funding since 2009 by 10 percent each year. Because the United States accounts for more than half of the global contributions to fight the disease, this decrease in funding has had wide-reaching effects (Tutu 2011).

The timing of these renewed challenges was sadly ironic, given that they were occurring the precise year Jacob Zuma replaced Mbeki. In other words, the end of denialism and a renewed political commitment on the part of the ANC government to addressing the scourge of HIV/AIDS occurred when the international arena was backtracking on funding and commitments to universal access on essential medicines. TAC has responded to these most recent developments by attempting to recommit itself to the promotion of health advocacy and education at the local, community level. It should be made clear, however, that TAC's commitment to community outreach and mobilization has mostly focused on treatment literacy and advocacy (where laypeople are trained in the science of HIV/AIDS and antiretrovirals), as well as monitoring the implementation of policy protocol on the rollout. In other words, the community-level activism was focused more on building health infrastructure and ensuring adequate supply, and less about the daily struggles people living with HIV/AIDS face in squatter conditions. This will become obvious later in this chapter when I explain the tensions that arise for people taking ARVs in conditions of extreme deprivation.

Throughout its history, TAC has framed its struggles within a human rights paradigm, arguing that equitable access to health care (and in particular medicines for HIV) is a human right that can be realized through the legal system, the strategic use of international conventions (such as those signed in Geneva and New York), and the South African constitution. As Mark Heywood explains: "the current global political conjuncture, despite the fact that the odds seem heavily stacked against the poor . . . [nonetheless provides] . . . opportunities for human rights approaches to the issue of poverty. . . . Rights can be the basis for a new politics that may enhance community struggles for development. They also allow civil society to create a new space for engagement with the state in emerging democracies" (Heywood 2009, 27, 29).

AIDS Science, Indigenous Healing, and the Myth of Modernization

Liz McGregor's book, *Khabzela* (2005), tells the story of a popular Y-FM radio DJ named Khabzela, who died in January 2004 of AIDS. Khabzela had openly disclosed his status on the radio, making him a hero in a country ravaged by stigma and silence. Despite this widely heralded decision, Khabzela made another decision that was not only publicly lamented, but that also became a common and troubling mystery.

Khabzela's premature death at the age of 35 could have been prevented. He was a modern, urban, cosmopolitan man, yet despite offers of and access to antiretroviral drugs—which may have given him another ten to twenty years of relatively healthy life—he refused them. (McGrane 2006)

Many South Africans go to a traditional healer before they will see a doctor. Khabzela's response was the norm. (*Observer* 2004)[13]

For many HIV/AIDS activists, scholars, and health-care professionals, this is the primary puzzle associated with HIV/AIDS in post-apartheid South Africa: why do people who have access to antiretrovirals eschew them and choose instead to pursue other remedies and most notably "traditional healing"? The most common explanation is that Mbeki's AIDS denialism caused what is usually referred to as "widespread confusion on the ground." As Nathan Geffen, longtime TAC activist, put it: "People are dying because of confusion. Tens of thousands of South Africans are dying because they are too confused and scared of being stigmatised to find out about their HIV status and get treatment" (Boseley 2005).

No matter the explanation, the solution to the puzzle, as it is posed in public sphere debates by scholars, activists, policy makers, and health care professionals, is: biomedical education. Because for so long,

South Africa was ravaged not only by the dual pandemics of poverty and AIDS but also by what Paula Treichler has labeled an "epidemic of signification" (Treichler 1999), there was constant reiteration of conflicting discourses and ideologies about the disease. Treatment activists believed it necessary to prevent the spread of signification, to fix the meaning of AIDS securely within a biomedical paradigm. For many, including activists associated with the TAC and ALP, biomedical solutions were the country's only salvation.

But, look . . . there is a confusion not amongst the healers but amongst the users of the healthcare system of what's appropriate . . . the confusion is mainly . . . with relation to HIV and AIDS . . . because HIV is potentially life threatening . . . the consequences are so much more real. So, if someone chooses—which I'm sure you know many people, as do I . . . I know people who've chosen not to go and take ARVs . . . the bottom line question is, why is there that type of confusion? Why isn't there a message to everybody from credible sources that say . . . clearly that you should not be doing this. The vitamins and these [indigenous] meds are not going to cure you. These are not cures. They are touted as cures. They are not going to have the same effect as ARVs. So, if you actually really are concerned about saving your life, you need to go on ARVs.[14]

And there was widespread hope that once denialism was defeated, this "confusion" would subside, and people would make the "rational choice" to begin ARV treatment *and* eschew all other forms of healing, including indigenous healing. During an interview I conducted in 2003, a nurse who worked at the Chris Hani Baragwanath Hospital in Soweto told me that the use of indigenous healing was declining; she was convinced that once antiretrovirals became readily available to the public sector, indigenous healing would become obsolete.[15] Policy associated with the rollout of antiretrovirals has attempted to turn this prophecy into a reality, as patients are told, in no uncertain terms, *not* to mix the two forms of healing or they risk undermining the entire ARV rollout program. ARVs have been available since 2004, and denialism was largely defeated by 2007, and yet most of the people I work with in Lawley and Sol Plaatjie continue to use indigenous healing—though many of them combine it with their ARVs. They do not suffer from any overwhelming sense of "confusion" about their health "choices." When the nurse made this prediction in 2003, I asked an HIV-infected community activist about it, and she laughed: "People will never stop going to traditional healers. That would be like suddenly abandoning your name because you are taking a new medication."[16]

There are two primary assumptions undergirding the nurse's beliefs about the relationship between biomedical and indigenous healing: (1) that indigenous healing actually serves as an obstacle to the uptake of biomedical treatment, and (2) that the two approaches are mutually exclusive and incommensurable. These two assumptions are consistently reiterated in the research conducted on health care practices *and* in health policy interventions in South Africa. One of my primary arguments has been that the symbolic struggles surrounding denialism helped to reify this myth of incommensurability. One of the denialists' key strategies was to paint biomedicine as anti-African and to pit it against more indigenous beliefs about healing. But this chapter will show how treatment activists and health professionals also contributed to this bifurcation. In fact, the rollout of antiretrovirals has played a significant role in reifying the myth of incommensurability, as patients enrolled in HAART are discouraged from using indigenous remedies for fear of adverse drug interactions.

From the National Antiretroviral Treatment Guidelines: "The patient must disclose any over-the-counter drugs and traditional medicines. Other medications as well as some traditional medicines cannot be taken concurrently with ART because they may cancel each other out or may lead to unacceptable adverse effects." (Department of Health 2004, 54)

From Department of Health Clinical Guidelines on ART: "Explain to patients how to avoid adverse drug-drug interactions. . . . The patient should understand the possible consequences of unknown content and the danger of . . . traditional medicines." (Department of Health 2010a, 18)

The following are some examples of how patients understand this admonition:

People living with HIV are advised that if they are on ARV treatment, they should not mix it with traditional medicine . . . because if they mix . . . the ARVs will be erased or undone.[17]

Where I take my treatment, I was told I mustn't use traditional medication anymore . . . Because they clean out the medication that you drink. They don't balance—the medical and traditional treatment.[18]

There's no way that you can use traditional healing and mix it with biomedical healing. Sometimes if you mix imbiza with the ARVs, then it makes you to be weak, in a weak state of health. . . . The consumption of both—the conventional medicine and the traditional medicine might lead you into complications of diarrhea, or you may be admitted to the hospital because of the complications of mixing.[19]

But if they are taking ARVs, we advise you mustn't mix. The ARV is for helping you to reduce HIV for the rest of your life. If you mix the ARVs, you kill that ARVs in your blood.[20]

As these comments make clear, the concerns associated with the mixing of biomedical and indigenous health practices and remedies are twofold: (1) the practices associated with indigenous healing often involve cleansing and purging, which might wash the drugs from the patient's system, thereby literally "erasing the drugs"; (2) certain interactions between biomedical pharmacopoeia and indigenous herbal remedies might cause ARVs to be ineffectual or weakened, or might result in diarrhea or other symptoms of toxicity. Both of these conditions could result in the development of drug resistance.[21] Because these drugs are a lifetime commitment—another catechism of "adherence counseling"—this essentially means patients are being forbidden from ever using indigenous health care again. There has been some effort made by the medical establishment of South Africa to scientifically test indigenous treatments for toxicity and potential adverse reactions between them and ARV treatment.[22]

The National Drug Policy sets out guidelines for the investigation of the "efficacy, safety and quality" of indigenous medicines "with a view to incorporating their use in the health care system. . . . Marketed traditional medicines will be established, and a national reference centre for traditional medicines will be registered and controlled" (Department of Health 1996, 26). Two separate institutions have been involved in this process. The first is the Medicines Control Council (MCC), which is a regulatory body (within the Department of Health) that mainly focuses on safety, quality, and the efficacy of medicines. In 1998 the government passed the South African Medicines and Medical Devices Regulatory Authority Act (no. 132), which requires *all* medicines, including indigenous herbs, to be registered with the MCC (Republic of South Africa 1998c). However, the MCC has been historically understaffed and underfunded, and it is far behind on the regulation and registration of biomedical treatments, including ARVs (Nattrass 2008b; Thom 2010; Gonzalez 2011). To date, it has done nothing by way of regulating or registering indigenous remedies.[23]

The Medical Research Council (MRC) has been slightly more active in this regard. The MRC is a "statutory science council formed through an act of Parliament to do biomedical research" (MRC 2003, 10). In 1997, the MRC set up a Traditional Medicines Research Unit, and in 2004, the Department of Health provided this unit with R4.5 million to test indigenous herbal remedies (Mills 2005). The MRC also set up the Indigenous Knowledge Systems of Health Unit, "a computer database of all South African plants and their possible medical benefits" (TAC 2005c). Finally, the MRC, Department of Health, and the Council for Scientific and Industrial Research developed a proposal for a South African National Reference Centre for African Traditional Medicines (NRCATM), based on a World Health Organization (WHO) policy initiative.

Very minimal testing of herbal remedies has actually been carried out by the South African state. In 2002, the Indigenous Knowledge Systems Division of the MRC tested the safety and effectiveness of *Sutherlandia microphylla*, an indigenous medicinal plant, for which there was anecdotal evidence that it delayed the onset of AIDS in HIV-positive patients. Vervet monkeys were given varying dosages of the plant in a controlled clinical setting for three months. No indication of toxicity was found (MRC 2002). This study was repeated with an herbal combination of African potato, milk thistle, and spirulina. Again, no conclusive evidence was found of the drug's toxicity *or* effectiveness (MRC 2004). There have been pharmacological studies on the activity and toxicity of indigenous plants in Southern Africa, which have shown that toxicity is most likely to occur when herbal remedies are misadministered or given in large quantities over a long period of time. "Of the nearly 4,000 ethnomedicinal plant taxa used in South African traditional healthcare, relatively few are considered likely to give rise to serious toxicity. Poisoning from traditional medicines is usually a consequence of misidentification, incorrect preparation or inappropriate administration and dosage, frequently due to self-administration rather than innate risks of using traditional healthcare" (Fennell et al. 2004, 212–13; see also Light et al. 2005 for an overview of some of these studies in South Africa).

However, the real problem with these clinical trials is that they assume an underlying translation between biomedical and indigenous epistemologies. In fact, each paradigm of healing differs greatly in its conceptualizations of disease categories, causation, and treatment; its assessment of what counts as reliable evidence; and its determination of which ingredients in drug combinations are considered most active.[24] Ashforth notes that "identifying medicinal properties of *muthi* is complicated because different plants are often combined in making *muthi*, they are prepared in infusions and decoctions with little regard for standardized dosage, and they are administered according to methods such as drinking and regurgitating, all of which makes it virtually impossible to determine their health-giving effects with any sort of scientific rigor" (2005, 152). The knowledge systems upon which these healing paradigms are based makes translation difficult, but the unequal distribution of resources and power (at the global level) means that "scientific knowledge practices . . . long after colonialism continue to serve as instruments for producing globalized medical 'truth'" (Adams 2002, 661).

Among the indigenous healers with whom I spoke, there was widespread skepticism about the scientific testing of indigenous "muthi":

Why should Western doctors test our medicines? What do they know about traditional healing? Will we get a chance to test *their* medicines, according to *our* standards? We have known about these medicines for centuries and knowledge about them has been passed down over the generations. Who are they to question our ancestors and their knowledge?[25]

Each indigenous healer uses different combinations of herbs to make his/her specialized remedies—this knowledge and the art of their usage is both secret and sacred. The remedies are often dreamed of or revealed by the ancestors themselves. Not only does this make testing the *muthi* difficult, it also makes it irreverent and suspect.

Our knowledge is so important, but they always refer to us as illiterate and who don't know anything. They have been to school for so many years, but we have also been in school—but in a different form of education. There are a lot of things we are doing that they don't want to recognize. Tablets are made out of muthi and herbs—that's where pharmaceuticals come from. They just give them fancy names—to market them and sell them. But they can't take our knowledge from us. . . . All modern medicines have their roots in traditional healing. . . . Before it was modern, it was traditional.[26]

Despite the admonitions of doctors and nurses to avoid the intermixing of the two forms of healing, biomedical scientists have not even been able to establish *scientific* evidence to support their concern that *muthi* negatively impacts ARV compliance and effectiveness. Rather, it seems to me biomedicine's admonition against health pluralism is an attempt to manage and contain uncertainty. Because fears of drug resistance are pervasive, but unknowable, and because indigenous forms of healing are sorely misunderstood, the biomedical establishment is attempting to simply erase it from the equation, thereby shoring up its privileged claim to medical "truth" and managing its own anxiety about the immeasurability of future risks. Using a completely different and in many ways more pragmatic approach, indigenous healers have come up with their own solutions to the possible complications that might arise from purging and cleansing rituals:

Then we say, "In the morning, you'll take your ARV. In the afternoon, in the evening, after eight hours, you'll take the traditional medicine." . . . we are saying a lot of doctors need to be taught that that is possible. Because this is immunostimulating, eight hours, it's dissolved in the system. You can then take something that is also immune boosting which will not contradict.[27]

For their part, TAC was for a time quite vociferous in advocating for the national testing of indigenous medicines. Their primary objective is of course to regulate the usage of potentially harmful natural herbs and to ensure they do not negatively interact with ARVs, but they also insist this testing is important because it will allow indigenous healers to claim financial remuneration, based on intellectual property rights (TAC 2005c).

The new initiatives to put—to push through certain traditional medicines through the Medicine Control Council and various clinical trials and all of that is more of the kind of thing we need because a lot of the traditional medicines that healers use have not been tested. So you don't really know what its side effects are, how it's going to interact with other drugs. So if you're really already on chronic medication, you don't know how certain herbal remedies are going to interact with that. And we do know herbal remedies can be very potent. So, *Sutherlandia*, for example, the African potato plant, which is recommended for strengthening your immune system for people who have HIV, has adverse, uh, reaction to ARVs. Right? So there has to be more information. There has to be more scientific study into the use of herbal remedies.[28]

This ALP lawyer's strong belief that the African potato has adverse reactions with ARVs stems not from evidence from clinical trials, but, rather, from an activist reaction against the promotion of the African potato by the minister of health, Manto Tshabalala-Msimang, who insinuated that it could be used as an alternative to ARVs.

The TAC's concerns with indigenous healing extend beyond the case of *muthi* safety and potential adverse drug interactions. Because the denialist state often wielded indigenous healing as a symbolic weapon aimed at orthodox science, the TAC was often put into a position of defending one against the other. This had horribly negative consequences for the profession of indigenous healing, which largely was uninvolved in the brawl. With one important exception. The Traditional Healers Organization (THO) entered the battle against the TAC when it took up with the Rath Foundation and even stood trial with Rath when the TAC took it to court for its gross public health violations. In part, this relationship developed out of a mutual dislike of the TAC. According to the TAC representatives I interviewed, as well as Phephsile Maseko (the acting chair of the THO), the TAC and THO held a joint workshop in the fall of 2004 to discuss their positions on treatment and possibilities of collaboration. The THO walked away feeling as though the TAC was patronizing them by using the opportunity to educate indigenous healers on the benefits of ARVs without listening to the healers' own concerns.[29] On November 24, 2004, the THO staged a massive rally against the TAC, in which they claimed that TAC only promotes antiretrovirals for HIV/AIDS treatment and that TAC ignores indigenous medicines and nutrition. The TAC responded: "The TAC believes that there are traditional medicines that work but proof of their safety and efficacy requires scientific data" (TAC 2004).

I was conducting interviews with treatment activists and indigenous healers throughout South Africa at the time of this public battle between TAC, Rath, and the THO. Most indigenous healers had no idea their profession and practice was being so hotly debated within the public sphere, and rank-and-file members of the THO did not even know who Rath was, let alone that their organization was engaged in a court battle with the Treatment Action Campaign. Among TAC members, there is some nuance in people's stances on indigenous beliefs and practices, but surprising uniformity when the question of "testing *muthi*" arose. The mother of Isaac Skhosana, provincial chairperson of TAC in Gauteng, is an indigenous healer. Despite the fact that Isaac grew up with indigenous healing and respected his mother, he believed indigenous herbs needed to be tested by biomedical scientists and was quite adamant about the possible negative effects of mixing indigenous and antiretroviral treatment. Xolani Kunene, TAC's provincial organizer in Gauteng, was the only person I interviewed within the TAC organization who recognized the fact that the scientific testing of indigenous *muthi* was problematic and suggested that indigenous healers needed to be actively involved in coming up with solutions about how to manage HIV more holistically.

In this section, I have provided evidence showing how the battle over treatment served to strengthen and reify the myth that indigenous and biomedical treatments are ideologically and empirically incommensurate. Treatment activists and health professionals readily employ the tropes of "modernity" and "traditionalism" (and their signifieds) to drive a symbolic wedge between two cultural approaches to healing and health, but in so doing, the battle over healing also served to buttress another important myth—the myth of modernization. The TAC's strong advocacy for a rational, legal, rights-based, and biomedical approach to redressing the legacy of apartheid and tackling the scourge of HIV/AIDS led them to embrace a vision of modernization that was directly at odds with the postcolonial state's. While the ANC (under Mbeki) promoted a fantasy of independence that was decidedly Africanist, the TAC's national imagining engaged a more normative, modernist narrative that incorporated a linear teleology of development achieved (at least in part) through biomedical and technological advancement.

For the Minister to say, we as a government are not going to prescribe to people and tell them what to do. People have choices. You can have this, you can have that. For me, that's not on. A state has to act rationally and reasonably. We have a constitution that must be abided. The state has to develop its health care policy on the basis of evidence. It has to be evidence based. We couldn't possibly develop an economic policy on the basis of the throwing of the bones. We couldn't do that. We have to monitor what we are putting into people's mouths—those *muthi* have to be scientifically tested . . . there's no getting around that. Because there is no equivalence between the systems, so the state can't pretend there is when there isn't. It has to be responsible.[30]

This quote is telling in a number of ways. The evident exasperation with a set of cultural beliefs at odds with "rationality" and "evidence-based," "scientifically tested" truths unveils the Westernized vision of modernity that epitomizes TAC's ideology. Put slightly differently, TAC activists' frustration with denialism reveals a certain modernist chauvinism that belies South Africa's position as a postcolonial state. This same sentiment is evident in the nurse's teleological assumption that the "traditional" will be abandoned once the "modern" is available to all. As Bruno Latour so brilliantly observed, modernity is premised on three myths: the teleology of time, the fundamental incommensurability between nature and the social, and the Great Divide between Us and Them, which is often accompanied by the assumption that only

Westerners have truly grasped what it means to be modern (1991). One of TAC's primary battles has been to "prove" that the developing world can also be "modern," but as Latour points out, the more we insist on incommensurability, the more we create its impossibility by allowing the creation and flow of hybrids. Modern society attempts to construct epistemological distinctions and categorical boundaries that disallow intermixture between nature and society, and yet such an ontology and the rules that police it are premised on the very hybridity that is disavowed. As such, "we have never been modern," or as one of the healers I quoted above put it: "before it was modern, it was traditional."

International Activism, Reframing Health Governance, and the Juridicalization of Struggle

Because of the valiant efforts of activists in Brazil, South Africa, Thailand, and India, the pharmaceutical industry has been forced to allow countries in the global South to bypass intellectual property right (IPR) protections on essential medications. I argue in this section that the development and success of these new health social movements and their historical battle for treatment served to reify neoliberal regulation in the global South and juridicalize activist struggles.

In 1995, when the World Trade Organization (WTO) was established, the Agreement on Trade-Related Intellectual Property Rights (TRIPS) came into effect. This agreement was meant to "level" the playing field by establishing an international policy on IPR protection, which confers patent rights for twenty years. In essence, TRIPS sets out guidelines for the establishment of *national* legislation on IPR. "Developing" countries were given four years to comply (until 2000). There were safeguard mechanisms written into the agreement. Article 31 authorizes the use of either parallel importing (where a country can import a drug sold by the patent holder for a cheaper price in another country) or compulsory licensing (whereby a country can produce generic medications without permission from the patent holder) only in the case of "national emergency or other circumstances of extreme urgency" (Hein 2007, 43) and only "after the failure to negotiate mutually acceptable terms with a patent holder" (Heimer 2007, 559). Initially, what constituted a national emergency was not clear, and compulsory licenses were never granted, but were rather, *claimed*, such that those that remained uncontested were eventually honored as precedent (Heimer 2007, 559).

However, most compulsory licenses *were* contested. The WTO Dispute Settlement Body and the US trade representative have repeatedly imposed trade sanctions (by implementing Section 301 of the US Trade Act) on Brazil, Thailand, and South Africa ('t Hoen 2002). In 1997, the South African government passed the Medicines and Related Substances Control Amendment Act (Republic of South Africa 1997), which provided the legislative framework for "generic substitution of off-patent medicines, transparent pricing for all medicines, and the parallel importation of patented medicines" ('t Hoen 2002, 30).[31] In 1998, the Pharmaceutical Manufacturing Association (PMA), an organization representing thirty-nine multinational pharmaceutical companies, sued the state of South Africa in an effort to remove the price reducing sections of this act (ibid.). The TAC joined the government as amicus curiae (friend of court) in January of 2000 and was able to draw prominent media attention to the case. TAC has claimed victory for the fact that the PMA subsequently withdrew its case in April 2000 (Heywood 2004b, 11; Mbali 2004, 107–8; Comaroff 2007, 211–12; Robins 2008a, 118). However, it would take several more years before the South African government would launch a Competition Commission case against pharmaceutical companies in order to secure low-cost treatment through the issuing of voluntary licenses. In other words, although the PMA withdrew its case, no steps were made to issue voluntary or compulsory licenses for several more years. Although not generally posited as a reason for the PMA's withdrawal, I do not think it coincidental that in 1999, South Africa signed a bilateral TRIPS Plus trade agreement with the United States (GRAIN 2001; Oxfam 2001).

Brazil was the first country to strike a compromise with the United States and the WTO—it would not *violate* TRIPS or pharmaceutical patents (without first getting the approval of the United States), but it would issue compulsory licenses. In 1996, Brazil became the first "developing" country able to offer ARVs within the public sector (which was enabled by a loan from the World Bank in 1992 meant to halt the "Africanization" of the AIDS epidemic in Brazil [Biehl 2006a, 212]). Brazil's AIDS program has been hailed as "proof that poor nations can do it" and "a model for treating AIDS worldwide" (Biehl 2004, 105). India was also able to produce generic medications because the state already had a patent law in place prior to TRIPS implementation, giving them an extended period of time to become compliant (Hein 2007, 57). However, generic producers in Brazil and India were forbidden (through bilateral trade agreements with the United States) from exporting generic essential medicines to other developing countries until the WTO passed the Doha Declaration in 2001, which not only lifted this ban on exports (Paragraph 6 of Article 31 [f] of the Agreement on Trade-Related Intellectual Property Rights) but also extended the date by which "least-developed countries" were obliged to implement patent law for pharmaceuticals until 2016.[32] Because of these struggles, the prices of ARVs have dropped significantly; in 2000, the price of first-line ARV treatment per patient per year was US$10,000 (Nattrass 2008b), and it is currently US$204 (WHO 2010a).[33]

During the 2003 court case the TAC launched against two major pharmaceutical corporations for patent abuse, the TAC gained international support and admiration from global justice activists who situate their own struggles within an antineoliberal framework. Vinh-Kim Nguyen argues that the year 2000 marked a historical convergence between HIV/AIDS and globalization activists (2010). When NGOs throughout the developing world took on the issue of treatment, this "resonated with broader concerns—and coalitions—that sprang up around a number of issues posed by globalization, in effect making access to treatment—and the global intellectual property laws thought to impede this—a signature issue for the antiglobalization movement" (ibid., 107). However, the TAC was criticized for the way in which the court case was settled—the two pharmaceutical companies granted *voluntary* licenses to South Africa, allowing them to produce or import generic medications. Global justice activists believed that the implementation of *compulsory* licensing would have better served the global struggle against international capital and better provided for all countries in the global South struggling against the pandemic.

While encouraging to those concerned with closing the access gap, these voluntary arrangements have thus far only involved one or two South African generic manufacturers and have been limited to a handful of antiretrovirals. Thus their impact is limited to a single disease (HIV/AIDS) in a single country (South Africa), and because they permit a limited number of generic manufacturers they appear unlikely to reduce prices as much as open competition between generics would. (Love 2005)

The TAC responded by stating that it was never their intention to fight global capitalism—it was simply trying to secure low-cost treatment for its own population.[34]

We're not attacking the patent system head on. We're saying we're not . . . we understand the issues . . . the question was, well, do we accept a settlement or do our clients,[35] because we took it back to the clients, accept a settlement that is actually going to have a massive impact immediately . . . or do we use this as a test case and fight it all the way through and get a judgment and maybe even lose? . . . We didn't get the precedent we wanted although I think to some extent we got a . . . precedent of sorts.[36]

In his work on Brazil, which underwent a similar global justice struggle and subsequent bargain with the WTO, the US government, and several pharmaceutical companies, João Biehl argues that these new social movements actually forged both a new relationship to the state and a reconfiguration of neoliberal policy on health care (2004; 2006a; 2007). "These committed AIDS professionals and activists were well aware of how to maximize equity within the neoliberalizing state" (Biehl 2004, 111). South African biomedical activists attempted to transform economic and political policy, from the inside out in two ways.

First, they attempted to use neoliberalism against the pharmaceutical industry and the developmental state:

You can't reverse globalization. You can't, as an economic or a social process. So therefore the question of social movements that are anti-capitalist is how do we check the excesses, how do we try to make sure that there's a global movement of poor people that constructs agendas that turn this irreversible process to the advantage of . . . of the people who are being cut out of it.[37]

Instead of fighting against the neoliberal order, the TAC has attempted to "exploit its incoherences . . . finding productive footholds within the aporias of the market system" (Comaroff 2007, 214). This is different from being "in the pockets of Big Pharma," which was a commonly reiterated critique made by the Rath Foundation (and Mbeki).[38]

This approach has distanced the TAC from other organizations in South Africa that linked their struggles to the fight against neoliberal restructuring, like the Anti-Privatisation Forum, the Landless People's Movement, and the Anti-Eviction Campaign—whom Mbeki had labeled "ultra-left," in part because they charged the ANC with "selling out" on their liberation promises when it adopted GEAR. In an effort to disassociate from such a label and convince the government they were still "card carrying members" of the ANC (Mbali 2005), the TAC avoided what it claimed were "ideological" positions on capitalism and preferred to work instead within the current economic and political arrangements. Although it was often seen as antagonistic to the government, TAC insisted it did so only to push the ANC to realize its democratic potential (Heywood 2004b). It has also preferred to partner with the Congress of South African Trade Unions (COSATU), which is part of the ANC tripartite alliance. Mark Heywood explained in an interview that TAC had decided not to couch their struggle within a necessarily anticapitalist framework:

Not because we think that capitalism is a good system or that capitalism can . . . deliver jobs or medicines or quality healthcare services, or whatever, but because we think that in South Africa, and not just in South Africa, in fact, globally, and some people will say we're naïve, but actually there is a space for mobilization and for winning social improvements and social reform. And it's important to occupy and mobilize in that space, because that course of mobilization will strengthen people's confidence in themselves, and will also lead to a certain amount of questioning around polices that deprive people of healthcare or deprive people of water and deprive people of electricity, etcetera.[39]

The second strategy the TAC deployed to transform political policy from the inside out involved the usage of a human rights framework and an attempt to force the government to live up to the promises outlined in the constitution, thereby constituting a "new epistemic community within the state" (Biehl 2004, 108).

We don't want to call for a regime change . . . we want to push the ANC and change the policies of the day. . . . We want policies to be changed, and if it means fighting, then we fight. But we use the right . . . we use the constitution as a weapon, we use courts as our home. . . . We use the constitution as a base. . . . If you can interpret the constitution to . . . to be able to give human rights back, then that's what we'll do.[40]

TAC operates from the political conviction that significant resources for social reform do exist in most countries of the world and that progressive policy shifts *can* be achieved within the current econo-legal framework—but only if they are fought for, described as rights, and linked to a more refined and legally development argument about the positive obligations of the state. (Heywood 2009, 23)

Heywood has also argued that though they only focus on the right to health (and particularly for those infected with HIV), their successes, in terms of economic and policy reform have benefited the poor more generally and have served to transfer wealth from the private to the public sector:

A campaign that successfully brings down the price of a medicine redistributes to poor communities a value that would otherwise have been claimed as profit by shareholders. Similarly, TAC's successful litigation to force the government to introduce a new health service . . . requires an investment in infrastructure and human resources that might otherwise not take place. This is a net gain for poor people which goes beyond the direct benefit received by the people in need of treatment. (Heywood 2009, 24)

TAC's attempts to formulate new economic and political praxis within neoliberal economics and in collaboration with the developmental state have had a number of consequences, which resonate globally. The first consequence is that struggles for social justice and redistribution have become increasingly juridicalized. The law has been fetishized and serves as the only means through which citizens can make claims on the polity (Comaroff and Comaroff 2000, 328–39). This conscripts people into fighting on the basis of constitutionally imbued rights as opposed to a broadened notion of citizenship based on communal struggles for sustainability.

The politics TAC and other global treatment activists engaged in has served to shift IPR policy on essential medicines, which has played an important role in reconstituting neoliberal governance at the global level. In other words, AIDS activists and their struggles for access to treatment for the poor in the global South have played a major role in the development of rollout neoliberalism and the social safety nets it inaugurated (Peck and Tickell 2002). In his article on the policy discussions surrounding the introduction of a Basic Income Grant (BIG)[41] in South Africa, James Ferguson argues that this ability of social movement and civil society organizations to use the language and logic of neoliberalism to fight for the expansion of social welfare "forces us to question conventional oppositions (e.g., neoliberal reasoning versus the interests of the poor; or ideologies of entrepreneurial risk-taking versus the security of state-guaranteed social payments) and conventional associations (e.g., the association of entrepreneurship with indifference to the poor; or the advocacy of state-funded social payments with ideologies of social democracy and 'safety nets')" (Ferguson 2007, 83). A "hybrid state" that combines neoliberalism and "developmental" features has emerged (ibid.). One is left to wonder: if neoliberalism can be so reconstituted as to extend social welfare and respond to the demands of civil society mobilization, then what makes it neoliberal? Is rollout neoliberalism simply a return to Fordist capitalism?

Throughout the book, I provide evidence that refutes such a conclusion. I argue, instead, that this new form of rollout neoliberalism leaves inequality largely intact, shifting the blame onto the shoulders of its victims, and circumscribes and provisionalizes citizenship on the basis of behavioral norms. As such, citizenship itself is privatized (as is social justice), and the logic of the "free market" prevails, but this time on the terrain of life itself: only those who are capable of self-entrepreneurialism and the maximization of their human capital are worthy of survival. This is indeed neoliberalism—in its most concentrated form. In fact, in the next section, I will show how biomedical citizenship becomes a primary tool of rollout neoliberalism at the global scale, promulgated through discourses of "responsibility." As such, a subtle biomedical imperialism is at work in the continued intensification and expansion of neoliberal regulatory regimes.

On the one hand, then, TAC successfully changed health care policy, used "wealth transfers" to relieve poverty and extend health care access, and fought against pharmaceutical profiteering in an effort to change essential medicines policy at the international level. In so doing, it helped to reconstitute neoliberalism at the global scale. On the other hand (and perhaps inadvertently), it restructured the basis upon which exclusion is allocated and contributed to the reification of neoliberalism, under its new purportedly "pro-poor" guise. It has also circumscribed subjectivities by linking citizenship rights to the embodiment of biomedical technologies of the self.

Therapeutic Governance and Biomedical Citizenship

As AIDS emerges as the foremost issue threatening economic and political futures in many countries around the world, the AIDS industry has become ever-more entangled with the development industry, a salient example of how humanitarian issues are quietly reconfiguring the contours of Bretton-Woods modernity. (NGUYEN 2005, 125)

In an eerie coincidence of global proportions, AIDS and neoliberalism share a common chronology and impact. AIDS and the industry that has grown up to manage, control, and capitalize on the disease is deeply implicated in neoliberalization efforts at multiple scales, even more so as biopolitical concerns are increasingly a focus of government at the international, national, and civil society levels. Nikolas Rose suggests that in the late twentieth and early twenty-first centuries, due to advances in biomedical technology and knowledge and the increasing spread of biomedical hegemony, a new biopolitics is emerging wherein biology plays a primary role in the constitution of subjectivities, in the regulation of populations, and in the economization of new forms of capital (2007). Likewise, a new set of theories has arisen exploring "biological citizenship" (Petryna 2002; Rose and Novas 2005; Rose 2007), which is generally used in two contexts: (1) when the body (or a biological condition, like HIV) becomes the basis for making rights-claims on either the state or the international community, or when biomedical categories are used to adjudicate claims for compensation (Petryna, 2002; Rose and Novas 2005; Nguyen 2005); and (2) when citizenry (or laypeople and patients) participate in the production of biomedical knowledge and get involved in key struggles over access to treatment and care (Rose and Novas 2005; Biehl 2004; Epstein 2007; Nguyen 2010).[42] In contrast, I use the more analytically specific term, "biomedical citizenship" to refer to the ways in which a biomedical industry made up of public health institutions, pharmaceutical corporations, NGOs, and various Western governments has imposed epistemic hegemony and disciplinary techniques onto subjects throughout the global South through the mechanism of social citizenship at the national scale. Certain citizenship rights, then, are only conferred on those who subscribe to a biomedical paradigm of "truth," which also entails the disciplining of bodies according to biomedical regulations and the creation of biomedical technologies of the self.

TAC's participation in global struggles for treatment access helped to initiate new forms of therapeutic governance and biomedical citizenship.[43] Once denialism was defeated, TAC and other treatment activists were able to take leadership positions in the development of health policy. This has institutionalized biomedicalized forms of citizenship and served to deeply embed South Africa into global circuits of public health "best practice."

The TAC sought to introduce biopolitical regulation over the population in order to maintain the health of the species body and thereby enhance the state's biological capital (Rose and Novas 2005; Rose 2007) through the provision of ARV medication. However, I will show how this necessitates disciplining the population—in part because 80 percent of South Africans utilize indigenous forms of healing (Department of Health 2003) and in part because biomedical technologies of the self must be learned. Toward this end, two disciplinary tactics have been deployed. First, citizenship rights are provided on the basis of the successful embodiment of the disciplined behavior necessary to adhere to ARV medication, thus contractualizing citizenship rights. Second, the discourse of responsibility urges citizens to become self-reliant entrepreneurs. "Patients on ARVs are not only told that they need to adhere to treatment protocols and change their behaviour in line with biomedical necessities in order, quite pragmatically, to stay alive, they are also told that these actions are 'their responsibility'" (Colvin and Robins 2009, 185). People living with AIDS are now asked to adopt certain survival discourses, adhere to disciplinary bodily practices defined and policed by a wide range of health care professionals, and constantly calculate the costs they are willing to pay in order to adhere to these difficult health regimens.

In the rest of the chapter, I explore the biomedical discipline required of those enrolled in the state's ARV program and the biomedical technologies of the self they are asked to embody. I then show how certain structural obstacles impede the poorest South Africans from assuming self-responsibility, ultimately marginalizing them from accessing the rights of citizenship. I argue that citizenship itself has become precarious in this new rollout neoliberal era of post-apartheid. Before moving forward with this argument, however, I want to briefly explain how members of the TAC were able to finally take part in health policy making after years of battling denialism and the pharmaceutical industry.

The production of scientific knowledge and the participation of "lay experts" (Epstein 1996) in scientific governance has dramatically changed over the past thirty years, and in many ways AIDS has been both the cause and effect of this shift toward "citizen science" (Irwin 1995). Steven Epstein has shown how the role of lay expertise in health policy making has shifted the contours of scientific competence and knowledge, which is one of the primary instigators of the proliferation of biomedical citizenship (1996). The radical US-based treatment activist organization, ACT UP (AIDS Coalition to Unleash Power) faced its own form of government denialism and forced the hands of reluctant pharmaceutical companies to invest in research and development costs for the creation and production of ARVs in the early years of the pandemic, in many ways changing the content and contours of scientific knowledge and governance forever. Almost two decades later, the TAC has followed quite closely in its footsteps—sometimes learning directly from ACT UP activists (through workshops and training sessions) and in other ways forging their own pathways toward "biomedical citizenship," as the geopolitical coordinates of the development of TAC's "lay expertification" were quite different. Like ACT UP, one of the TAC's largest mobilizing efforts has been the proliferation of citizen expertise through treatment literacy programs—a subject to which I will return later in this chapter. But the TAC has also waged a long and arduous battle against the state to finally win a seat at the policy-making table, through the South African National AIDS Council (SANAC).

SANAC was established in January 2000 as a multisectoral advisory council (made up of representatives from different government ministries and civil society organizations) focusing on HIV/AIDS (Department of Health 2000; SANAC 2010). It was also meant to monitor and organize resources for the implementation of the HIV/AIDS and STD Strategic Plan for South Africa, 2000–2005 (Department of Health 2000). From its inception, however, the council lacked transparency, public accountability, and broad representation, and it also appeared to meet too irregularly to accomplish much (Nattrass 2004, 50). No scientists, medical practitioners, representatives of the MCC or MRC, and especially no TAC or ALP members were included. "It thus appears to have been set up as a lame duck and behaved as such" (ibid.). SANAC was restructured in 2003 to include more civil society organizations (including the TAC), and civil society constituencies were able to elect their own representatives to SANAC (whereas previously the ANC chose which civil society organizations and members would participate, thus controlling the council's policy recommendations) (Baccaro and Papadakis 2009, 263). The reshuffling that took place in the Department of Health after Tshabalala-Msimang's beetroot and lemon display at the International AIDS Conference in Toronto in 2006 instigated a second major overhauling of SANAC, which also coincided with a renewed National Strategic Plan, 2007–2011 (Nattrass 2008a, 175; Department of Health 2007).[44]

This second restructuring has facilitated the ascendency of TAC to a leadership role in SANAC policy making. SANAC is cochaired by the deputy president of the ANC and a representative of civil society. In 2007, Mark Heywood (of the TAC and ALP) assumed the position of SANAC deputy chairperson. But other TAC leaders have at one point taken active roles in SANAC: Nomfundo Eland (who is chairperson of SANAC's Women's Sector and TAC's national women's rights coordinator), Nonkosi Khumalo (who is the TAC national chairperson and sits on SANAC's plenary board), and Victor Lakay (TAC's head of Community Health Advocacy who has also worked in one of SANAC's Sectoral Coordinating Committees).[45] And TAC and the ALP credit themselves with having drafted some of the most important policies SANAC approved, including the most recent HIV/AIDS National Strategic Plan (Department of Health 2007):

SANAC has really come as far as it has come because Mark Heywood has basically run the show . . . since before he became Deputy Chair because the ALP was involved in drafting the National Strategic Plan. . . . I mean, we literally wrote things into the National Strategic Plan. And even wrote things in that we knew we were to be called to court on later, so that we could rely on . . . [laughs] rely on the NSP, which we did for our cases. It was quite nice that we wrote those few sentences that we quoted. It was fine because it was now in that official policy document. So it was driven by civil society. It continues to be driven by civil society, SANAC.[46]

The problem with this, according to the ALP lawyer who provided this information, is that the TAC and the ALP lack the resources and administrative capacity to be running the policy-making initiatives for the South African Department of Health. Although steps have been taken to rectify these infrastructural setbacks (the successes of which remain to be seen), what is absolutely clear is that the TAC has been able to use SANAC to become indispensable players in the writing and implementation of health policy in South Africa since at least 2007— which incidentally is also the year that the last nail in the denialist coffin was secured.

I would like to provide a brief example of how this shift in TAC's political capacity has served to institutionalize biomedical citizenship in the post-apartheid era. Because of the controversies spawned by the disability grant (and the de facto policy of making people choose between it and ARV medication, which was discussed in the previous chapter), there have been recent discussions around amending the eligibility requirements set out in the Social Assistance Act. These renewed conversations have prompted the TAC and ALP to advocate for the introduction of a chronic illness grant, which they have submitted to the Department of Social Development for consideration in the new amendment. A chronic illness grant would no longer punish people (by refusing them welfare support) for being on ARVs, but rather *require* people to be on ARVs in order to receive welfare provisions.[47] In other words, only people who are enrolled in the state's ARV program would be eligible for a chronic illness grant. These discussions around the introduction of the chronic illness grant have all taken place in and through SANAC: "The general feeling is that the grant should be about three to five hundred rand a month [US$43–$71]. Just as a bit of a stipend to encourage you to get to the facilities to pick up your medication and just to adhere and a little bit of food money aside."[48] On September 16–17, 2010, a group of civil society HIV/AIDS organizations and trade unions met to discuss how best to promote the human right to health through SANAC (ALP 2010a). One of the primary agenda items was the chronic illness grant proposal, which had been rejected during the public hearings on the Social Assistance Amendment Bill (PMG 2010). The group proposed that SANAC play a key role in drafting policy for the chronic illness grant to be included in the social assistance system based on Section 27(1)(c) of the constitution (ALP 2010a). The chronic illness grant is far from being implemented, but it does represent a shift in health governance, which parallels economic shifts toward rollout neoliberalism. This grant provisionalizes citizenship rights by requiring people infected with HIV to be enrolled in an ARV treatment program in order to receive social welfare—thus linking biomedical hegemony to citizenship entitlements.

In the end, TAC's involvement in health care policy making in South Africa provides the ideal lens for analyzing the operations of global public health in a localized context. Theirs is a perfect case for illustrating the destatization of both international and national health governance, the circulation and inculcation of international "best practice" expertise, and the marketization of humanitarian aid. Both Nguyen (2010) and Fassin (2007a; 2011) argue that not unlike colonialism before it, humanitarian aid has become a new means of intervening in sovereign relations and the valuation of life itself, thereby reconfiguring geopolitical boundaries and producing new subjects who are called into being in order to be saved.

In the rest of this chapter, I discuss the kinds of subjectivities being drafted as best practice by global policy makers and imposed on the poor by a whole host of state and nonstate actors (like clinic nurses and NGO staff) through the implementation of disciplinary biomedical techniques. My data calls into question the viability and feasibility of such inscriptions and prescriptions in everyday squatter conditions. I focus my attention on the shifting contours of inclusion and exclusion. My data show very clearly how the provision of individualized salvation based on people's capacity to assume a series of disciplinary behaviors and norms in structurally uncertain conditions simply absolves the state and global governmental agencies from responsibility for their exclusion and death.

Biomedical Discipline

Patients begin the process of enrolling in the state ARV program by having their CD4 count checked through blood work. One's CD4 count must be under 200, but if it's too low or the patient is also suffering from an opportunistic infection (OI), s/he may be discouraged from beginning HAART until the OI has been treated. Patients with very low CD4 counts are sometimes considered risky because they may be too ill to sustain the potent drugs. Once the patient is considered eligible for HAART, s/he is put onto a waiting list at the closest rollout site (people can wait for extended periods of time, depending on the availability of the drug supply in the province in which s/he lives).[49] Once it is the patient's turn to begin treatment, s/he must have her/his CD4 count checked again (in conditions of extreme poverty, people's CD4 counts can drop quickly). The patient will begin pretreatment and adherence counseling. Each patient may go through as many as three sessions of counseling. "We don't rush them. We make it a point to wait until the patient is ready, and firstly we want to know if she is or he is really committed to taking the drugs."[50] While the patient is going through adherence counseling, s/he is also booked for a series of screenings, which may include blood tests, a TB test, and a pap smear. The patient is asked to select an adherence partner (a family member generally) who is meant to help the patient take the drugs on time and monitor her/his progress. There are a series of follow-up visits (at first every two weeks and then monthly) in which the patient sees her/his doctor who checks on any side effects or adherence issues and asks about OIs or other ailments that may have developed. The patient must attend these follow-up appointments to receive the next month's supply of ARVs. The patient has blood work done every six months to monitor the viral load.[51]

Although it depends on the province, there are a series of standards intended to ensure that a patient complies with the ARV treatment program.[52] Patients receive training on HAART and adherence counseling from nurses (and sometimes lay health workers) at the closest clinics. Adherence counselors sometimes ask patients to sign a contract of agreement,[53] and all develop a treatment "plan" with the patient to be reviewed on follow-up visits (Department of Health 2004). In fact, it has been suggested that a treatment "contract" between providers and clients might encourage patients to become self-reliant and responsible for their own health care in a way that avoids more paternalistic programs like "directly observed therapy," which is often used for TB treatment compliance (Schneider and Coetzee 2003). The language of contract and responsibility is directly in line with the forms of citizenship I argue are being promoted through the ARV treatment program:

The evidence from pilot projects is that high levels of adherence stem from a new kind of contract between providers and clients. This contract is premised on very high levels of understanding, treatment literacy and preparation on the part of the users, the establishment of explicit support systems around users and community advocacy processes that promote the rights of people living with HIV/AIDS. The responsibility for adherence is given to the client within a clear framework of empowerment and support. (Schneider and Coetzee 2003, 772)

Ideally, a strong support system, made up of doctors, treatment counselors, and community social support systems (including home-based caregivers) are supposed to help the patient comply. In addition, patients can negotiate for access to nutritional support, pillboxes, and dosing diaries. Counselors are encouraged to be open and honest about the difficulties of taking ARVs, especially in poor living conditions, including engaging in discussions with the patient on questions of stigma, depression, side effects, drug and alcohol usage, access to sustained nutritious food sources, and the patient's capacity to follow the disciplinary requirements for compliance. Here is a list of "deterrents" counselors are encouraged to discuss with potential ARV users before they begin treatment:

From Department of Health Adherence Manual (2010b)
Some deterrents against taking ART (DISADVANTAGES):

· Patients must adhere to the timing, frequency, and dosage of the drug regimen for a lifelong treatment period
· Dosing regimens may be complex
· There are differing dietary requirements
· Some drugs require refrigeration
· Some require preparation
· Multidrug regimens require taking numerous pills per day
· Certain drugs may interact
· There is a high possibility of experiencing drug side effects
· Loss of confidentiality as a result of being seen taking the drugs
· Risk of drug resistance and, therefore, limitations of future ART choices including: too low CD4 counts, too many opportunistic infections, alcohol or drug use, or insufficient social support.

In the minds of policy makers, one of the primary concerns is drug resistance (especially given the scarcity of drug combinations available within the public sector). Therefore, those who are not able to adhere to a strict drug regimen might pose a risk to the sanctity of the ARV roll-out by introducing drug-resistant strands of the virus within already vulnerable communities. However, establishing contractual disciplinary standards for life-saving medications effectively demarcates those who are deserving of citizenship rights from those who are not. Here is an exchange from a focus group discussion held in Lawley:

Woman 1: First, they take us and tell us how to take the ARVs—they train us. Then, they ask us if we are ready. Then, they test us whether we understand how the tablets have to be taken. If they see you will mix them, or default on treatment, then they won't get them. If you cannot follow the instructions on taking them, then they won't give them to you.

Woman 2: They gave me a test. I failed. I got sick and had to go to the hospital because I failed the test and could not get the ARVs. That's the reason I got so sick in the first place because I couldn't pass the test and get the treatment when I needed it.

Man: Many are failing the test. They have to come back without drugs—even if they are still sick.[54]

Under a model of biomedical citizenship, survival is premised on the ability (or desire) to adhere to a strict biomedical drug regimen, which includes not only a calculus of the number of pills and their time-tables but also food intake, social support, and an agreement not to engage in other forms of healing—most specifically, indigenous forms of healing.

Patients are told that some "life-adjustments" may be required for compliance with HAART (Department of Health 2010b, 6). People I spoke with who are taking ARVs discussed some of the associated challenges, which include avoiding alcohol and cigarette usage, openly disclosing their status to their families, seeking out nutritious food sources, and making sure to keep clinic appointments. But beyond the adjustments in everyday activities, people's subjectivities are being refashioned.

Biomedical Technologies of the Self

Treatment testimonies—with their references to CD4 counts, viral loads and the role of TAC in giving "new life"—seem to blur the lines between science and religion, medicine and spirituality, and technology and magic. Even though TAC is a modernist and secular organization, the quasi-religious quality of these testimonies is evident. (ROBINS 2008A, 136)

Since the beginning of the AIDS epidemic, the global therapeutic economy, operating through NGO-sponsored support groups, has attempted to forge responsibilized subjects. Prior to the introduction of ARVs, engaging in a "healthy lifestyle" and "living positively" entailed public disclosure of one's status, a commitment not to infect others, and making funeral and child-care arrangements. In 2002–2003 and 2004–2005, I volunteered with a major NGO operating in multiple township communities in South Africa. I witnessed the various confessional techniques deployed in one support group after another, and I sat in on countless reiterative lessons on how to "live positively" by eating healthfully, abstaining from alcohol and drug use, and engaging in safer sex practices. I was often shown support group members' memory boxes or diaries, which were keepsakes for their children but which also included wills detailing their wishes for the children they were soon to leave behind. Vinh-Kim Nguyen suggests that the development of these techniques of the self emerged out of a complicated process of bricolage whereby NGOs and community-based organizations (CBOs) served as hybridized institutional forms allowing for the intermixture of global therapeutic strategies with local evangelical cultural practices (2005, 129).

These processes are magnified with the introduction of ARVs, when new subjectivities are forged through "local economies of salvation" (Biehl 2006b, 459). Given the fact that ARVs do, in a sense, bring people back from the dead, biomedical narratives have, in a way, been evangelized:

Look at me, Claire. Thanks to my ARVs, I have my life back. And we had a second baby. You remember, I was so sick. Now my whole family is healthy and strong. You remember I told you I'm a fighter . . . we survived.[55]

I drink these tablets. I'm on the ART program. When I started to drink these tablets, I was critically ill. I could not walk or do anything. After I use these tablets, its me. Nothing is painful in me. They are treating me well. No problem. I have no problems . . . now I'm Agnes[56] again.[57]

I was living in Sparrow [in hospice] for five years. And there, I was sick, and people [in the community] laughed at me. But when I stayed at Sparrow, I took medication from Helen Joseph [ARVs]. . . . Then I was discharged from Sparrow—I was told I was better and that I can take care of myself . . . there are a lot of them who laughed at me, but now I'm walking on top of them—they are all dead.[58]

In 2006, my wife, Elizabeth, got really sick . . . her CD4 count was 10. She got put on ARVs at Helen Joseph hospital, but then was admitted to Baragwanath.[59] . . .

She didn't have strength. Her body was shaking and she felt like sometimes she was losing power. And then she lost weight. That lasted for three or four months. Then, she came back but she was admitted again because she couldn't eat. Well, she would eat, but then have to spit it out. But now, her CD4 count is 342—it's over mine! And she had a baby, and she's so strong now. You would never know.[60]

TAC activism has contributed to these discourses of biomedical salvation in three ways: (1) its treatment literacy programs have extended biomedical knowledge, such that people use medical terminology to describe their subjectivities; (2) the social capital accumulated through attachment with an NGO like TAC and the ARVs themselves can lead to economic salvation; and (3) TAC activism has given rise to a new form of "responsibilized citizenry." I will explore each of these in turn.

TAC was the first AIDS activist organization to pioneer treatment literacy in the global South, based on models created by ACT UP and the Gay Men's Health Clinic (GMHC)—members of whom actually traveled to South Africa in 1999 to train the first cadre of TAC activists (Heywood 2009, 17). Treatment literacy involves undergoing training on the science of HIV (what it is, how it affects the body, what kinds of opportunistic infections it generates) and on ARVs (the different classifications of drugs, how they attack the virus) and other HIV-related treatments. Once TAC volunteers have been trained and have passed an exam, they are called treatment literacy practitioners, or TLPs, and they are given a small bursary and are assigned to clinics, hospitals, and community organizations where they train others (ibid.). Although TAC's treatment literacy programs are often overlooked, they are "the largest part of TAC's apparatus . . . and also the largest part of TAC's budget" (ibid., 18). "Treatment literacy is the base for both self-help and self-mobilization" (ibid.). And it directly puts biomedical knowledge into the hands of its users, as opposed to experts and professionals.[61]

In addition to "treatment literacy" and thus biomedical orthodoxy, the TAC advocates a certain discourse of "positive living," which means, at least as a first step, publicly disclosing one's status. In this way, people identify themselves as a population that needs servicing: "In these contexts, claiming positive identity can be tantamount to a conversion experience: quite literally, a path to salvation, since identification can begin access to medication and material support" (Comaroff 2007, 204). In order to be saved, one needs to adopt biomedical orthodoxy and attempt to embody a biomedical technology of the self. For Foucault, "technologies of the self" are a means by which individuals pull on prevailing moral codes, discourses, disciplines, and techniques of subjection as a means of fashioning oneself (1988). It is a process of subjectivation whereby subjects cultivate identities, which then shape their experiences as citizens and believers. For example, Nguyen notes that before ARVs were more widely available in African countries, the only means by which the poor could self-identify as someone in need of treatment (and thus receive medication from donors and NGOs) would be to become adept at telling his/her illness narrative, which served as a "confessional technology" (2010, chapter 2). In the contemporary South African context, the way in which people describe themselves through recourse to their CD4 count or viral load is a means of self-identifying as an AIDS sufferer, who has embodied a biomedical understanding of his/her subjectivity. Robins notes that "conversion rituals" are a primary way in which TAC reaches out to isolated HIV-positive South Africans and provides them with a means of joining an activist community, which also serves to responsibilize them (Robins 2006, 321; Robins 2008a).

"Now using AIDS drugs and on their own, these patient citizens face the daily challenge of translating medical investments into social capital and wage-earning power" (Biehl 2006b, 472). Many HIV-positive community members join the TAC or other NGOs because it gives them access to material resources and social and cultural capital. As such, people purchase social mobility by becoming involved in an organization and rising through its hierarchical positions.

Look, I'm concerned about the programs that the TAC implements on the ground. . . . Support is given to the people who can access their offices that date, and be organizers doing, whatever, doing important jobs. For many people, joining the TAC is a moneymaking scheme. People get into the organization hoping they will be hired, that they will find employment. But there is also some prestige. Some members get to travel to Cape Town . . . and they help people get things from the government. If you are a member of TAC, though, you have to follow their mandate. You have to agree with their rules. Because they don't listen to the communities. They don't respond to what we suggest because they think they already have all the answers.[62]

In addition, biological salvation is linked to economic rebirth as promises of employment opportunities and productive livelihoods abound.

If people are on ARVs, then the government has to invest in them for that period, but then you have a person who is now beginning to take control of his or her own life in terms of health, right? And then of course the knock-on effects of that is being able to find a job . . . being able to be strong enough to go and look for work.[63]

Finally, through their promotion of biomedical embodiment, which has accompanied the successful rollout of antiretrovirals, TAC has also taken part in a campaign to responsibilize South African citizens. According to Nikolas Rose (1999), neoliberalism is an art of government premised on freedom whereby certain rationalities of rule guide the conduct of citizens without seeming to do so. Experts, who act as knowledge workers, help to provide the information necessary, for example, in the form of risk assessments that enable and empower individuals to self-govern (Rose 1999, 147; Ferguson and Gupta 2002, 989). Rather than making claims on the state, the neoliberal subject becomes "an entrepreneur of himself" (Ong 2006, 14; Foucault 2008, 226), as s/he attempts to maximize his/her own human capital (Foucault 2008, 224). The subject of neoliberalism is both responsibilized and entrepreneurialized, and citizens act as consumers of public goods such that their rights are constantly contractualized (Rose 1999, 139, 165). However, for those who are deemed socially pathological and unable (or unwilling) to self-discipline, a whole host of policies and agencies have emerged to help teach civility and self-determination (Rose 1999, 86–89). One of the primary ways in which rollout neoliberalism functions, therefore, is through the responsibilization of citizens, which also serves to privatize blame. Most of the literature on neoliberal governmentality avoids the question of those unable to assume responsibility and self-entrepreneurialism—those who are undisciplinable. In this chapter, I argue that structural inequality often impedes certain subjects of the late neoliberal era from fashioning responsible subjectivities. The state and civil society are able to relieve themselves of responsibility for these subjects, constituting a new form of exclusionary inclusion.

In his book, Robins (2008a) argues that the "near death" experiences associated with living with "full-blown AIDS" and the "social death" associated with the stigma attached to having this condition "produce the conditions for AIDS survivors' commitment to forms of 'responsibilized citizenship'" (127). According to this account, TAC helps people living with the virus recast their trauma in new light and also welcomes them into a new sociality—a new social community associated with AIDS. Part of this transformation, which Robins terms "rights passage," is the "miraculous recovery that ARV treatment provides" (131). Robins claims that this transformation and the fact that people are learning to take responsibility for their own health does not necessarily need to be understood as utilitarian, individualistic, and apolitical. He argues that most theorists of neoliberal governance critique emergent discourses of responsibility because they ask citizens to take responsibility for services the state should provide. He suggests that TAC is calling for something different: "They argue that what is needed for AIDS treatment prevention programmes to succeed is a well-resourced and responsible public health sector health system *and* empowered, knowledgeable and 'responsibilized' client-citizens. They are calling for an effective health system together with new forms of community participation and citizenship, or . . . 'governance from below'" (142).

There is no doubt that the discourses of "living positively" and the new politics of survival generated by the TAC have salvaged countless South Africans' lives and livelihoods. But its reliance on neoliberal modes of governance and regulation remains problematic for five reasons. First, I have argued that discourses of responsibility serve to privatize blame. This practice has a long history in the case of HIV/AIDS, as "irresponsible sexual behavior" was often used to blame the victims of the epidemic for their own vulnerability to infection. Obviously, the analysis most commonly leveled at discourses of responsibility refers to the retraction of the state from its social welfare responsibilities, as social services, health care, pensions, and prisons are privatized. However, as Robins points out, the TAC has not abdicated its responsibility for the care of the destitute, nor is it relieving the state of its own obligations in this regard. In fact, rollout neoliberalism reinstates social safety nets, usually provided through civil society organizations or through some contractualized form of social support. And this is the key. In the age of rollout neoliberalism, the individual is blamed for his/her own failure to seize the opportunities made available by social institutions and the state—not because of some innate trait rooted in the individualized body, but rather for her/his incapacity to self-regulate or capitalize on her/his human capital. As mentioned in the previous chapter, this has redefined the contours of exclusion, such that it is no longer premised on a binary construction of self/other, but rather on a normal curve, where those on the margins simply fall off the edges of the social because their grasp on the body politic is so tenuous and provisional. Some people with HIV are saved, they are blessed with the rights of citizenship, but only because they happen to be lucky enough to garner some minimal form of social capital, or convincing enough in their performance of the requisite technologies of the self, or savvy enough in the way they work the system. And the fact that some are

149

saved provides the necessary "proof" that the problem is not systemic. As such, "the dystopic implications of neoliberalism [are projected] onto the victims themselves" (Comaroff 2007, 199).

A second problem is that this form of "triage" enables a "government-by-exception" whereby "sometimes the only way to survive is by having a fatal illness called HIV" (Nguyen 2010, 186, 182). In other words, only some people are eligible for state support because of chronic conditions, whereas others are left to fend for themselves. This is particularly true in South Africa where there is no social support based on income or indigence—one must be elderly, caring for a vulnerable child, or disabled to be eligible for a grant. "People gave their lives to achieve sovereignty in these postcolonial lands. Today, it seems, the only way to maintain that sovereignty would be to let themselves die" (ibid., 187).

Third, at the margins, social citizenship[64] is contingent on the successful exercise of biomedical practices and the embodiment of disciplinary norms. I borrow the term "exclusionary inclusion" from Giorgio Agamben, who uses it to detail the ways in which neoliberalism's disposable populations are managed. They exist in a juridical threshold—they are internal to the nation-state and yet do not enjoy all of its rights. Aihwa Ong (2006) takes issue with Agamben's rather haunting description of contemporary biopolitics:

Increasingly, a diversity of multilateral systems—multinational companies, religious organizations, UN agencies, and other NGOs—intervenes to deal with specific, situated and practical problems of abused, naked, and flawed bodies. The nonstate administration of excluded humanity is an emergent transnational phenomenon, despite its discontinuous, disjointed, and contingent nature. (24)

Countering Ong's intervention, I argue that even these humanitarian efforts are thanatopolitical in the end, as those who cannot assume entrepreneurialized and biomedicalized selves are "let die" while the state and the administrators of the "therapeutic economy" (Nguyen 2010) are absolved of the responsibility of having invoked the sovereign decision.

The people in this study can access the rights of citizenship and are important to the very definition and political legitimacy of the state. In fact, in the most recent presidential elections (in 2009), the poor showed their tremendous political power by overthrowing Mbeki and replacing him with Jacob Zuma—a leader they believed was more likely to deliver services and jobs. However, the social rights the poor can access are contingent on their capabilities of embodying or at least correctly performing certain technologies of the self, which are very difficult to sustain in squatter conditions and which require them to abandon indigenous healing practices. In my analysis, "exclusionary inclusion" is used to describe this threshold state where disease is both the basis of citizenship and serves to redefine it in the neoliberal age. In other words, being HIV-infected becomes a means of accessing the rights of citizenship (in this case, antiretrovirals), but also becomes the basis for the institution of a new form of exclusionary citizenship premised on the incorporation of biomedical subjectivities.

The fourth way in which TAC's approach is problematic is that it fails to contend with the hybrid nature of people's health beliefs and practices. When I explained the debates around the chronic illness grant to the HIV-infected residents of Lawley, Nomachina Makalo responded: "but, that's blackmail!"[65] She wasn't the only respondent who pointed out that this policy blackmails poor South Africans into accepting biomedical doctrine by linking it to citizenship rights. Biomedicine may be applied through universal "best practices," but it is received, interpreted, and utilized in very localized ways—often through combination with other forms of healing and through engagement with various expert cultures. Thulani refuses to use antiretrovirals because he fears that they will require him to forsake his identity. First, because the doctors will ask him to avoid using indigenous forms of healing—a contract he is not willing to abide by. But he also fears becoming a "machine" that must follow a rigid timetable and adhere to a regimen he finds not only somewhat ridiculous, given his living conditions, but also undesirable and burdensome. "I just imagine being programmed. That's what they do—they program you. I don't want to be programmed like that."[66] Thulani is keenly aware of the price he is being asked to pay for inclusion in the body politic—not only will he be "programmed" by biomedical discipline, but should his performance fail, the responsibility for his abandonment will be his alone to bear.

While the TAC has won significant battles for health care and treatment, their reception at the community level is surprisingly ambiguous. During the height of the struggle against denialism, antiretrovirals were often viewed as yet another possible treatment option in a long line of available sources of health care. In the interviews I held with community members, antiretrovirals were sometimes understood to be manufactured and produced *by* the TAC.[67] Vitamins, indigenous *muthi*, micronutrients, and antiretrovirals were *all* touted as miracle cures in townships throughout South Africa. Like so many others, TAC activists attempted to "sell hope" to the masses, and as such, for community members, all treatment options became a matter of ideological choice.

From my birth until now, I've been cautious about medicines. I didn't use multivitamins or *muthis* because it's confusing because each and every person is coming with a product. What are you supposed to do? Buy all of them in order to be ok? No, I don't use anything. . . . As long as I can walk, eat, sleep, I'm ok. I'm not going to use anything. . . . I've got a problem with the very same ARVs. My concern is that each and everyone will rush to say you should get onto the ARV program, but I'm worried. If one is subjected to that treatment, one has to do it for life. Sometimes they could have prescribed something that could assist someone without pushing everyone to getting on ARV. It is a one-size fit all treatment. But that's what the other ones do too. How can I tell the difference?[68]

This comment was actually made in an FGD held in 2009—long after the debate over denialism had ended. Despite the fears and confusion, people living in informal settlements (which charlatans pushing every conceivable miracle cure have targeted) have begun to take ARVs, and they no longer (if they ever did) associate them with the TAC. But they do mix them with other forms of treatment (despite the admonitions from biomedical staff)—which will be the topic of chapter 5. The point I want to stress here is simply that the plural and hybrid nature of people's sense of self is not accommodated by the biomedical technologies treatment protocol requires.

The final and perhaps most glaring problem with biomedicalized citizenship is that structural obstacles often make the embodiment of biomedical technologies of the self impossible. Modernizing public health initiatives always included the provision of water, sanitation, and health care. Such a model has been replaced, in the neoliberal era, with an individualized, contractualized, and commodified approach to treating individuals with highly technologized and biomedicalized interventions, without regard for the safety, sanitation, or sustainability of the community in which they live.

Infrastructural Constraints

Some of the obstacles to a successful ARV rollout are infrastructural, and these are the problems the TAC and ALP have begun to tackle since they restructured their organizational focus in 2003/2004 toward monitoring and evaluating the rollout. I begin by explaining some of these ongoing administrative and economic challenges. But then I go on to show that living in an informal settlement presents its own set of challenges for ARV provisioning, and these are largely being ignored in the promotion of responsible citizenship.

One of the most serious challenges to maintaining the ARV rollout has been shortages in drug supply. There was a moratorium on the rollout of ARVs in the Free State (one of South Africa's nine provinces) from November 2008 through February 2009 (TAC 2009c), which resulted in thirty deaths (TAC 2009c, 11). "The province's Department of Health stopped initiating new patients on ARVs because of out-of-stock drugs and lack of funds. . . . The moratorium will increase morbidity and mortality, but the loss of trust in the health system and the potential impact of the ARV crisis on existing patient adherence also need to be considered" (El-Khatib and Richter 2009, 412).

There was no discussion with civil society or with the national health department about what could be done. Rather, they just issued a moratorium and cut other services. The problem doesn't go away, unless you just let the patients die. Now, they are going to be sicker because of the lack of ARVs. This is simply not cost effective in the long run. . . . This is going to happen in other provinces because of poor budgeting and poor use of funds by provincial government. The recession also certainly won't help matters.[69]

Then again, in June 2009, a primary location in KwaZulu-Natal was unable to provide ARVs for a brief period because of a lack of pharmacists.[70]

The official policy is that when this happens, those who are already on the rollout will continue to access it, but new patients can't begin their treatment. But . . . we found . . . that even those who were on treatment . . . were affected . . . It's drilled into you that you *have* to take it morning, noon, and night and with the meals, and at this time, always at the same time. And this thing is just bloody drilled into you and then this is what happens . . . And so it undermines your entire adherence counseling and, you know, the entire program.[71]

When moratoriums on the rollout occur, it has also been reported that patients who are already enrolled in the ARV program share their drugs with family members, neighbors, and friends who cannot receive the drugs because of the shortage (Campero et al. 2007). Obviously, with the economic recession and decreases in international funding and political commitment for ARV provision, these shortages are likely to continue.

Another major infrastructural problem that affects long-term ARV provisioning is the shortage of health-care workers. The public sector serves 82 percent of the population but has only 27 percent of the country's general practitioners (TAC 2005a).

The biggest obstacle is too much workload and a shortage of staff. Every morning the clinic is full. It doesn't matter how many you are, you have to man this clinic, and the department is saying, don't turn away patients. . . . And there are shortages, drastic shortages of resources, human resources, material resources . . . drugs, um . . . drugs are being ordered, but mainly because you cannot predict the number of patients that you can see. It's never enough. And even if you have ordered it, there is no guarantee that you . . . you will get what you have ordered.[72]

South Africa is suffering from a severe "brain-drain"—more and more health workers (both doctors and nurses) are abandoning the public health sector for the private sector, or they are leaving South Africa altogether. Nearly one in three public health positions are constantly vacant, and three hundred nurses leave South Africa every month (TAC 2005a).[73]

Nurses are moving from the public to the private health sector in droves. In the private sector, they are paid much better and their working conditions are much better. Their nurse to patient ratio is like 1:3, but here, at Bara, it's like 1:100! In the private sector, there's less hours, less stress, and more pay. There is no incentive to stay in the public health sector. The turnover for nurses in the public sector is only 3 to 6 months.[74]

Between 1996 and 2004, South Africa produced just over 34,000 nurses, but over 27,000 were "lost to the system" (TAC 2005a). It is estimated that there is a 54 percent shortage of nurses in all primary health clinics in South Africa (*Mail and Guardian* 2007a). Due to severe nursing shortages and growing numbers of patients, the nurse-patient ratio in the public health system is shocking. In 1998, there were 149 registered nurses per 100,000 population, which dropped to 110 per 100,000 by 2007 (Coovadia et al. 2009, 830). The burden the HIV/AIDS pandemic has had on the health sector also includes a high infection rate among nursing staff—16 percent of the profession (ibid.).

Public clinics and hospitals are not only understaffed and underresourced, they are also immensely overcrowded—a problem made even more acute by the rising numbers of sick and dying AIDS patients. In 2006, one nurse reported:

In my ward, people have full-blown AIDS. I think that 99 percent of my patients have HIV. I'm being honest. And I think it's getting worse instead of improving, despite these ARVs. There are more and more patients every day, and they are getting more and more sick. So the statistics are going up.[75]

The problem has shifted with the increasing provision of ARVs, but mortality rates are still high, and now nurses face the additional burden of staffing the complex rollout program.

There have been two highly publicized public service workers strikes in South Africa in recent years. The first was held in June 2007, and the second from July through August of 2010. Public service workers, including doctors and nurses, teachers, police, and government bureaucrats, numbering approximately 1.3 million, were represented by various unions under the rubric of COSATU (*BBC News* 2010). Due to the strikes, workers were able to get 7.5 percent wage increases on both occasions (*Mail and Guardian* 2007b; *Mail and Guardian* 2010). During the 2007 strike, three thousand workers, mainly in the health sector, were given dismissal notices (*Mail and Guardian* 2007c). One of twelve nurses fired in the Eastern Cape had this to say: "We work with broken equipment, inadequate facilities, not enough drugs for our patients, and we're paid pathetic salaries. Thousands of qualified nurses are leaving the country, doubling our workload. And the only words our president has for us is to condemn vandalism and violence" (Emilia Maloi, quoted in *Mail and Guardian* 2007a).

One final infrastructural issue is that housing and service delivery is meant to be the responsibility of municipal government, but health care delivery is a provincial matter. Grants are managed by a separate national entity, titled the South African Social Security Agency. People often get stuck between different levels of the state and between different departments (Health, Social Development, and Housing). There is often conflict between national, provincial, and local policy and priorities, which is exacerbated by limited budgets. And people end up being volleyed back and forth between different governmental departments as they try to apply for grants, ARVs, housing, and other social provisions. SANAC is supposed to operate in a multisectoral way to promote coordination between governmental units on issues associated with HIV/AIDS, but it hasn't been very effective in this capacity.[76]

Since the beginning of the ARV rollout in 2004, the TAC and ALP have focused on monitoring the rollout and addressing problems associated with infrastructure and capacity.[77] However, the challenges associated with ARV provision, especially in conditions of abject poverty, extend far beyond the infrastructural. Systemic inequality and the conditions of living in squatter communities present their own set of severe obstacles to the rollout program.

The Contingencies of Citizenship

Many of the predictors of poor adherence listed in the Department of Health's manual on adherence counseling are associated with living in squatter conditions (Department of Health 2010b, 7). The simple lack of resources to purchase food or pay for transportation to the clinic was mentioned again and again in interviews and focus group discussions:

I don't even know when I'm going to have a healthy meal from one day to the next. How can I take these ARVs, when I can't even afford to eat right?[78]

I have five kids, and I'm also living with HIV. There's a problem with regard to checking the CD4 count. Every six months, you have to go to check. Sometimes when you go, you are automatically disqualified from receiving a grant. But I'm taking ARVs, and you are supposed to eat good food when you are taking ARVs—all the time. So, how am I supposed to eat without any money?[79]

But the biggest problem we have? It's the stress. Because we don't possess money. We don't get grants. . . . And we are still expected to take the medication. And you don't have money for transportation. You don't have money for food. And you still have to go there, you know, and sometimes if you miss one or two, then you affect the whole program.[80]

Pheello and his family earn R250 ($36) per month from a child support grant. It costs him R28 ($4) and his wife R68 ($10) just to cover transportation to the clinics where they receive their monthly ARV allotments—that's almost half of their entire earnings for the month. And if one of them (or one of their children) is sick, they will have additional transportation costs to cover. Patients at public hospitals, informal settlement clinics, and rural clinics spend on average R120 ($17) per visit to obtain their "free" ARVs, which includes transportation, clinic fees, nonprescription medicines, special foods, and other medical care fees (Rosen et al. 2007).

In addition, people are supposed to have fully disclosed their status to their families and communities before beginning ART; however, most of the people I met in Lawley and Sol Plaatjie, who are taking ARVs, do so silently and clandestinely because the stigma associated with HIV/AIDS is still quite high in informal settlements. This can augment the stress of attending the clinic on a monthly basis to receive new supplies, because one might be seen or because one might need to ask neighbors for financial help for transportation.

People are also deemed likely to default on HAART if they cannot identify their medications. "I have become a small pharmacy,"[81] Pheello proudly told me one day as he brought out his box full of medicines. He knew which pills were his ARVs, when he needed to take them, and which were most difficult to take. Yet Pheello has scores of other medications in plastic bags, vials, and boxes. Upon questioning, he was quite confused about the drugs' purposes, dosage requirements, and expiration dates. Pheello does not speak or read English—not that his English skills are the only obstacle toward understanding the biomedical language used on the packages. Presumably, the doctor had explained each pill when it was first prescribed; however, I have often accompanied Pheello to the clinic and hospital, and there is rarely a Sotho interpreter on hand. Pheello often does not understand his diagnosis or prescription. In the seven years I've known Pheello, he has been extremely sick—he has suffered from numerous opportunistic infections (including cytomegalovirus, neuropathy, and thrush), has often been coinfected with TB, suffers from almost constant diarrhea—this and his ongoing battle against flus and colds keeps him on continual antibiotics. But because he has been to the clinic so often over the years, he has collected a wide array of medications he no longer knows how to use. This doesn't keep him from self-diagnosing and mixing these pharmaceuticals with his ARVs when he feels sick. It is important not to misconstrue this story—Pheello is one of the best informed, dedicated, and proactive patients I have ever met. He not only takes his ARV treatment seriously, but he also tries to convince other people in his community to begin the treatment and counsels them on how to remain compliant. I tell this story simply to show that even those with the best of intentions face serious challenges in adhering to the biomedical requirements for HAART.

In each of the communities, I was told that some people are so desperate for food that they are forced to sell their ARV medications to buy groceries:

We sell ARVs so that we can buy paraffin. We don't have food, so we buy food. If they give us ARVs, we sell those to get supplies.[82]

Because people are starving, they see the business from the ARVs. They get the medications for free and then they sell it for R30 to the kids, who then use it as a drug. With that R30, a woman can buy veggies, sugar, etc.[83]

Because of poverty, people who are taking ARVs at times you find that they don't have anything, no food, no money, then they'll be tempted to sell the tablets to the boys who mix it with other drugs. It's either they'll sell tablets, one, two, or three, or at times the whole book . . . but it's only the one drug, the one we take at night, that they use to make *nyawupe*.[84]

Efavirenz is a strong non-nucleoside reverse transcriptase inhibitor[85] that has hallucinatory side effects. In some locations in South Africa (including both Sol Plaatjie and Lawley), it has been reported that a market in the drug has developed among teenagers who grind it up and smoke it to get high (Marwaha 2008; Hull 2010). The resultant drug is referred to as either *whoonga* or *nyawupe*—the latter because it causes the user to become itchy, *unwaya* being the Zulu verb "to scratch."[86] I have heard people pragmatically calculate between the costs and benefits of selling one ARV to buy groceries, telling themselves that they are still taking two out of the three antiretrovirals that makeup their "cocktail" therapy. Whereas triple antiretroviral therapy completely suppresses HIV replication, double therapy does not, allowing the virus to become resistant to not just the two drugs themselves but to other drugs in the same class (Nguyen 2010, 196–97nn9–10). As such, this gamble compromises the drug rollout more than patients realize.

And there are other gambles people in squatter camps are forced to make in order to attempt to comply with the drug regimen despite the structural conditions in which they live. Sandra Mkhwanazi is originally from Zimbabwe, and she has faced severe xenophobia and HIV-related stigma in Lawley. Sandra's husband bought them a plot of land in Lawley in 2000. He then passed away in 2002. She did not know her own status until 2008 when she got extraordinarily sick and almost died. Even though she is not a South African citizen, she was put onto the ARV program. But she cannot receive a disability grant, and she has no income to support herself and her two children.

I had an ordeal last month because, I mean, I didn't have money for transport to go and fetch my treatment. . . . I woke up very early at around four thirty so that

I could walk because people normally walk . . . across this empty field between Lawley and Lenasia . . . if they don't have money for transport. It takes people one hour to walk, but it takes me two because I have this serious pain in my feet. . . . So as I was walking and approaching, there's a dam. And then four men actually came from the field, you know. And then they all raped me. And all of them slept with me . . . [crying] . . . I think it happens quite often because, I mean, before my ordeal, a lot of people had already reported that these incidents that are happening, especially around that road.[87]

Sandra still went to the clinic that day, because she said she had to. I asked her if she told the nurses what had happened to her, and she said that they simply listened and then gave her the next month's supply of ARVs. Sandra's story unveils the invisible boundaries that circumscribe the South African body politic—the literal void she must traverse to access the privileges of the polis and the price she must pay for the passage, before returning to her precarious position as one who has been abandoned to the margins of the social.

The logic associated with biomedical citizenship is that if people cannot adhere to the strict regimens outlined by the Department of

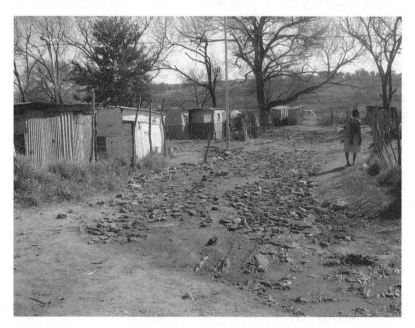

FIGURE 18.   Sol Plaatjie. Photo taken by the author in 2005.

Health, they are responsible for their own failure and their subsequent loss of citizenship rights, like the disability grant. Obviously there are many nurses, doctors, and health activists who are aware of and do not personally punish the individuals in their care for the difficulties they face in complying with ARV protocol because they live in squatter conditions. But the system is set up so that people often do default. Their options are to remain silent about their defaulting and hope that they do not become resistant to the medications (or spread a resistant strand of the virus on to someone else), or to stop treatment. Either way, they suffer in silence, as their conditions of existence and the neoliberal policies that sustain them remain largely unchanged.

Exclusive Inclusion

In the political decisions that administer the scientific, technological, and social resources to respond to the epidemic of AIDS . . . the lives to be saved are insidiously demarcated from those who will be left to die. . . . But this demarcation is, of course, largely implicit; modern power "administers" life in part through the silent withdrawal of its resources. In this way politics can achieve the goal of death, can target its own population, under the very sign of the administration of life. This "inversion" of power performs the work of death under the very signs of life, scientific progress, technological advance. (BUTLER 1996, 73)

During the struggle against denialism, TAC often engaged in a radical biopolitics that directly targeted Mbeki's thanatopolitical regime. It did so by literalizing the deaths denialism caused—it staged "die-ins" whereby people in the final stages of AIDS would lie on the ground (and sometimes in hospital beds) at the entrances of Department of Health buildings holding signs saying, "The South African Government's Neglect Is Causing 600 Deaths Per Day." Agamben argues that the target of thanatopolitics is *homo sacer*—a character who exists in a threshold state because he cannot be sacrificed, but his death would go unpunished (1998). TAC made AIDS deaths sacrificial once more (Comaroff 2007, 207). But the political and biological salvation they sought was based on a biosociality, which was *exclusively* biomedical—one that not everyone would want or be able to assume. And they won that battle through the inculcation of a neoliberal governmentality of rule. In the end, then, TAC's approach paradoxically hid a politics of death, as Butler explains in the quote above, "under the very sign of the administration of life."

As Foucault himself once declared, "I have tried to understand power by looking at its extremities, at where its exercise became less and less juridical" (1997, 28). Those who become targets of this new form of "letting die" exist in an ambiguous political realm—they are inside the juridical order; the state is responsible for their lives. And because of their radical potential for resistance, they are even essential for the legitimation of state power. And yet, the various tenuous lifelines they have been thrown are fragile, reliant as they are on people's capacities to assume new bodily regimes and new technologies of the self. Worse yet, people must navigate precipitous and arduous structural obstacles simply to survive on a daily basis. By dolling out pills without providing sustainable living conditions, the poor have been abandoned. By granting minimal inclusionary provisions on the basis of behavioral change, the state and civil society are absolved of responsibility—they have washed their hands. If people die, it's their own fault.

My contribution to the literature on biomedical citizenship comes from analyzing the ways in which certain structural barriers make assuming biomedical subjectivity impossible, such that severe systemic poverty coupled with the privatization of blame leads to a situation in which biopolitics blurs into thanatopolitics, at the threshold of citizenship. Scheper-Hughes refers to a globalized "apartheid medicine" where those who receive medical attention are recognized as patients, whereas those who do not are rendered obsolete or invisible (2005, 149). Fassin refers to the ways in which humanitarian aid and the politics of life it plays relies upon a "complex ontology of inequality [that] unfolds . . . in a hierarchical manner [in order to] value lives" (2007a, 519). Nguyen refers to these "triage" decisions as "government by exception" (2010, 186–87). My contribution builds on but differs from these accounts by showing that even those who are "lucky enough" to be targeted by biomedicine and are extended the opportunity for biomedical citizenship live in a state of uncertainty, their citizenship rendered precarious and contingent, reliant on the capacity to convincingly perform "responsible" and "positive living." I also show how the technologies of the self required in the neoliberal age are not only entrepreneurial but also increasingly *biomedical*, thereby contributing to an imperialistic expansion of biomedical hegemony.

The intention of this chapter is not to imply that antiretrovirals should cease to be provided in resource-poor settings. Rather, it is to point out a certain logic that undergirds treatment governance throughout the global South—a logic that individualizes blame, contractualizes rights, and utilizes technological interventions (like antiretrovirals) in an attempt to responsibilize undesirable populations. New forms of biomedicalized citizenship reconfigure the contours and technologies of exclusion in this new age of rollout neoliberalism. Endemic structural inequality, deeply entrenched patterns of neoliberal regulation, and the ongoing privatization of "responsibility," are the causal factors that lead to the "letting die" of the poorest of the poor.

FOUR

The Politicization
of Sexuality

The image in figure 19 accompanied an *Economist* article
from January 9, 2010, titled "A President Who Promotes
Tradition":

Decked out in a leopard-skin mantle and an animal-pelt loincloth
together with white designer sneakers, South Africa's 67-year-old
president, Jacob Zuma, celebrated his marriage to his third concurrent wife (and fifth bride in all) in a grand Zulu ceremony attended
by some 3,000 guests at his family home deep in rural KwaZulu-
Natal. . . . Mike Siluma, a former editor of the *Sowetan*, a daily that is
read mainly by blacks, points out that South Africa is not the Western
country so many take it to be, but a "dynamic kaleidoscope of cultures, religions, and traditions." Many black South African Christians
still also worship their ancestors, he notes. Most weddings mix the
traditional with the Christian. Many people practise customary law
alongside the Western kind and take traditional as well as Western
medicine. Mr Siluma thinks the elevation of a Zulu from a peasant
background to the presidency of sub-Saharan Africa's most sophisticated country may help revive some of the mores and cultures that
had been sadly fading. (*Economist* 2010)

Jacob Zuma's "retraditioning of the postcolony"[1] is perhaps
best described as a mirrored reflection of Mbeki's attempts
to manage the postcolonial paradox. Whereas Mbeki used
"traditional" healing and racial/indigenous "authenticity,"
Zuma draws on clearly gendered mores and performs a
particular version of "traditional" Zulu sexuality.[2] On the

163

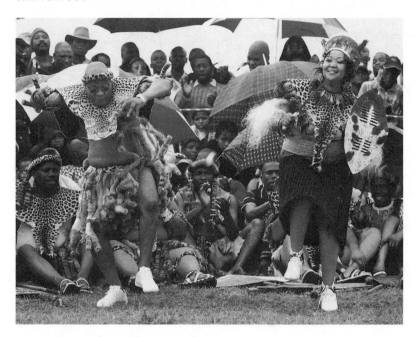

FIGURE 19. President Zuma. Getty.

other hand, Mbeki embraced "modern," rights-based gender policies, and Zuma has gone out of his way to champion orthodox biomedical health care. This juxtapositioning illustrates the very slippery nature of signification: the tropes of "tradition" call forth custom, race, and culture, whereas "modernity" is meant to represent rights, freedom, and development—and yet each are deployed in novel articulations that often defy such simple classification. Their binary opposition yields them power in symbolic struggle, but the paradoxes of their articulation unveil an underlying hybridity. This chapter will compare the hegemonic masculinities performed by Thabo Mbeki and Jacob Zuma, but will also discuss other state and nonstate actors' interventions in the postapartheid politicization of sexuality. I show how the tropes of "tradition" and "modernity" get deployed and (re)signified in and through discursive struggles over masculinity and sexuality in an attempt to manage anxieties about South Africa's national identity and position in the global economy.

Several scholars have recently argued that the post-apartheid era is marked by a generalized "sexualisation of politics and . . . politicisation of sexuality" (Robins 2008b, 412; Posel 2005). According to Deborah Posel, from the end of apartheid through the early years of the new democracy, public discussions about gender and sexuality were slowly on the rise, peaking in 2001–2002 with a very public discussion of the pervasiveness of rape and domestic violence triggered by a spate of "baby rapes'" (Posel 2005). In October 2001, a case of an infant who was sexually abused by six adult family members became the source of national moral outcry, which turned into national panic and horror, when subsequent news footage began uncovering the pervasiveness of the sexual abuse of children in post-apartheid South Africa (ibid.).

The most prominent and scandalous explanation given for this national trend was that men believed they would be cured of AIDS if they had sex with a virgin (Leclerc-Madlala 1997; *Sunday Times* 1999; Smith 2005). In an effort to show that this "baby rape" discourse is not unique to South Africa, Helen Epstein (2007) has uncovered the "myth about the myth," situating its antecedent in nineteenth-century America, where rumors were circulated about recent European immigrants who were said to believe they could cure themselves of syphilis if they had sex with a virgin. While it is certainly questionable that this myth is actually a causal factor for the high incidences of sexual violence in South Africa, the "baby rape" controversy did mark the beginning of a very public debate about sexuality and violence. According to Posel, these debates about sexuality unveiled a widespread fear about the moral state of the nation.

The association of sex with death has been perhaps one of the most mundane and at the same time traumatic legacies of the AIDS epidemic in South Africa. As such, the politicization of sexuality is hardly surprising. However, the arrival of AIDS was accompanied (and exacerbated) by other crises that have unsettled South Africa's gender orders. Because sexuality is situated in a material economy of gift exchange, neoliberalism has had a profound impact on the institution of the family and gender relations in the post-apartheid era. I argue in this chapter that Jacob Zuma's performance of masculinity quelled the sentiments of precariousness instigated by the unmooring of gender identity in the post-apartheid era. He rose to power by exploiting the crisis of state legitimacy the poor felt so profoundly under Mbeki's reign. I will show how gender has become a primary terrain upon which the paradoxes of postcolonialism are navigated.

This chapter begins by exploring debates over the social construction of gender in the public sphere, and specifically the starkly different masculinities performed by South Africa's two most recent presidents. It then moves to the squatter camp, examining the reception of these representations at the local level, but also the shifting terrain of gender ideologies and sexual practices.³ Finally, the chapter explains the "messianic" rise of Jacob Zuma (Kondlo 2010, 1) by describing the unique combination of political tools he has deployed in an attempt to resolve the postcolonial paradox.

The Social Construction of Gender

Post-apartheid South Africa has been widely celebrated for the various ways in which its democratization has been marked by a transforma- tion of the relationship between the state and gender/sexuality (Nie- haus 2000). South Africa's constitution, ratified in 1996, was the first in the world to outlaw discrimination on the basis of sexual prefer- ence (*BBC News* 2005). On December 1, 2005, the Constitutional Court ruled in favor of same-sex marriages, and exactly one year later they be- came legal (*BBC News* 2005; Timberg 2005; Nullis 2006). In 1996, abor- tion was legalized through the Choice on Termination of Pregnancy Act (Republic of South Africa 1996a). The 1998 Employment Equity Act provides federal legislation outlawing sexual harassment, which is quite ambitiously defined and severely punished (Republic of South Af- rica 1998a). And as of 1997, the Commission for Gender Equality (an institution established to meet the constitutional mandate to promote and protect gender equality) has been working to transform South Af- rica by "exposing gender discrimination in laws, policies and practices; advocating changes in sexist attitudes and gender stereotypes; and in- stilling respect for women's rights as human rights" (Commission for Gender Equality 2000).

Yet, some have been critical of the ways in which gendered citizen- ship was "rendered in the grammar of liberal democracy" (Manicom 2005, 32; quoted in Hunter 2011, 1123), which left intact many struc- tural gender inequalities (Hassim 2006). As I demonstrate in this chap- ter, this focus on "rights" is often problematically positioned in opposi- tion to gendered "traditions" (Hunter 2010). Such polarizing discourses not only feed the myth of incommensurability but also serve to shift attention away from foundational crises occurring in the economic and gender systems in the post-apartheid era. The politicization of sex- uality, then, both signifies and masks a concern about the "success" of liberation.

As mentioned in Chapter 2, Thabo Mbeki embraced "modern," lib- eral, gender rights—despite his attempts to "retradition" health care. In part, this endorsement of rights-based gender policy was a response to the racist assumptions he believed undergirded much of the international health policy on HIV/AIDS—as this excerpt from the controversial "Castro Hlongwane" article (discussed at length in chapter 2) makes clear:

The answer lies in the reality that the hypotheses about ourselves, that are presented as facts, rest on an age-old definition, by others of what and who we are as Africans. . . . For their part, the Africans believe this story, as told by their friends. They too shout the message that—yes, indeed, we are as you say we are!

Yes, we are sex-crazy! Yes, we are diseased!

Yes, we spread the deadly HI Virus through our uncontrolled heterosexual sex! In this regard, yes we are different from the US and Western Europe!

Yes, we, the men, abuse women and the girl-child with gay abandon! Yes, among us rape is endemic because of our culture!

Yes, we do believe that sleeping with young virgins will cure us of AIDS! Yes, as a result of all this, we are threatened with destruction by the HIV/AIDS pandemic!

Yes, what we need, and cannot afford, because we are poor, are condoms and antiretroviral drugs!

Help!" (ANC 2002)

In an *ANC Today* article, Mbeki (2004c) challenged an "internationally recognized expert" on sexual violence who blamed "African traditions, indigenous religions and culture [for] prescrib[ing] and institutionalis[ing] rape." Mbeki went on to expose this expert's assumptions: "Given this view, which defines the African people as barbaric savages, it should come as no surprise that . . . 'South Africa has the highest rates of rape in the world' . . . because, after all, we are an African country, and therefore have the men conditioned by African culture, tradition and religion to commit rape."

Mbeki's criticisms are not unwarranted. Public health campaigns have often focused so fully on the practices of "unsafe sex" or "risk groups" that not only is blame for the spread of the virus problematically individualized (Katz 2002), but sexuality (and particularly African sexuality and nonheteronormative sexuality) has been both exoticized and demonized in the process.[4] However, some TAC activists claimed that when Mbeki criticized the racist colonial assumptions associating Africanness and promiscuity, he contributed to the silence and shame surrounding sexuality. Jonathan Berger, advocate for the AIDS Law Project, explained this point in an interview: "I see these inherent contradictions in the president's . . . views on sex and sexuality, and how if you say we have lots of sex, it's a bad thing. Who said sex is a bad thing? Queen Victoria might have, but maybe it's not part of African culture that looks at sex and sexuality and the body as inherently evil and disgusting!"[5] Some have argued that instead of engaging with Mbeki's critique of the racist assumptions regarding African sexuality, TAC attempted to reclaim and celebrate sexuality (Berger 2004; Cameron 2005). "TAC has adopted a very different approach to these representational questions. Instead of resorting to a defensive, and potentially lethal, response of AIDS denial, TAC AIDS activists have sought to destigmatize and depathologise African sexualities" (Robins 2004, 660n17). And yet, this is no simple task, as nationally renowned AIDS activists and Supreme Court of Appeals justice Edwin Cameron[6] explains:

I think it is a conscious tactic on the part of HIV activists. And . . . the underlying issue really is the problem of . . . of the stigmatization of the sexually transmitted disease. And the fact is . . . that even 20 years after acquiring the virus, and 19 years this month after my diagnosis, I think I still feel at some level that my illness is different because I acquired it sexually. And what the TAC activists have tried to do is to . . . render that more indifferent. And it's been very difficult because I think at some profound level . . . people do think it's different to get a disease sexually. . . . One cannot really say that the ways in which people have sex, transact with sex, negotiate with sex, and, in fact engage in sex, is . . . is a matter of indifference. One can't say that.[7]

TAC's efforts to depathologize sexuality are laudatory. However, because a series of crises have recently disrupted South Africa's gender orders, rendering gender norms and sexual practices unstable, people's relationship to their sexuality is, indeed, anything but indifferent. This will be the focus of the next section of this chapter.

Mbeki did not simply instill a regime of gender "rights," he also actively promoted and performed a particular masculinity. This masculinity played a role in his dreams of an African renaissance and support for Black Economic Empowerment (BEE).[8] The African renaissance man gains status from economic wealth and a "modern" outlook on gender relations (e.g., willingness to change diapers or cook a meal) but remains head of the household (Hunter 2010, 159–60). In other words, wealth and the maintenance of certain patriarchal norms of masculinity, such as being the primary breadwinner who is capable of providing for a family, allows for "transcendence" of other '"traditional" roles and the assumption of certain "modern" gender practices.

Mbeki's concerns over the racialization of sexuality may have contributed to the stigmatization of the virus, but he also questioned the medicalization of sexuality. Jacob Zuma uses some of the same symbolic weaponry, but deploys it quite differently. Zuma's version of sexuality is both biomedicalized and "traditional." As such, the articulation of the "tradition"/"modern" binary is not only reversed, but its relationship to the biomedical is reconfigured.

Jacob Zuma was deputy president of the country (under Mbeki's leadership) until 2005, when he was implicated in a corruption scandal involving his financial advisor, businessman and ANC activist Schabir Shaik. As a result, Mbeki asked Zuma to resign. "Zuma's sacking . . . instantly became a rallying ground for disgruntled ANC members"— many of whom had been ousted from politics for disagreeing with Mbeki (Gumede 2008, 264). At the 2005 National General Council, these "walking wounded" joined together and forced Mbeki to keep Zuma as deputy president of the ANC (ibid.). In addition to corruption, Zuma was accused of raping an HIV-positive woman who was a long-time family friend. Zuma admitted that he had unprotected sex with the woman, but claimed it was consensual. His trial and acquittal of rape took place in May 2006. The tensions within the ranks of the ANC continued until December 2007, when Zuma was elected president of the ANC (even though Thabo Mbeki was still president of the country) at the National Conference of the ANC held in Polokwane, Limpopo. In September 2008, Mbeki resigned from the presidency (after the ANC declared him unfit to govern) and was replaced, temporarily, by Kgalema Motlanthe (deputy president of the ANC and current deputy president of the country). In April 2009, Jacob Zuma was acquitted of all corruption charges and won the national presidency in a landslide victory—securing 66 percent of the vote.

During the rape trial, the sexual and personal history of the woman who accused Zuma of rape was used as evidence to delegitimize her charge. Zuma claimed she led him on and was engaging in sexually provocative behavior because she wore "revealing clothes."[9] Zuma claimed that "traditional" Zulu culture justified his behavior. "'If she had said no, I would have stopped there and got up and left.' But, he claimed: 'I know as we grew up in the Zulu culture you don't leave a woman in that situation, because if you do then she will even have you arrested and say that you are a rapist'" (Soros 2006). In addition, Zuma invoked outrage by claiming that he reduced his chances of being infected with HIV because he took a shower after intercourse.

I was in South Africa in May 2006 and watched the rape trial unfold on television. I was struck by the elusive way in which the victim's HIV status was alluded to. There seemed to be a quiet assumption that people infected with HIV should remain celibate. In fact, Zuma's position as chairperson of the South African National AIDS Council (SANAC) was often invoked to signify that he should have "known better" than to declare that showers were preventative, but also, perhaps, that he should have known *not* to sleep with someone infected with HIV. And so, despite the fact that she was the victim, blame for her active sexuality lurked in the subtext.

The Zuma rape trial is the perfect example of the way in which the tropes of "traditionalism" and "modernity" are pitted against each other in public sphere debates about sexuality. Throughout the entire ordeal, images of "traditional" Zulu culture (and of Zulu masculinity in particular) were contrasted with images of "women's rights activists" protesting outside of the courthouse (figs. 20 and 21).

Many of Zuma's supporters, sporting "100% Zulu Boy" t-shirts, burned photographs of the rape accuser, singing "burn the bitch" (Vetten 2007, 439; Robins 2008b, 418).

"A young man stood up, [and] . . . declared that Zuma was his leader and that from now on he would no longer be wearing a condom, to laughter and applause from many of the young men who filled the back benches and the upstairs gallery." Zulu men who did speak out against the misogyny were portrayed as not being quite Zulu. (Terreblanche 2006)

In addition, several social analysts have pointed out that Zuma's signature song, "Umshini Wami" ("Bring Me My Machine Gun") relies on a "masculinist conception of militarism and nationalism" (Gunner 2008, 40; see also Suttner 2009).[10] Zuma was supported by African women as well as men (Hunter 2010, 2) and not simply within the Zulu population (Hunter 2011). Mark Hunter suggests this is because the masculinity he performs is a marker of respectability—he has paid *ilobolo* (bride wealth) for each of his wives, he understands the gendered nature of HIV/AIDS, and he has responded to South Africa's "crisis of social reproduction" (Hunter 2010 and 2011). "Zuma's 'traditionalism' was partly understood . . . not as Zulu chauvinism . . . but . . . as a reaction to Mbeki's apparent elitism; as a signifier of 'the poor' in an era of rising class divisions; and as a sign of 'family' and 'kinship' at a time when an unprecedented number of people are unmarried" (Hunter 2011, 1109). I will return to this analysis later in the chapter.

In their outrage, many women's rights activists employed dehumanizing terminology to bemoan the way in which they felt "modern"

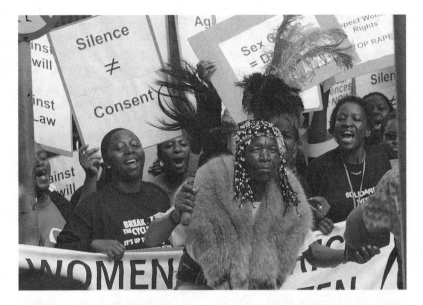

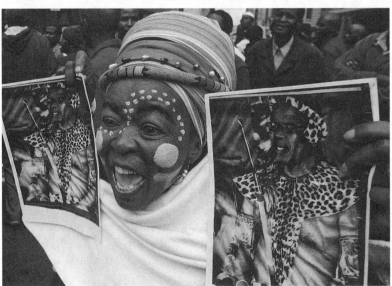

FIGURES 20 AND 21. Protesters at Zuma rape trial. Figure 20, Getty/Soros. Figure 21, AP/BBC.

rights were being reversed or undermined: "Zuma's testimony revealed his *Neanderthal* attitudes to women and sexual violence" (Robinson, Tabane, and Haffajee 2006; my emphasis). It is for this reason that Zuma's performance of "traditionalism" irreparably linked, in the public's imaginary, Zulu culture and misogynistic sexual behavior, leading many social commentators to interpret Zuma's rise to power as simply a return to sexual conservatism (Robins 2008b, 413).

Still, Zuma's performance of Zulu identity is highly contested.[11] Many have warned against Zuma's particular version of "traditionalism." An editorial in the *Sowetan* newspaper warned: "During his rape trial, ANC president Jacob Zuma . . . testified that according to the Zulu culture he is not allowed to leave a woman unattended if she is ready for sex. Why are we degrading and humiliating our cultural heritage to suit our own reckless lifestyles?" (Mmila 2009). In late 2008, Zuma confirmed publicly that he had recently fathered a child out of wedlock. Polygamy is a historic practice within Zulu culture (which Zuma engages in),[12] but extramarital sex is not. Although many Africans engage in extramarital sexual relations, they often do so (at least in part) because of their inability to pay for *ilobolo*.[13] Because Zuma can afford to pay *ilobolo* and already has a number of wives, many suggested that Zuma's behavior (once again) dragged Zulu identity through the mud:

"This is my culture," said Zuma tongue-in-cheek. But people should not use culture selectively, utilising only aspects of that culture or interpretations thereof which suit their personal situation. According to the traditions of the Zulus and African culture as a whole, premarital and extramarital sex are taboo. Even a man who chooses to be polygamous cannot have sex with the woman until they are married as per tradition. (Bofelo 2010; written by a political commissar from KZN)

In our present day, it seems that those prejudiced against Africans need not even lift a finger to do their dirty job—Africans themselves appear to be doing it on their behalf. . . . As someone who projects himself to the world as a custodian of African culture, Zuma should know . . . that Africans believe in children being born in marriage, to give them a sense of security and identity. (Sesanti 2010; written by a professor from Stellenbosh University)

Steven Robins suggests that it was Zuma's performance of "traditional" Zulu masculinity, juxtaposed and positioned in opposition to Mbeki's "modernism," that won Zuma the presidency (Robins 2008b, 423). In other words, Zuma strategically deployed this "traditionalist'" persona in order to position himself as everything that Mbeki was not.

However, such an analysis assumes that Zuma's performance of "traditionalism" is coherent and consistent. Rather, Zuma manipulates the tropes of "modernity'" and "traditionalism" to fit his political needs—much as Mbeki did. Zuma uses "traditionalism" to call for a reconstitution of sexuality, thereby sanctioning certain cultural practices while simultaneously "modernizing" them. For example, Zuma approached the Zulu king, Goodwill Zwelithini, to discuss the policy of restoring the "tradition" of male circumcision among the Zulu people in an effort to curb HIV transmission (Dugger 2010a). The practice had been outlawed by King Shaka in the nineteenth century because his warriors were spending too much time recovering from the surgery (Mazrui 1975, 74–75; *BBC News* 2009). Zuma is calling for the reinstallation of more "traditional" norms as part of the government's effort to scale-up HIV testing, prevention, and treatment efforts in South Africa (Dugger 2010b). One of the reasons, then, for Zuma's sexualization of politics has to do with the way in which the AIDS pandemic has necessitated a shift in the governmentality of biopolitics. It remains to be seen whether or not Zuma's rearticulation of the "tradition"/"modernity" tropes will succeed in resolving the crisis of liberation the poor are facing.

It has not been my intention to reify the idealized constructs of "modernity" and "traditionalism," but rather to show that while they are powerful ideological tools wielded in symbolic struggles for hegemony, they are replete with contradictions and inconsistencies. Mbeki and Zuma have recoded the *colonial* tropes of "traditionalism" and "modernity" to deal with the *post*colonial dilemma of satisfying the demands of neoliberal capital while simultaneously convincing the masses that their liberation is imminent. Mbeki and Zuma perform this subtle political maneuver in different ways, but for both of them, the AIDS epidemic has been the primary political terrain upon which these battles are played out.

Gender Insecurity and the Informalization of the Sexual Economy

In this chapter, I deploy a theory of gender inspired by Raewyn Connell's scholarship, tweaked slightly to accommodate a postcolonial perspective. Connell's theory of gender is particularly relevant to an analysis of postcolonial gender structures and practices for several reasons: (1) in her decidedly materialist account, gender both structures and is structuring (1987, 95); (2) there is a bidirectional relationship between gendered performances/practices and gendered structures, which can account for historical transformations; (3) gender is processual, historically contingent, and internally differentiated and contradictory (ibid., 96); (4) femininities and masculinities are always multiple and relational, but they are hierarchically organized, and different performances of gender are yielded more or less power and value (Connell 1995; 2005). However, Connell's theory of crisis tendencies (which are fueled by contradictions in different sets of gender relations) can only help explain disruptions to *coherent* gender orders and must be amended to account for the overwhelmingly destabilizing effects of colonial and neocolonial forces on gender systems in the global South (Silberschmidt 2005; Sideris 2005). In the postcolonial context, I argue, there are multiple (often competing or conflicting) gender orders at play, which operate within systems of extreme structural inequality. Postcolonial gender theory[14] must be able to grasp the simultaneous processes of colonial coercion and its epistemic ruptures *as well as* the processes of hybridization, subversion, and uncertainty that emerge out of the postcolonial condition.

The fall of apartheid, the onslaught of AIDS, and the introduction of neoliberal economic reform (in its multiple modalities) have all had profound impacts on the conjuncture of gender orders that characterize post-apartheid South Africa. These conjunctural crises have served to render gender insecure and informalize the sexual economy. In this section, I begin by providing background on the destabilization of marriage and the rise of "transactional" forms of sexuality. I show how deindustrialization and AIDS have challenged idealized notions of masculinity and contributed to poor men's experiences of emasculation. I then detail the ambiguous impact of neoliberalism on women, illustrating the ways in which new configurations of the family and sexuality present both possibilities and challenges for women in the post-apartheid era.

In much of his work, Mark Hunter has detailed the ways in which changes in the political economy and the state instigated shifts in gender ideologies, sexual practices, and the institution of the family from the colonial to the post-apartheid eras (2002; 2004; 2007; 2010). The forced migration required to sustain the mining industry under apartheid disrupted the pre-apartheid institution of the family and the taboo on extramarital sexual relations. *Ilobolo*, the custom of the groom's family providing cows (or the monetary equivalent) to the bride's family, a stable accompaniment of marriage until the post-apartheid period, has been undermined by the stagnation of the formal economy. A precipitous drop in marriage rates has accompanied deindustrialization. Only 30 percent of the African population is currently married (half the rate of marriage in the same population in the 1960s) (Hunter 2011, 1114 and 1124).[15] This is, in part, because of the growing economic independence of women and in part because of men's inability to secure *ilobolo* (ibid.). "Marriage today is, in many respects, a middle-class institution" (Hunter 2007, 695). However, sexual double standards persist since idealized masculinity is defined by the ability to engage in multiple, simultaneous sexual partnerships, whereas idealized femininity is still expressed through monogamy.[16]

And sexuality is still linked to a material economy of gift exchange. The cultural expectation that men should provide some form of subsistence to the women with whom they are engaged in sexual relations is usually referred to as "transactional sex."[17] Hunter refers to this practice as the "materiality of everyday sex" in order to avoid representing sex as overly commodified and therefore distanced from feelings of love and reciprocity (2010, 6). This practice is in no way related to the institution or profession of prostitution (Hunter 2002; Epstein 2007), nor is it necessarily related to concurrency—engagement in more than one sexual relationship at a time (Dunkle et al. 2004; Epstein 2007). However, with unemployment and poverty rates as high as they are, women *are* often forced to engage in more than one "transactional" relationship at a time in order to provide for their families. This situation is exacerbated by the fact that women are generally expected to raise any children that result from sexual relations (though men's dignity is also linked to providing something for their children, even those with whom they do not live [Hunter 2010, 170]).

Because of the material economy of gift exchange, men must have purchasing power in order to have sex. But men who simply have sex with women, without being able to make their partners' lives and the lives of their children secure, are not considered respectable (Hunter 2004). But neither are poor men who cannot afford to engage in sexual relationships. As Thulani explains:

When I lost my job, I had a lovely wife, you know. But since there was no income, she . . . she left. She took my two kids with her. And she went. I couldn't afford to keep her because I didn't have an income. For a while, she was working when I couldn't find work. She used to bring in food, you know, but . . . it is not the custom. There is this mentality, the mentality that you have to pay in order to be a man. It is so fixed—that idea. . . . People looked down on me in the community. They said, like, "Wow, you're useless," and it was partially because I didn't have a woman. If you're a bachelor, you don't have a dignity.[18]

Poor men's masculinities are as precarious as their opportunities for work and pay (Silberschmidt 2005, 195)—the insecurity that plagues their lives has been embodied into their very senses of self. "Men who don't work . . . can't have a relationship. They laugh at you if you are unemployed. When you start working, even in a piece job, you start now wanting to enjoy yourself and you want women next to you. You start now spending your money on women, and that is how men contract the disease."[19]

As illustrated in chapter 1, there is considerable variation in the incomes of residents living in informal settlements (Smit 2006, 111, 113). This creates a lot of class tension among (especially male) residents, as only those with income are able to secure girlfriends. In an interview with a resident from Sol Plaatjie, she explained that a lot of women go to the neighboring town of Roodepoort in order to find working men with whom they can begin relationships because the men in Sol Plaatjie are too poor.[20]

As a consequence of the increasingly winner-takes-all sexual economy—in which wealth can secure many girlfriends and poverty none—men marginalized from the productive economy also face marginalization from the sexual economy. Indeed, poorer men can be extremely resentful of richer men, not simply because disposable income drives conspicuous consumption, but because richer men consume many of the area's women. (Hunter 2010, 167)

In an FGD held on July 4, 2009, in Sol Plaatjie, I asked those present to comment on the immigrants who had been moving into the community in increasing numbers since it had been upgraded. I had heard rumors that during the eruption of xenophobic violence that had seized the country in May and June of 2008, Sol Plaatjie was a primary site of brutality. Tension arose in the FGD because several of the women indicated that they preferred to carry on relations with immigrants who they claimed were more likely to have stable incomes. One man was angered at the insinuation and explained that immigrant men were willing to work for very little, and a women responded: "well, they treat us right—giving us nice presents and good money. Unlike you local boys. They don't leave women behind or change women." And so, not only are immigrants charged with taking domestic jobs (a somewhat ludicrous stereotype given the high rates of unemployment), they are also suspected of monopolizing the sexual economy.

AIDS contributes to poor men's loss of dignity, as "real men don't get sick." Throughout the world, studies have shown that men are less likely to admit to being sick or to seek care,[21] but as Hunter points out, because of its devastating toll on the body, "AIDS is [also] both emasculating and de-masculinizing" (2010, 221). Rachel Snow (2007) has found evidence suggesting that South African women are more likely to test for HIV, and not just because they attend antenatal (prenatal) clinics. They are also more likely to utilize national Voluntary Counseling and Testing (VCT) services (Snow 2007; see also UN IRIN 2005). Men are also likely to start antiretroviral treatment later.[22] "Women are closer to the clinics. They always attend the clinic. It is easier for them. They go for contraceptives. It's easy, then, for them to access testing and treatment that is available."[23] Shifts in the political economy, the definitions of idealized masculinity, and the institution of the family have all contributed to the insecurity of masculinity, in its multifarious iterations.

It has been well documented that neoliberalism's impact on women is ambiguous—contributing on the one hand to a certain feminization of the labor market (though in largely low-paid, insecure forms of employment) but also an erosion of the welfare state (see, for example, Bakker 1994; Sassen 1998; Benería 2003; Barker and Feiner 2004). In South Africa, because of deindustrialization, the rise of the NGO sector, and the fact that the minimal state welfare still provided is often linked to child care, very poor women sometimes have more recourse to some money than very poor men. However, scholars have suggested that these forms of social welfare (disability grants, child grants, and pensions) have institutionalized a gendered burden of care without providing women with sufficient financial revenue to support their households (Susser 2009, 136). With huge declines in marriage, the gendered expectation that women care for children from all sexual unions, not to mention the elderly and the sick, and heightened unemployment, women are carrying the burden of both production and social reproduction. In South Africa, 42.4 percent of all households are currently female-headed (Department of Health, Medical Research Council, and OrcMacro 2007).

In addition, the focus on drastic increases in men's unemployment and unemployability obscures the fact that "many more women are excluded from the formal economy" (Susser 2009, 135). In the late 1990s, the number of women seeking work in the labor market was twice the increase in the female population of working age (Casale and Posel 2002). Because of this considerable increase in the number of economically active women and the institutionalized gender division of labor, women are employed for far lower wages than men and have minimal access to assets. Women earn a ratio of 0.656:1 what men earn (Casale 2004). "Those women who are [formally] employed find themselves in the worst paid sectors of the labor market, notably in domestic and retail work" (Hassim 2005).[24] In addition to domestic work, women can often only find employment in the poorly remunerated and unstable informal sector. Therefore, women's median income has fallen significantly in the post-apartheid period (Casale 2004). From 1995 to 2001, the nominal median earning for women decreased by 16.5 percent but for men increased by 19.3 percent (ibid.). As of 2005, 72 percent of women and 58 percent of men between the ages of fifteen and twenty-four were unemployed (Hunter 2010, 5; Department of Labour 2006, 18).

Although under apartheid it was much more common for men to migrate in search of work, leaving women behind in rural areas, the urbanization that has accompanied deindustrialization and the escalation of unemployment has generated a large increase in the number of female migrants (Hunter 2007). Many women explained to me that they moved to informal settlements to escape stigma and the strict control of their families:

Some of them leave their formal houses to come here, running away from stigma. Then, they feel free here. Because I was married and went to live with my husband away from Lawley, after I was diagnosed with HIV/AIDS. I had a lot of nurses visiting me to see if I'm ok. The neighbors put pressure on me—asking why nurses were visiting me. The stigma made me leave. . . . The best thing was to leave and come . . . here.[25]

In many instances, women who move to informal settlements can only survive through dependence on the "transactional" sexual economy—especially in the beginning (Hunter 2007, 158).

A lot of people come to informal settlements from a family house where there are aunties, grannies, everyone . . . and maybe there is no unity or support in the house, and so you go and stay in the squatter camp to make a future or better life for yourself. . . . Then when she comes to stay here, she don't find any job. She starts changing or rooming around with different men . . . maybe she will find something like a man in order to buy some food . . . or to provide the family. Yeah, so I think the situation there in the squatter camp is just like that.[26]

Hunter (2010) points out that post-apartheid housing policy (which entailed the "technocratic" allocation of two-room housing units) failed to integrate domestic and economic considerations and thus contributed to the feminization of households, the splitting of family units, and the rise of shack settlements (110–11). In fact, he suggests that the term for shack, "*umjondolo*[,] evolved from the word *umjendevu* (a spinster) signifying the association between shifting gender norms (with lots of single women) and the growth of informal settlements" (ibid., 142).

Neoliberal economic policies have had a profound impact on people's capacity to engage in sexual behaviors that protect them from HIV transmission. Because it is increasingly likely that at least one if not both sexual partners are in concurrent relationships, "transactional sex" is one of the primary mechanisms of HIV transmission (Morris and Kretzschmar 1997; Wojcicki and Malala 2001; Kaufman and Stavrou 2002; Dunkle et al. 2004). In a demographic study on "transactional sex" in Soweto, Dunkle and colleagues found that "transactional sex was associated with HIV seropositivity after controlling for lifetime number of male partners and length of time a woman had been sexually active" (2004, 1581).[27]

Consider the fact that we are focusing on culture and we want to respect it. We are saying it's a democracy, but some women are still following their culture where the man is the head of the house, and they have to bow to whatever the man is saying. Think about it—if I've already disclosed to my partner about my HIV status, and he refuses to use a condom, then what option do I have? I'm not working— because that's another problem—unemployment. And I have children. What will happen if he kicks me out of the house? Because I ask him to use a condom. Because most women depend on their man for income, so I would agree with whatever the man says. Because he's the person who's maintaining me and looking after me. I have no choice but to accept his decision, even if I know it's putting my life in danger.[28]

With regards to AIDS, sometimes us as women, we are afraid to disclose to our men. Firstly because we are not working and we are highly dependent on them. Sometimes the man will not want to use a condom even if you ask him. Because you are dependent on this person, you will just accept and submit. You don't know how he is going to respond if you tell him about your status.[29]

Ukuphanda is Zulu slang meaning "to get by," to survive in times of constraint; however, it has taken on new meaning in the era of neoliberalism. It is often used to refer to illegal means of making ends meet (Motsemme 2007, 389), but I have also found that the word is strongly gendered. It is often used to explain the practice of "transactional sex" (Wojcicki 2002).

It's poverty. Whilst we are hungry, we go out and *phanda*—to forage—to find anything you can to survive.[30]

Our kids are going out to *phanda*. But in times of de Klerk [under apartheid], we didn't have any grants. Instead, there was more employment. I used to be a machinist, and I used to go from one company to another because employment was ripe. That didn't allow us to go out and *phanda*. But today, there is no employment.[31]

I can't stand hunger as a woman. And there's the kids here also. And there you are, the man, sitting there on the bed. You can't go anywhere to look for anything to do so that you can come and feed us. I take it in my hands to do something in order for my kids especially to get something to eat. Yes. Then I go out. There's working men outside I meet.[32]

There is a serious problem that makes women vulnerable—poverty. Some women get casual work, for a few days. But then once that work is over, they look around and find they have no work. And they still have to feed their kids and make sure they have a roof over their head and food on the table. So, then, maybe she will exchange sex for money. Others, they don't do it because they like it, but because they have no choice. Maybe if the government could assist people to find work, then they wouldn't need to do this. Then the practice would diminish.[33]

Nthabiseng Motsemme has argued that through *ukuphanda* poor women construct a "viable identity amidst social chaos" (2007, 370).

It is important not to misconstrue the practice of "transactional" relationships. They are usually enduring, they often involve cohabitation and the sharing of child-rearing responsibilities, and women exercise agency in choosing their partners (Hunter 2002 and 2010). For many women, "transactional sex" actually allows for greater freedom than marriage. It allows a woman to choose her sexual partners, leave them when she wants, negotiate safer sex practices (sometimes), and perhaps most importantly, the money comes directly to her as opposed to her family (ibid.). "Transactional" sexual relationships may be monogamous and are quite often experienced as loving and enduring.[34]

One of the women with whom I was close in Lawley, Nomachina Makalo, explained that she used to live in Soweto, with her family. Her brother and one of her sisters died of AIDS. When Nomachina found out she was infected with HIV as well, her remaining family was very "judgmental—they were embarrassed of having to face this situation again." They made her life very difficult. One of her sisters had moved away to Lawley and had secured her own shack. Nomachina often visited her sister and was impressed with her independence and strength. When the situation in Soweto became unbearable (compounded by the collapse of a romantic relationship), Nomachina moved to Lawley— her sister was moving away and gave her the shack. Her sister was concerned Nomachina would not "make it because she's not working and life this side is tough." But a neighbor stood up for Nomachina, insisting: "she's a real woman. She'll survive." This neighbor became a "mother" to Nomachina after she moved in.

I came here because I wanted to have my independence and a place of my own, where no one will give me problems . . . [where I can] exercise my independence. Where I come from, other people would want to make me miserable because they know my [HIV] status. This is the reason I wanted to have my own place.[35]

Nomachina is very open about her HIV status. In the focus group discussions I held with HIV-positive support group members, she would openly chide anyone who would not disclose publicly. She is also adamant about her own sexual expression and rights to engage in multiple relationships with men. As another woman in an FGD put it:

People are more free in informal settlement to do as they please—they will have sex with everyone. In the rural areas or at home, where there is formal housing, there is law and principles, you have to adhere to and observe. But here, there is no such thing. Here I'm free. I can get a stand and live alone, and no one will tell me how to act. I can have more than one relationship, and no one will say anything.[36]

Gender relations and sexual practices are transforming in poor communities throughout South Africa in response to shifts in the terrains of culture and political economy. With the increasing informalization of the economy and the growing precariousness of survival, the sexual economy has become one of the only means of survival for many women and has further destabilized masculinity. As such, gender identities have become unmoored. Motsemme suggests that this is, in part, because of the very complex ways in which national and global policies are entering into poor communities' "subjective constructions of intimacy" (2007, 388). These changes in gender norms and sexual practices invoke a wide range of responses from community members.

"Women's Rights" and "50/50"

When I first began conducting interviews focusing on gender practices and ideologies in Sol Plaatjie and Lawley, I would ask people the following question: "In your opinion, is there a connection between gender oppression and HIV/AIDS?" When my interpreter, Torong, would repeat the question, a long discussion would almost inevitably ensue. He would provide a lengthy explanation of what the question meant, the respondent would ask questions, and finally an answer would emerge. Almost every time, the answer would include the term "women's rights," which was referred to with derision. I soon learned that the language I used to discuss gender relations was considered "Western" and was therefore met with anger.

In fact, my presence in the community (especially in the beginning) was occasionally interpreted and experienced as a threat, and it was often the women in the community who were most suspicious of my intentions. Torong, as well as Thulani and Pheello (who introduced me and my research into the communities), are all men. My association with them, along with my race, class, and education, my lack of children, and the fact that I was always alone (or accompanied by Torong) when I visited, meant my life was starkly different from the lives of the women in the community, and my presence was confusing and strange. People often insinuated or assumed that I was carrying on a sexual relationship with Torong, Pheello, or Thulani. This is because of the strong correlation between sexuality, friendship, and trust on the one hand and material exchange on the other. It took me much longer to forge lasting friendships with the women in Lawley and Sol Plaatjie than the men, and language and cultural barriers often continuously strained these friendships.

In addition, the language I used to discuss gender relations was deeply contested. The men and women with whom I worked felt very strongly that it was precisely the imposition of liberal definitions of gender (what they refer to as "women's rights" or "50/50") that was directly responsible for destabilizing gender norms in their community, leading to high rates of HIV infection:

If a woman says "no, this is my right," this encourages the husband or boyfriend to go out and seek other avenues for receiving pleasure or sex. As a result, this causes the spread of disease.[37]

Marriage is not happening anymore because of this 50/50 thing.[38]

Yes, men have lost their sense of manhood. Men are undermined now. Because of "women's rights," men is [sic] no longer the head of the family, and men can no longer do anything.[39]

I feel that women also abuse men—because of this thing of 50/50 and "women's rights." . . . The women are losing sight of what their role is. Our president is giving more power to women, and this makes women disrespect men. The president should teach women about their rights *and* their responsibilities.[40]

Unlike Leclerc-Madlala (2001b) and Kimmel (1987), both of whom suggest that women initiate change and men cling to "tradition," I have found that both men and women express anger at the imposition of "women's rights"—because they suspect the intention is the erasure of their sense of identity. By defining progress and development as an abandonment of "traditionalism" in the move toward liberal or constitutional definitions of gender and sexuality, an unquestioned cultural imperialism is at work in the popular, media discourses on masculinity.

This thing of "rights" has changed our culture and our value systems, and how people should conduct themselves. The manner in which it happened—it just came and nullified who the men are. These things only promoted the rights of women.

Culture is culture . . . Claire, where you are from, you have your *own* culture, and we have our own culture. In fact, by assuming we will just adopt other people's culture and nullify our own culture, this is a problem. This is where we are going to lose ourselves. . . . Now, we are taking other people's cultures more seriously than our own, and so we are going to lose our culture, and lose ourselves.[41]

I think that one of the problems is that we adopted too much of white people's cultures and everything because we think that everything the white people are doing is right. We forgot what was originally ours.
CD: During apartheid?
No, this happened after.[42]

Even if the judgment of "modern" rights is homogenizing and simplistic, the underlying critique of the operations of power is significant. "Tradition" is often invoked within these communities as a protest against a threat of cultural imperialism and erasure. But just as it does in public sphere discourses, "tradition" has a loose signification. It is often used to resurrect an idealized (and impossible) past untainted by colonialism, but it is just as often used to critique contemporary economic and political realities. For many, the past signifies horrific racism, violence, and oppression, but also the glory of struggle and the hope for freedom—and many of the participants in this research were an integral part of that battle. Yet the rewards of liberation were distributed unequally. As such, "tradition" is often summoned in an attempt to control the uncertainty that has accompanied millennial capitalism—an uncertainty that the poor feel most profoundly (Comaroff and Comaroff 2000). In many ways, the condemnation of "women's rights" is an expression of exasperation over having been left behind on the road to freedom. It is the poors' way of dealing with the postcolonial paradox.

Many women do, however, welcome the promises of "women's rights." A woman in Lawley told me that she was forced to abandon her children in order to escape her husband who beat her so brutally he almost killed her. The courts ruled in favor of her husband. "Now I need to know where those women's rights exist because I have not seen them. And the government is not doing anything about it."[43] She escaped her husband by moving to an informal settlement. Another woman explained: "I love these rights because they have helped a lot of women. Because previously our mothers and our grannies were ill-treated by our fathers and grandfathers. Today we are able to stand up and take up our fights from wrong treatment from our spouses."[44] Mark Hunter also discusses the ways in which women often embrace the discourse of "rights" in order to break down the sexual double standard and insist that if masculinity is now defined by multiple sexual conquests, then women, too, should have the "right" to be involved with several men. Some even insist they require several men to meet all of their needs: "one for money, one for food, and one for rent" (2010, 147–48).

Many scholars have attempted to explain the shifting terrain of gender norms and a certain "return" to "traditionalism" by suggesting that either masculinity or social reproduction is in crisis. I find both of these explanations problematic. The "crisis of masculinity" thesis suggests that because of the historical linkages between the sexual and political economies, rising unemployment has undermined respectable masculinity, which has caused poor men to act out their frustrations on women's bodies. This theory is used to explain everything from high rates of violence against women, to stigmatizing behaviors and sexual promiscuity. Although economic conditions are often listed as causal factors, when possible policies are suggested, the focus shifts from economic reforms to solutions aimed at "modernizing" gender norms. Some of the academic literature promoting this thesis upholds a kind of binaristic "clash of civilizations" thesis whereby "modern" and "traditional" gender orders are presumed to be mutually exclusive. For example, Walker (2005) claims that liberal versions of sexuality, embodied in the constitution and popularized by public discourses on rights, have come in conflict with "traditional" notions of gender and sexual relations, thereby destabilizing masculinity. Leclerc-Madlala (2001b) argues that while women in South Africa are more likely to celebrate changes in gender dynamics brought by the proliferation of "liberal" feminist ideology, men are more likely to pine for the strictness imposed by "tradition." She notes that this differentiation in men and women's abilities and willingness to adapt to ideological shifts has brought on a crisis of gender politics. Sideris (2005) reports on a group of men who have embraced a human rights framework in order to reject the use of violence as a conflict resolution strategy in their own homes, thereby coming to define themselves as "different" from the rest of the men in their communities. These studies are laudable for the way in which they illustrate the multiplicity of masculinities at play in the postcolonial context, but they tend to homogenize and demonize "traditional" masculinity by situating it firmly within the African population and by characterizing it as violent and misogynistic.[45] In addition, such an approach assumes a cultural teleology whereby liberal gender rights are not only heralded but are presumed to be "winning" an anachronistic battle of civilizations.

Taking up a postcolonial perspective, I argue that South Africa's multiple, conjunctural gender orders are riddled with contradictions and conflicts, but they are not the outcome of a simplistic colonial confrontation between "traditional" and "modern" gender orders. Such an approach not only ignores the processes of hybridization that have occurred throughout the past four-hundred-plus years of South Africa's colonial history, but it also discounts the complex ways in which "tradition" and "modernity" are constantly being (re)invented. I agree that the transition to democracy instigated a series of transformations in South Africa's gender orders, which served to seriously destabilize hegemonic masculinity, so that sexuality has become a primary site of symbolic struggle in the post-apartheid era. However, the data presented here shows how the tropes of "traditionalism" and "modernity" are utilized as political weapons in contestations over hegemonic masculinity[46] and to manage the contradictions of postcolonialism rather than as legitimate stages in a teleological development of more democratic configurations of gender relations.

Scholars of social reproduction argue that a crisis was initiated under apartheid and exacerbated by neoliberal restructuring. The racial capitalism that epitomized apartheid shifted the burden of social reproduction to the household; wives who were left at home in Bantustans[47] (while men traveled to work in the mines) had some recourse to agriculture to supplement the household, which allowed employers to pay workers lower wages (Wolpe 1972; Legassick and Wolpe 1976). Bezuidenhout and Fakier (2006) argue that this logic also underpins the outsourcing that accompanies neoliberalization because the lowering of wages, lack of benefits, and privatization of social services forces poor people to subsidize their household budgets with their own labor (for example, by growing vegetables or slaughtering meat), which also increases the time put into domestic labor (479). In addition, the poor are forced to subsidize their incomes by doing work at home (bringing in sewing, ironing, or washing, and selling vegetables or other foodstuffs), thus blurring the lines between production and reproduction. Fakier and Cock (2009) note that increasing unemployment makes it necessary for all household members to seek out paid work, which is generally insecure and unprotected, and yet the burden of social reproduction is still borne largely by women (361). Hunter (2011) argues that because of the breakdown of marriage and loss of employment, the sexual economy has been transformed from one of paying *ilobolo* and institutionalizing households, to one where families are smaller or transitional and rely, instead, on a series of gift exchanges. As already mentioned, he argues that Zuma's rise to power can partially be explained by this crisis of social reproduction.

While it is certainly important to pay heed to the gendered dynamics of racial capitalism, I contend that the language of social reproduction obscures rather than clarifies the impact of neoliberalism, the shift in the institution of the family, and the informalization of the sexual economy on gender relations and sexual practices. Although I recognize that scholars of social reproduction attempt to avoid making simplistic causal analyses that explain the shifting terrain of gender relations and practices through recourse to changes in the relations of capital, this is often the unintended consequence of such approaches. Further, crises of reproduction occur at the scale of the household, which individualizes what is experienced as a community-level crisis. Consider this man's contribution to a focus group discussion about rights:

These rights have ruined so many things and have destroyed a lot of people's lives. Previously, it was not that women were not beaten by their men, but . . . families would come together to discuss and solve the problem. . . . But today, the introduction of women's rights, it has made people stay away from engaging and assisting the family to build each other. Also other communities would come together to help each family get along, but now people just worry about themselves. We have lost our social cohesion. . . . Our very leaders, they grew up under the same tradition, in the same way. They were given the same training, but they themselves are passing laws that are taking us away from our tradition.[48]

According to this man, the problem with post-apartheid is that it has destroyed "tradition" and in so doing, the community. Rights discourses privatize agency, which many residents feel destabilizes communities and contributes to social disintegration.

Rather than a crisis of masculinity or social reproduction, I argue that poor South Africans are suffering from a serious crisis of liberation. The data in this chapter show how people struggle to make sense of the radical disturbances South Africa's gender orders have undergone in a relatively short historical period. Some pine for an idealized and constructed sense of gender stability and others bemoan the uneven way in which the rewards of "modernity" have been distributed. These crises of postcolonial identity are articulated in and through the (re)configuration of gendered meanings and relations.

The Multiple "Economies" of Exchange

It is easy to misrecognize "transactional sex" as purely economic and even utilitarian; however, "transactional sex" also involves symbolic, cultural, and spiritual transactions and creates potential for reconfiguring other circuits of exchange. It is possible to understand these multiple exchanges as exchanges of different forms of "capital," in the Bourdieusian sense (1980; 1984; 1986). Within a "transactional" sexual relationship, men exchange money for cultural and social capital. They accrue cultural capital in the sense of an affirmation of their masculinity and social capital[49] in the prestige they gain by accruing people to whom they are both economically and sexually responsible. "Men seek to demonstrate their 'wealth in people' by becoming patrons to poorer women" (Swidler and Watkins 2007, 152).

Women are also involved in various markets of exchange. First, some young women use "transactional sex" to achieve a higher status in particular youth cultures, thereby accruing cultural capital (Leclerc-Madlala 2001a; Nyanzi, Pool, and Kinsman 2001; Hunter 2002; Kaufman and Stavrou 2002; Luke 2003). Second, "transactional sex" is increasingly utilized by young women as a means of securing luxury or fashion items. Hunter explains that because neither men nor women are using income to invest in "home building," any funds not used to maintain the home are used to "stylize the self" (Hunter 2010, 140–41, quoting Nuttall 2004).[50] Third, "transactional sex" can also lend women a kind of autonomy from marriage constraints and a certain access to power and resources that they deploy strategically in order to survive the constraints posed by abject poverty and ever-increasing unemployment (Hunter 2002 and 2007). In addition to lending economic agency to poor women, "transactional sex" can be tied to women's sense of self-respect (Caldwell, Caldwell, and Quiggin 1989; Wight et al. 2006; Johnson-Hanks 2006; Swidler and Watkins 2007). Some women with whom I spoke not only felt empowered by their ability to engage in "transactional sex" but also found that they were better able to negotiate the *terms* of this sexual encounter.

Below, I have provided a long quote from an interview with Dr. Robert Tshabalala—an indigenous healer with whom I conducted multiple in-depth interviews over the course of several years. In it, he pines for an idealized past when sex was the site of symbolic, as opposed to economic, exchange:

RT: This notion of girls expecting gifts from their boyfriends, it comes with these new laws . . . the *new rights of women and everything*. And now it has become a notion or trend where a lot of girls are expecting something from men before maybe they have sex. They don't actually respect their bodies. . . . A woman is someone who is very respected and these bodies that they have, they are not even theirs. They should respect their flesh. If nothing is exchanged, they will . . . they will think that "this man doesn't love me, because he isn't actually buy me x, y and z." And then that thing, it's a problem. There was no such thing before . . .

Now they want to make it like sex is a money-making scheme or the employment bureau. I used to come from town and look in the taxi, and there were so many girls, little girls, counting their money and asking each other, "how much did you make?" And then I'm wondering where do these kids come from? You know, and that thing *is busy killing the nation.*

CD: What did you mean when you said that women's bodies are not their own?

RT: They are pillars of the house . . . of the family. The woman's vagina is not hers. It's the gift for her to build her family or home. Supposing a woman disrespects her vagina, then there is no way that she can build a house and a home. And no way she can satisfy anyone. . . . And everyone will just isolate her. Because this vagina, it produces here at home. *And then actually bears the nation,* you know. And then the

family and the nation, or the community. It produces . . . it's a production. [laughs]
It's a company.[51]

I have quoted this long explanation because it illustrates a number of
the complicated aspects of contemporary sexuality in South Africa.
First, Dr. Tshabalala holds that historically, women's role in the economy was limited to domestic production and reproduction. With the
rise of "transactional sex," women began using their bodies to enter
the labor market. According to Dr. Tshabalala, this is antithetical to the
very definition and purpose of female sexuality. The economy is not
the space for sex. Sex is not a commodity to be exchanged for material
wealth or even survival. Its value is *symbolic*.

He blames "women's rights" for this shift, and earlier in the same interview, he had equated "transactional sex" with women entering the
labor market more generally. According to this viewpoint, in becoming
breadwinners (and often household heads) in their own right, women
are transgressing social hierarchies and "traditional" identities. And in
so doing, they are not respecting the *symbolic* quality of sexuality.

Obviously, Dr. Tshabalala's idealization of a past in which social hierarchies were always clear and respected, identities were well-bounded,
and there were distinct demarcations between gendered spaces of production and reproduction (and between the public and private spheres)
is fantastical. Colonialism and apartheid disrupted such customs centuries ago, if they ever existed in the first place. Despite Tshabalala's
concerns, contemporary sexual practices are still deeply implicated in
indigenous, cultural conceptualizations of the body and identity. But
today, it is clear that sexuality has been hybridized—it has become a
point of convergence for spiritual, social, cultural, *and* economic transactions, which had previously been conceptualized as distinct or, at
least, circumscribed—each with its own particular logic of exchange
and conversion.

However, the form and content of sexual exchange in contemporary
South Africa cannot be fully captured by a Bourdieusian framework of
"capital." One of the most understudied aspects of "transactional sex"
is the way in which gift exchange is accompanied by a whole host of
exchanges of "substance." Because the act of sex also allows ancestral
communication, sexual relations and their material base are the nexus
of spiritual, social, *and* economic exchange.

This flow of goods replicates the flow of sexual substance in that it "goes both ways"
and represents a social and economic flow of good symbolising "respect" and "fili-

ation" both of which create social identities and imbue them with *cultural capital*. The parallel flow of sexual substance similarly *constitutes the "persons"* of those who share these substances, and thus generate the blood that flows into the next generation. Just as sex that involves flow of semen and vaginal fluid helps to constitute the body and person of both partners as well as their offspring, the flow of material goods constitutes the social context in which the relationship is validated and the child grows. (Thornton 2002; my emphasis)

The flow of substances, linked through sexual relations, moves in two directions: vertically, through time (i.e., through the generations); and horizontally, across space through social networks (Thornton 2008, 205). In addition, because the ancestors (and the history they represent) are embodied, the sexual act is essentially one of historical and social exchange. In other words, sexual exchange allows the ancestors to communicate with one another.[52] Sex is also constitutive of identity—through procreation, recreation, and role creation; in fact, this is the way in which people become gendered selves (Thornton 2008, 217). Because gifts are linked to identity and the self is multiple (as explained in chapter 1), people are literally accruing (or adding on to their) identities through sexual exchange.

In addition to important ancestral exchanges (and therefore, historical, social, and communal affiliations), trust, prestige, and respect are established through these various "flows of substances" (Thornton 2002) that accompany sexual relations. For instance, when men provide gifts or cash to a "transactional" partner, it is understood as a sign of respect. Because sex is now affiliated with possible contagion (not only with HIV, but also with other forms of pollution), sex without a condom signifies trust and respect for the sexual partner (ibid.).

Therefore, sex draws on and instantiates complex social networks in which various forms of "capital" are transacted, and thus legitimated and valued: economic (money/gifts), social ("wealth in people"), and symbolic (trust, honor, prestige). Spiritual "substances" (auras, blood) are also "transacted" and accrued. If the self is conceptualized as contiguous with both the ancestral and social world, but also incremented through the interactions one has throughout one's life, then these sexual "exchanges" are also the building blocks of identity. Through these sexual "transactions," then, subjects forge their hybrid, gender identities.

Thornton's interventions into the scholarship on sexuality are absolutely unique and essential, but he posits a rather static theory of sexual networks in order to explain why South Africans are so vulnerable to

HIV infection. He does not, however, explore the ways in which AIDS and neoliberalism have caused major shifts in the constitution of gender identity and the operation of the sexual economy. I argue that AIDS has fragmented the connectivity of sexual networks, thereby rendering identities themselves extremely vulnerable and precarious. Since the onset of AIDS, identities are at risk from multiple sources. There are additional threats associated with pollution, jealousy, and witchcraft, but expectations of reciprocity have also been unmoored, as have bonds of social cohesion. Anomie, the privatization of care and trust, stigma, and the informalization of the sexual economy have all served to destabilize gender identities in the post-apartheid era. The ways in which the respondents in this study bemoan the loss of "tradition" signifies all of these other losses of trust, culture, and identity.

Bourdieu challenges us to present our research participants' perspectives "as they are in reality, not to relativize them in an infinite number of cross-cutting images, but, quite to the contrary, through simple juxtaposition, to bring out everything that results when different and antagonistic visions of the world confront each other" (Bourdieu 1999, 3; quoted in Auyero and Swistun 2009, 65). In this chapter I have tried to show how "tradition" is used in different contexts, by different actors, toward different ends. Rather than illustrating that there is any one "traditional" gender identity, I have showed the tremendous flexibility and hybridity of gender ideologies and sexual practices. Still, "tradition" is mobilized as a *discursive formation* (Foucault 1972) to manage the paradoxes of postcolonialism. Because thanatopolitics and biomedical exclusion have often been cloaked in discourses of "rights," in the squatter camps, "tradition" is deployed as a form of resistance, against symbolic extermination and the destabilization of gender identities. I contend, then, that this perceived loss or devaluation of "tradition" played a key role in the "messianic" rise of Jacob Zuma.

The "Zunami"

Zuma's success in capturing the ANC presidency has been based on carefully riding the wave of popular dissatisfaction. (GUMEDE 2008, 265)

Throughout this chapter, I have explained the various ways in which Zuma marshaled popular disillusionment with and within the ANC to promote himself as a radically different alternative to Mbeki, as a new kind of leader with a different vision for the future of South Africa.[53] While Mbeki is Xhosa, highly educated, and comes from a long history with the ANC—one that required him to be raised in exile, Zuma is Zulu, has no formal education, and was part of Umkhonto we Sizwe (MK), the military wing of the ANC. Whereas Mbeki drew on the symbolism of the African renaissance, Zuma has embodied the "rags to riches" fairy tale, which has ensured his popularity among the poor. These differences mean that each represents different ANC lineages but also speaks to different South African populations.

As Liz Gunner notes (2008), Zuma's trademark song, "Umshini Wami" ("Bring Me My Machine Gun") "captured the structure of feeling in the body politic" (33) and even served to bridge "different constituencies in a fragmented and plural polity" (29), thus forging a new (heterogeneous but united) public.[54] In part, this is due to Zuma's presentation of a new national imagination—one that has thus far had the capacity to overcome alien-nation, as the Comaroffs describe it (2000). They argue that the more diverse the nation-state becomes, the higher level of abstraction needed to theorize or imagine the nation. This is due, in part, to the ways in which states have been undermined by market forces, but also due to the levels of inequality sustained and exacerbated by millennial capitalism. As such, the "magical" power of "hyphen-nation"—or national imagining—must forge a sense of community that is capable of speaking across class, racial, and other structural divides.

Zuma's performance of "Umshini Wami" and his guerilla warrior persona recall the apartheid-era struggle—foregrounding the popular sentiment of Africans united in struggle against a racist and unjust government. But beyond simply reminiscing a latent political unconscious of the nation and simultaneously offering a resolution to the nation's anomie, Zuma reactivated apartheid-era organizing to canvass votes. In other words, he not only remobilized the sensation of people working together to forge a collective spirit and democratic nation, but he also reactivated dormant ANC grassroots structures, which had been used when the organization was banned, to communicate messages and organize meetings and mass actions.[55] As such, the poor not only felt included in the body politic, through the nation's resymbolization, but they also felt more active in promoting the needs of their own communities. Finally, he promised to confront poverty, deliver services, and address the material needs of the poor.

I believe in him as a true leader of the poor people of our country. Yes . . . He's a president for everyone, rich or poor, but he's a true leader of poor people.[56]

There's hope in Zuma's administration because he comes to see us, to see us in the conditions where we live, so he knows what we face . . . the challenges we face. . . . So that's why we still have that hope . . . he has made priorities that are being set up to address key issues that are affecting poor people . . . even the people living with HIV.[57]

Zuma's rise to power can be explained by a conjuncture of events: the split within the ANC (and particularly, growing resentment of Mbeki's centralized and autocratic leadership style), the crisis of liberation felt so acutely by the poor, and the faltering of new social movements. Once in power, however, Zuma needed to convince the poor (who were largely responsible for his overwhelming success in the polls) that he would deliver on his campaign promises. With the build-up to the World Cup in 2010, he also needed to persuade a very skeptical international audience of his capacity to quell the frustrations of the poor while simultaneously ensuring economic stability and growth within a neoliberal frame. As for Mbeki, this juggling of the postcolonial paradox required Zuma to deploy the tropes of "modernity" and "traditionalism" in contradictory ways. Yet his articulation of the myth of incommensurability was a complete reversal of Mbeki's. Zuma used "traditional" sexuality (instead of healing) to promote Third Way politics while garnering legitimacy with the poor; however, his AIDS politics have been nothing if not biomedically orthodox.

Within five months of becoming president, Zuma gave what AIDS activists and health professionals have heralded as a "landmark speech,"[58] in which he "left no doubt about the decisive departure from the previous government's stance of denialism and indifference" (*Lancet* 2009). His health minister, Dr. Aaron Mostoaledi, donned a TAC t-shirt (with the "HIV-positive" logo emblazoned across the chest) at the 2009 International AIDS Society Conference in Cape Town and told a "cheering crowd" that the "government would honour its obligations on HIV treatment and prevention" (Kapp 2009). Later that same year, Zuma announced a massive expansion of both treatment and prevention efforts by vowing to cut new infections in half and scale up treatment to 80 percent of those who need it by 2011 (Sidibé 2009).

On World AIDS Day, December 1, 2009, Zuma launched the "I am responsible; we are responsible; South Africa is taking responsibility" campaign. The "I am responsible" component of the campaign asks people to take HIV tests and to engage in safer sex practices; the "we are responsible" component asks communities and families to take responsibility not to spread the virus and to support those who are already infected; and the "South Africa is taking responsibility" component of the campaign promises that the government (through SANAC) will take responsibility in scaling up prevention and treatment efforts (Republic of South Africa 2009).

Today we join millions of people across the globe to mark World AIDS Day. . . . We join millions who understand that the epidemic is not merely a health challenge. It is a challenge with profound social, cultural and economic consequences. It is an epidemic that affects entire nations. Yet it touches on matters that are intensely personal and private. Unlike many others, HIV and AIDS cannot be overcome simply by improving the quality of drinking water, or eradicating mosquitoes, or mass immunisation. It can only be overcome by individuals taking responsibility for their own lives and the lives of those around them. . . . We have to overcome HIV the same that it spreads—one individual at a time. We have to really show that all of us are responsible. (Zuma 2009)

In this same speech he insisted that the country must face the epidemic in its full reality and not attempt to "downplay the statistics." He promised to take an HIV test to set an example: "I am making arrangements for my own test. I have taken tests before, and I know my status. I will do another test soon as part of this new campaign. I urge you to start planning for your own tests" (ibid.). He also initiated several new policies: HIV-positive children under one year of age would be issued treatment regardless of CD4 counts; patients coinfected with HIV and TB would be given antiretrovirals when their CD4 count is under 350 (as opposed to 200); all pregnant women with a CD4 count less than 350 (as opposed to 200) would have access to treatment; all health institutions will be capacitated to provide counseling, testing, and treatment (as opposed to a few accredited ARV rollout sites) by April 2010.

This campaign is interesting in its redeployment of the discourse of responsibilization. The campaign represents an effort to not simply individualize responsibility, but to denote the collective effort and "extraordinary measures [required] to reverse the trends we are seeing in the health profile of our people" (Zuma 2009). At the same time, however, it highlights some of the key features of Zuma's particular brand of Third Way politics.

Zuma's administration has adopted the label of a "developmental state": "the idea of a developmental state . . . appeared as a cornerstone of the ANC's election manifesto during the 2009 general elections. When Zuma delivered his State of the Nation address on 3 June 2009, he made reference to a developmental state and the creation of an economically inclusive society in South Africa" (Kondlo 2010, 6). Yet there exist certain tensions under the signifier "developmental." On the one hand, it signals a pro-working-class agenda, promoted especially by the Congress of South African Trade Unions (COSATU). On the other, it involves a multiclass project focusing on the further development of the Black middle and upper classes through programs like Black Economic Empowerment (BEE) (ibid.). In many ways, this has forced Zuma to adopt Mbeki's focus on the two economies—where those who are poor are targets of "service delivery" and those who are more economically stable or part of the skilled work force are privileged with tax cuts and other incentives (Mashigo 2010, 111). Although he has embraced the label "developmental" (which Mbeki never did to avoid the insinuation of dependence), Zuma's so-called pro-poor policies are actually simply carryovers from the Mbeki regime. Many large development projects (including, for example, the upgrading of Sol Plaatjie) were initiated under the Mbeki administration, and so while Zuma's administration has been heralded as *the* "delivery administration" (Kondlo 2010, 8) and there was a definite scaling-up of development projects in the run-up to the 2010 World Cup, the Third Way policies of the two administrations are not as different as the media pundits and Zuma supporters would have us believe. Zuma has scaled up largely technocratic service delivery initiatives to quell protests and cover up for a lack of more integrative or radical forms of structural redistribution. As discussed in chapter 3 (regarding ARV provision), such efforts leave deep-rooted inequalities largely intact.

Often, the poor adopt the technocratic language of "development" and "service delivery," which unveils the ways in which they, too, are embroiled in the paradoxes of postcolonialism. Here is how Thulani understands the shift in politics under Zuma—the new age he has ushered in:

Zuma has a mandate from us and the people have spoken through their casting of votes . . . but the government is for the people by the people . . . gone are the days that we sit back and just say, "the government is doing nothing" . . . If Zuma doesn't do anything for the people, what are we going to do in the next election? You know. That is the responsibility of every one of us to make sure that the ANC manifestos are implemented . . . but we'll have to wait and see. The hope is not rest-assured in Zuma. It's rest-assured on each and every individual of South Africa to work together. In these next five years, we are not running politics, we are running the development of our people.[59]

Throughout the post-apartheid era, poor living conditions in squatter camps have sparked violent uprisings, generally in the run-up to local government elections. There were widespread "basic service protests" just after Zuma was elected, in July 2009, leaving many to wonder how successful Zuma would be in addressing the needs of those who were responsible for putting him in power.

Another tension Zuma must manage is his relationship to COSATU—the trade union arm of the ANC alliance, which played a huge role in rallying support for Zuma at the end of the Mbeki regime. "They won the public relations battle, successfully blaming the ANC government's failure to sufficiently share South Africa's remarkable prosperity with the poor masses directly on Mbeki's centrist economic and social reforms, known as GEAR" (Gumede 2008, 265). But Zuma has not repealed GEAR—in fact, he has managed to fit his vision of South Africa as a "developmental state" within the confines outlined in GEAR. In late 2010 and early 2011, Zuma launched a New Growth Plan, which is meant to create five million jobs by 2020, but which has been heavily criticized and rejected by COSATU because it looks so similar to Mbeki's GEAR (Rossouw 2011). Economists (both internationally and nationally) have been relieved by Zuma's ability to meet some of the demands of COSATU while maintaining a largely neoliberal macroeconomic approach (Govender 2011). However, there have been times when these tensions have erupted in protests—for example, the public sector strikes (of 1.3 million government employees, nurses, doctors, and teachers) that seized the country for two months from August through October 2010. As a *Time* story reports: "The strikes represent a political conundrum for President Jacob Zuma, whose rise to power in 2009 involved heavy political and financial backing from the unions. But caving in to their demands would imperil his government's efforts to create an economic growth environment that could begin to reverse South Africa's chronic unemployment" (Perry 2010).

In many ways, Zuma's politics are ambiguous—he has successfully juggled the contradictory demands of postcolonialism both within and outside the borders of South Africa. He has done so, in part, through the deployment of a national fantasy of independence that is wildly divergent from Mbeki's African renaissance. By claiming the label of the "developmental state" and embracing biomedical orthodoxy, Zuma has embedded South Africa more firmly within the global economic system rather than declaring independence from Western capital. For him, the independence comes in the form of cultural identity—through the "retraditioning" of the postcolony. And it is through his performance of "traditional" sexuality and his embodiment of the "rags to riches" ethos that he has resignified the national imaginary and attempted to convince the poor that they have finally been incorporated into the body politic.

When I returned to South Africa in June 2012, I found that Zuma's popularity among the poor was already declining. People joked openly about the fact that he seemed to care more about finding new wives than addressing the needs of the poor—a reference to the fact that in April 2012, Zuma married for the sixth time, his second marriage while in office. After discussing all of the various economic struggles they face, I asked a focus group of women in Lawley to explain the desperate economic situation in South Africa. This is how they responded:

Woman 1: Black people are there as leaders, but the white people still control the money and don't want to share with Black populations.

Woman 2: Another problem is that the government wants power for themselves and they are corrupt, and they end up fighting amongst themselves and they don't think about people at the grassroots level—they don't think about developing us and helping us. And they just fight amongst themselves and help themselves.

Woman 3: Once we vote for them they forget about us. They come only during elections times.

Woman 4: Zuma just takes a new wife every year. . . . Maybe if he was interested in marrying *me*, he would address my needs, but only then . . . [*laughs*].[60]

And so, the excitement Zuma inspired among the poor lasted less than three years, and the crisis of liberation they feel so acutely has only deepened.

In a trenchant editorial published in *Business Day* at the end of 2009, Jonny Steinberg suggested that the public had been quick to label Thabo Mbeki an "ogre" because he was plagued by the ills of post-apartheid, whereas Zuma invoked an era of appeasement and calmness. "Whatever Zuma's flaws, it was a relief to have a president who seemed to feel at ease with himself and comfortable among his people. And with that relief came great anger towards Mbeki. . . . We have made [Mbeki] into an ogre, I think, because we wish that what has departed with him is a country ill at ease with itself." Still, one is left to ponder whether or not this signals a widespread acceptance of structural inequality, as the harbinger of what post-apartheid has come to signify. This would certainly explain, more than anything else, why the poor were so hopeful about a president who has largely ensured that the more things change, the more they stay the same.

The Crisis of Liberation

In response to economic deterministic analyses that suggest that Zuma's rise to power was simply a smokescreen for neoliberal "business-as-usual," Gillian Hart suggests that we ignore the implications of what Zuma's popularity meant for the nation and liberation at our own peril (2008, 700). In other words, Zuma's election constituted a fundamental critique of the policies of Mbeki's administration. With their vote, the populace was certainly protesting against the failure of the ANC to redistribute wealth after the end of apartheid, but they were also protesting against cultural imperialism, the way in which the politics of recognition have been used to symbolically exclude certain populations from the nation's imaginary, and the way in which cultural "traditions" were being besmirched in the name of progress.

Zuma *did* respond to the call for recognition and to a certain extent gave people hope that liberation is still in their future. And for a while the poor were willing to give him the benefit of the doubt, in part, because they have seen some service delivery and development. However, with certain nods and acquiescences to pressure from COSATU, Zuma has largely reinstated the neoliberal policies characteristic of the Mbeki era. So like Mbeki before him, Zuma has attempted a politically complicated sleight of hand, which has entailed a new articulation of the tropes of "tradition" and "modernity"—on gendered terrains. This reveals the powerful way in which these tropes can be mobilized to dole out differential material rewards and thereby resignify the relationship between racial, gender, and class identities. However, the tropes are also deployed by communities who have been relegated to the margins of citizenship in order to engage in oppositional resistance. Because these tropes have been utilized to support such a varied array of political projects, they reveal, in a certain way, the hybridity that underpins them. And yet, these mythical tropes also serve to both signify and deflect attention away from fundamental contradictions in the relations of power and production, thereby signaling, more than anything else, an ongoing crisis of liberation.

FIVE

Hybridity

"Ellen"[1] is an indigenous healer, and she also owns and operates a *shebeen* (tavern) from her home—making her both a business and community leader in Alexandra, a township located in the heart of Johannesburg. Both Ellen and her husband are HIV positive. Ellen's husband has a full-time job that provides him and his entire family with comprehensive private health care—a rare privilege in most African townships. Following the advice of his doctor, Ellen's husband began antiretroviral treatment while I was conducting in-depth interviews with her in 2005. At this time, ARVs were just beginning to be rolled out in the public health sector, and they were met with a lot of fear and skepticism. Ellen was very wary of the course of therapy her husband had chosen to follow—especially when he began refusing his wife's *muthi* because his doctor had told him they would interfere with his drug regimen. She informed me that she surreptitiously infused his tea with *muthi* despite his objections. Then, at the urging of her husband, she visited his doctor who recommended she begin antiretroviral treatment as well. She was very conflicted and scared. Ellen had always trusted in her own herbal remedies, but the doctor had told her that her CD4 count was low enough that he would strongly encourage her to start ART. She called me to get my advice, she spoke with her husband, she consulted her colleagues, and she communicated with her ancestors. In the end, she did begin triple cocktail therapy, which she took in conjunction with her own indigenous treatments. When I asked her what finally made her decide to mix the two kinds of methods, she said that she had spoken with her ancestors and that they had guided her toward this hybrid approach. "In an ideal world, everyone would take both kinds of treatment."[2]

"Tebogho" works as a project manager for a respected NGO where I conducted ten months of participant observation research in Soweto.[3] Tebogho earns her living by trying to convince HIV-infected people in her township to follow the regimens prescribed by their doctors and health care professionals, including promoting the use of antiretroviral medication. Because of the habitus her NGO job requires, Tebogho often parrots common Western ideologies about "traditionalism," equating indigenous healing with ruralism, backwardness, and lack of education. However, I realized after some time that she was engaging in what Homi Bhabha might refer to as performative mockery (1994). Because of *my* identity, Tebogho was performing her "Westernness" and therefore proving her ability to do her job well; however, as time progressed and we got to know each other better, I came to find out that she refuses to take antiretrovirals herself. She believes, instead, in "positive living." She told me that she exercises, eats right, and maintains a healthy lifestyle. "This is the best medicine for me. Those drugs have so many side effects and sometimes they don't even work. I don't need them. I'd rather stick with natural remedies and *muthi* than put all those toxins into my system."[4]

From the time I first met Pheello Limapo, he was a strong advocate of biomedical treatment and rejected indigenous healing completely. "I believe that traditional healing is part of our culture. I do believe that. I'm just not convinced that traditional healers can deal with HIV/AIDS, especially at the present moment. They've got no knowledge of this disease . . . it's a problem."[5]

Instead, Pheello is a firm believer in the power of antiretroviral therapy. Pheello expended a great deal of his energy and resources trying to get onto the ART program in the early years of the rollout. It took six months and a near-death health emergency to get a referral to one of the ARV sites, in which he finally enrolled in October 2005. But he was unable to get his wife, Elizabeth, onto ARVs because she is not a South African citizen. Pheello was very sick and in and out of the hospital for most of 2005, but his wife and child remained quite healthy. Suddenly, however, in March 2006, they both became quite ill, and Elizabeth almost died. After a harrowing few months when Pheello's every bit of energy and money was spent visiting them both in the hos-

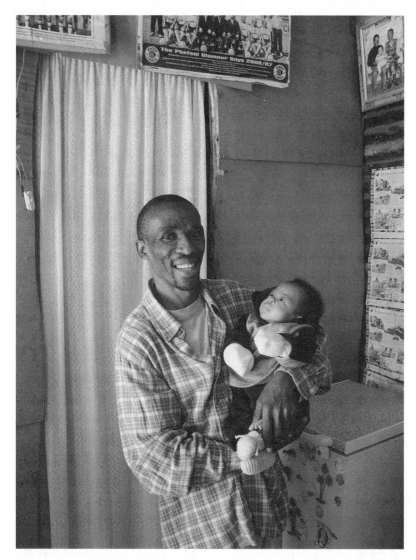

FIGURE 22.   Pheello Limapo with his son, Tshepo. Photo taken by the author in June 2009.

pital every day, they all returned home. Elizabeth's CD4 count was 10. When I next saw Pheello, he pulled me aside and whispered, "Claire, remember how I told you I don't trust traditional healers? Well, I'm using them now." When I asked him why, he said: "Because I need help, and I don't know what else to do."[6] Elizabeth was eventually put onto

ARVs (through connections with the Treatment Action Campaign), and she and Pheello are doing quite well today. When I asked Pheello in 2009 if he was still utilizing the services of indigenous healers, he said that he was not.

But in fact, I came to find out that Pheello has always mixed methods—though he does not use *muthi* or *sangomas*. Rather, he uses the cleansing rituals of the Zion Christian Church (ZCC). He joined right after he first tested HIV positive, before he publicly disclosed his status.[7] The ZCC use natural mediums like water, coffee, and tea to cleanse the body of pollutants and evil spirits. Therefore, even though Pheello only seeks out the services of a *sangoma* in times of crisis, his beliefs about health and healing incorporate spiritual healing and notions of the occult.

Nozipho Dlamini was in a serious car accident in 2000, and while she was in the hospital, they told her HIV-testing was compulsory. She found out she was infected, but didn't believe the diagnosis because "I was a little bit ignorant about the HIV itself . . . I thought someone with HIV . . . was very skinny and very critically ill . . . and I didn't feel sick and I have a large body structure."[8] But then in 2004, Nozipho started to get very sick—with one illness after another—first pneumonia, then thrush . . . "And then I started to remember that . . . by the way, I was diagnosed with HIV." Nozipho was scared to go to the clinic, but eventually her knee injury from her 2000 accident started bothering her, and she was forced to go to the hospital. This time, they tested her CD4 count, and it was 74. She was referred to the Lillian Ngoyi clinic to begin ART. At first, she had a few side effects, but since then the drugs have "treated her well." Each time she went to the doctor, her CD4 count was higher, and she was feeling better and better. Thulani, who is Nozipho's partner, first met her when she was very sick. He thought she was surely dying, and then suddenly she began attending the support group meetings looking healthy, strong, and rejuvenated.

Nozipho had never used indigenous healing until *after* she started taking antiretrovirals. Some of her fellow support group members encouraged her to try some *muthi* to boost her immune system, and she was convinced of its capacity to supplement her ARVs. Now she is a strong advocate of mixing the two, despite the fact that the people at the clinic have told her not to. "There are certain things they are failing to address at the clinic . . . but if you go to the traditional healers, you get rid of that thing . . . [the two kinds of healing] complement each other. . . . According to me, I think the two can work together. I drink the *muthi* together with the ARVs."

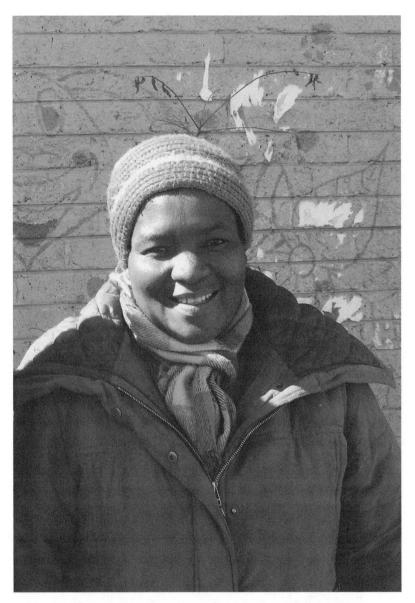

FIGURE 23.   Nozihpo Dlamini. Photo taken by the author in July 2009.

Interestingly, Thulani himself is a strong advocate of using *only* indigenous healing. As he proudly declared in a focus group discussion:

If I'm told I have to go to the clinic, I don't want to go. I haven't liked the clinic since I was young. Even today, I'm HIV positive, and don't attend the clinic. And I still don't attend the clinic. I'm living proof. . . . There is so much speculation about the ARVs. . . . I don't want anyone to tell me that I have to live like this, and if I don't live like that, I'll die. I don't like discipline. . . . Every day, I can't swallow something at the same time. I'm not a machine. That's my feeling. I don't have to take ARVs for now. Because I'm not ill. I can't get ill because I know how to take care of myself—living a healthy, positive life, instead of being programmed into something that you might fail or that might fail you. You can't fail yourself. But I always encourage people to take ARVs whenever they are sick. But me, I don't take any medication—even a Panado.[9] I don't take it.[10]

Thulani's stance may have something to do with the fact that he has been lucky enough to remain relatively healthy. His CD4 count has stayed above 200, making him thus far ineligible for ARVs. He and I had a long conversation in 2009 about what he would do once his CD4 dropped—he is anxious about the changes he might have to make in his life to remain compliant with the ARV program, but he is also scared of being sick all the time—it is what he fears most.

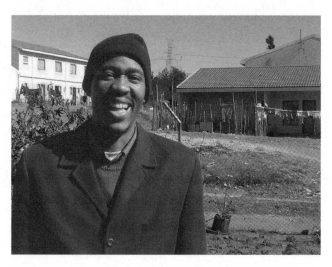

FIGURE 24.   Thulani Skhosana. Photo taken by the author in July 2009.

Thulani's reaction when he actually faces an acute illness is much more hybrid than he admits. In the fall of 2005, a rash began to develop on Thulani's hands, feet, and face. He visited his local *sangoma* to determine the cause of the infection and was prescribed an indigenous unguent, which he rubbed into his skin every day. However, he also spent the money, time, and energy to travel to the closest clinic, wait in line all day, and visit the doctor. He walked away with antibiotics, aspirin, and vitamin supplements dispensed by the Department of Health.[11] When faced with a medical emergency, Thulani's first impulse was to combine biomedical and indigenous treatments. Thulani stores all of the numerous remedies he has received and taken over the years in a box. In it, an entire cornucopia of treatments lie side by side: natural herbs and roots, biomedical prescriptions, spiritual amulets and candles, aspirins, several miracle cures, immune boosters, and the government-endorsed vitamins. Thulani's medicine chest is a material incarnation of the hybrid nature of South Africans' healing regimens and ideologies.

These case studies are just a few examples of the hybridity that has come to mark the landscape of healing politics and practices in postapartheid South Africa. Several nurses at the Chris Hani Baragwanath Hospital commented on the various ways in which patients continue to use indigenous healing during their hospitalizations—from the surreptitious usage of *muthi* to boldly inviting their *sangomas* to conduct rituals at their bedsides.[12] At the very apex of the Rath scandal, Khayelitsha—the site where the Rath Foundation set up its clinic, most likely because it is also a stronghold of the TAC—was a virtual war zone between the two camps. However, many of the community members with whom I spoke were using both Rath's vitamins *and* antiretrovirals. When I asked them about this, they seemed nonchalant, as if it only made sense to try them both.[13] There were even rumors circulating that the nurses in some of the clinics providing antiretrovirals were selling Rath vitamins to their clients under the table.[14] Indigenous healers often discuss the way in which current African leaders and doctors have betrayed their culture by "passing over to the side of Western medicine."[15] According to many indigenous healers, the African bourgeoisie disavow indigenous healing and attempt to suppress its influence in an effort to thrive in the new "modern" South Africa. While this is understood to be the worst kind of betrayal, these very same African elite "secretly come knocking on our doors at night to get treated."[16] Therefore, what seems from the outside like incommensurable paradigms is custom in most townships in South Africa, and people traverse these multivocal and discordant healing ideologies and systems for a wide range of purposes.

The hybridity articulated in and through my respondents' health-seeking behavior is informed by historical patterns of health pluralism. In fact, indigenous forms of healing survived the racial capitalism of the apartheid era through processes of adaptation and hybridization. Therefore, the fact that people continue to subscribe to hybrid health practices to manage and survive the AIDS epidemic is hardly surprising. What is surprising is that people do not claim this hybridity. Again and again, when asked what kinds of healing they use, or what forms of treatment they prefer, the people in my study told me, often quite emphatically, that they *only* used either biomedical or indigenous forms of healing. Yet through my ethnographies of their health trajectories, I came to discover that despite what they *claimed*, they still *practiced* hybridity. In the rare cases when people openly shared with me their decisions to mix treatments (as in the case of Ellen and Nozipho), it was clear that this was a decision with which they struggled and a practice about which they keep quiet in their communities. What accounts for this disjuncture between what people say and what they do?

To understand this, I begin by providing a history of the uneven historical development of health hybridity in South Africa.[17] Since the beginning of the colonial enterprise and throughout the apartheid era, while biomedical healers resisted amalgamation with other forms of healing and insisted on monotherapeutic practices and ideologies, indigenous healing accommodated not only biomedical healing but also invited pluralism within and across cultural and ethnic differences (Digby 2006, 346). This asymmetrical system turned acrimonious in the post-apartheid era, especially in debates over how to manage HIV/AIDS. Although some initial efforts were made to pluralize South Africa's health system as a whole,[18] the tremendous power of the international biomedical industry and its efforts to expand medical hegemony have flourished in the era of AIDS. In this chapter, I show how the conjuncture of events that marked the transition to post-apartheid and especially the onset of AIDS served to radically unsettle and ultimately transform the South African field of health and healing, so that today it is marked by a disjuncture between the layout and structure of the field, and the actions of those who negotiate it. I illustrate how it is this simultaneous bifurcation (in terms of health production) and hybridity (in terms of health consumption) that explains people's healing beliefs and practices, and I end the chapter by offering a theory of action that takes radical disjunction into account.

The South African Field of Health and Healing

Field theory elegantly handles as fundamentally the same two social phenomena usually considered to be antithetical, namely the feeling that there is some social force which constrains individuals externally and the feeling that we act on the basis of our motivations.

(MARTIN 2003, 36–37)

Pierre Bourdieu's field theory insists the social system is comprised of a relationship between objective social relations and schemas of perception (the "vision and division" of society) and their incorporation into subjects' habitus. In this way, his analysis insists on the important relationship *between* material structures, signifying systems, and embodied practice. Causality is always historically and socially contingent, as well as bidirectional. Further, hegemony is secured through conflict, and as such, always tends toward rupture. For all of these reasons field theory is a helpful theoretical tool oriented toward explaining the historical relationship between biomedical and indigenous healing in South Africa and its impact on subjects' health strategies and action.

"Fields present themselves synchronically as structured spaces of positions (or posts) whose properties depend on their position within these spaces and which can be analysed independently of the characteristics of their occupants (which are partly determined by them)" (Bourdieu 1993, 72). Members of any field are always in constant competition for legitimacy, for the ability to define which forms of capital are dominant in the field (which therefore determines the hierarchization of the field), and for the accumulation of this valued capital. "A species of capital is what is efficacious in a given field, both as a weapon and as a stake of struggle, that which allows its possessors to wield a power, and influence, and thus to *exist*, in the field under consideration, instead of being considered a negligible quantity" (Bourdieu and Wacquant 1992, 98). However, the struggle is in no way utilitarian because capital is often misrecognized as capital, and the struggles that are an intrinsic property of every field are symbolic as well as material.

According to Bourdieu, there are a variety of "invariant laws of functioning" for each field (Bourdieu 1993, 72): all occupants of a field share a primary belief in the interests and stakes of the "game" (Bourdieu 1993; 1984; 1996a); there are criteria of eligibility for those playing the game, policed by adherence to codified membership credentials

(1996a; 1996b); the value, composition, and exchange rate between different forms of capital invested in the field are a primary site of struggle among the participants (Bourdieu 1984); the participants in the field have to have the correct "habitus" to play the "game," which means they are endowed with the proper knowledge to play (1993); fields are autonomous—though they often reproduce and serve to sustain national class hierarchies (1996a; 1996b). All of these laws of functioning exist in the South African field of health and healing—for both biomedical and indigenous health care (Decoteau 2008), and yet the field has changed dramatically over time. In this section, I apply Bourdieu's field theory to a historical account of the uneven development of South Africa's field of health and healing.

Anthropological and historical accounts of colonial and apartheid South Africa are rife with tales of religious and health syncretism—most of which highlight the contestation inherent in the colonial encounter. In South Africa, as in other parts of the world, colonizers often used biomedicine as a "tool of empire" (Flint 2008, 119).[19] From the beginning of the colonial enterprise, biomedicine set itself up in antagonistic opposition to indigenous healers. Early missionaries (with and without medical training) viewed both witchcraft and divination to be "incompatible with Christianity' (Digby 2006, 308)—though there was some early interest in African botany (ibid, 311, 346). Similarly, British imperial authorities recognized biomedicine as the only plausible and effective healing system, but did not begrudge Africans using herbal remedies "provided they do not indulge in malicious practices" (Witchcraft Proclamation Act of 1927; quoted in Digby 2006, 321). As such, herbalists' practices were tolerated, whereas witchcraft was banned.[20] Missionaries held that religious conversion necessitated cultural transformation, so Christianity was bound up with expectations of the acceptance of Western biomedicine (ibid., 334). Digby (2006) explains how this elicited a bifurcated and parallel system of health care:

Medical cultures were shaped by larger patterns of estrangement in a segregated society, so that among whites a sense of racial superiority tended to filter—sometimes obscure—indigenous practices. There were therefore strong macro influences producing cultural resistance to the assimilation of indigenous ideas and practices, and this contributed to parallelism rather than pluralism in medicine. (346)

To the dismay of many a colonist, Christian conversion and the criminalization of African healing did little to delimit the power or prevalence of African cosmology (Comaroff and Comaroff 1991; Flint 2008). Although white, biomedical practitioners remained resistant (if not hostile) toward indigenous healing, indigenous healers and African patients were more syncretic in their beliefs and practices. For example, biomedical doctors risked losing their licenses from the South African Medical and Dental Council if they collaborated with or referred patients to indigenous healers, and yet indigenous healers regularly referred patients to biomedical clinics, especially for diseases perceived as "Western," like tuberculosis (Digby 2006, 354).

According to Karen Flint, biomedical doctors were introduced to the African population (in the middle of the nineteenth century) for three reasons: first, to diminish the power of indigenous healers and thus chiefs; second, to combat the dependence on "superstition" and beliefs in witchcraft among the colonized; and third, to maintain African health in order to protect the white population—this latter motivation became particularly prominent with the growth of industry in the twentieth century (Flint 2008). The need to provide adequate primary health care to the African labor force on the diamond and gold mines was the primary motivation for the establishment of biomedical clinics in urban townships.[21]

As a result of the expansion of biomedical services to the African populations, indigenous healing transformed as healers incorporated influences from colonial medicine and from other ethnic traditions. This partially occurred because of the new opportunities that mining communities, for example, offered healers: to learn from one another *and* to treat new "white men's diseases" (Digby 2006, 278–80). Herbs were mixed with biomedicines to increase their potency or to treat new emerging diseases. "A melting pot of healing practices was found on the Rand[22] as a result of large-scale labour mobility to the gold mines. . . . Healers were drawn into the area since it offered a buoyant medical market" (ibid., 279).[23] As they incorporated biomedical elements into their healing practices, healers were faced with a paradoxical situation, as they were also forced to perform the cultural continuity expected of those engaged in "traditional" therapeutics (ibid.). This paradox remains one of the primary features of indigenous health care in the contemporary era.

In the early twentieth century, there was growing concern about widespread malnutrition in rural areas, and in 1942, a commission was set up under Henry Gluckman, who proposed radical reforms that would unite and centralize health service under one health authority (for all South African citizens) (Digby 2006, 413–19). The National Party election in 1948, which marked the inauguration of the apartheid era, made these "liberal ideas incongruent with political realities" (ibid., 419). Although Dutch- and later Afrikaans-speaking populations had initially relied upon folk and herbal remedies (sometimes combining them with local African remedies), mostly because these populations were geographically removed from British, colonial medical services (ibid., 374–80), this shifted under apartheid. Apartheid segregation insured the development of starkly different health systems partitioned along racial lines and etched severe health inequalities into the landscape of South African society.[24]

The apartheid government transferred oversight for "homeland" health services to the Department of Bantu Administration and Development, and later each "homeland" developed its own individualized department of health (Digby 2006, 423). This meant that the national government could wash its hands of responsibility for "homeland" health. As a result, over half the African population (who lived in Bantustans) "suffered diseases of an impoverished indigenous economy that had been worsened by their function as reservoirs for migrant labour" (ibid., 424). However, the deficiencies in the provision of biomedical health services were filled by indigenous healers, who lacked proper resources and whose movements were circumscribed, but who nonetheless attempted to fill the void left by a racist social order.

Under apartheid, the Witchcraft Suppression Act 3 of 1957 and the Amended Act 50 of 1970, made it illegal for "any person to exercise supernatural powers" or "to impute the cause of certain occurrences to another person" (Xaba 2002, 9).[25] According to Thokozani Xaba (2005), the apartheid state was more successful at restricting the use of indigenous practices and medicines than previous governments had been (123). The ban was on the practice of divination, but because the distinction between herbalists (*inyangas*) and diviners (*sangomas*) was not properly understood, both groups faced repression, especially in urban areas (124). The legislation banned divination only within the confines of "white South Africa," meaning it was still legal in rural areas and Bantustans (121). The imposition of influx controls further stifled the practice in urban regions, and especially the abilities of healers to gather herbs and import them into the cities. Initially *inyangas* could register and receive a license to practice indigenous medicine (which had to be approved by the Ministry of Health or Secretary of

Bantu Administration and Development), but in 1967 a Government Gazette declared that no *new* licenses would be issued, but already existing licenses could be renewed (155–56). Often, *sangomas* registered as *inyangas* in order to avoid attracting the penalizing gaze of apartheid authorities (163).

Prior to apartheid, *inyangas* relied on knowledge of herbs passed down from generations, and some *sangomas* would collect their own herbs through the intervention of the ancestors. For both, the process involved prayer, rituals, and entailed a complex and selective harvesting process. However, under apartheid, due to hard economic conditions in rural areas, more and more women turned to the informal economy,[26] which included trading, preparing, and producing indigenous medicines (Xaba 2005, 183–84). This rise in an informal trade in indigenous herbs as well as extremely restrictive property laws and pass laws further transformed the profession of *inyangas*. "The entry of these women changed the nature of harvesting indigenous plants and the manner in which medicines were sold. Anyone could then buy medicines from the women in . . . established Muthi Market[s] and then set themselves up as indigenous healers. The sale of indigenous medicines proved very lucrative for many sellers" (ibid., 183–84). Today, indigenous healers of all shades are now forced to buy their herbs at sanitized market places where predominantly female gatherers sell natural herbs and roots, and animal bones, skins, and unguents. In Johannesburg, this market is called Faraday (figs. 25a–d).[27]

Today, it is difficult for the traditional healers. It used to be that if my patient came to me, and the ancestors gave me a prescription for my patient, then I would go immediately to the *veld*[28] and harvest that plant or *muthi* myself. But today, I need to have a permit. Because if I come with a bunch of branches, you know, of *muthi*, they will ask me, "Where's your permit?" So, apartheid has had a really long-term effect on our profession.[29]

I hate being forced to use Faraday market to buy my herbs. They aren't fresh, and the people who sell them don't even know anything about where they came from. They weren't collected with prayer, and so it's not even the correct process [i.e. harvesting was done incorrectly]. And the herbs are so expensive. But we don't have any other choice.[30]

As under colonialism, the criminalization of indigenous forms of healing under apartheid did not dissuade people from using it. In fact,

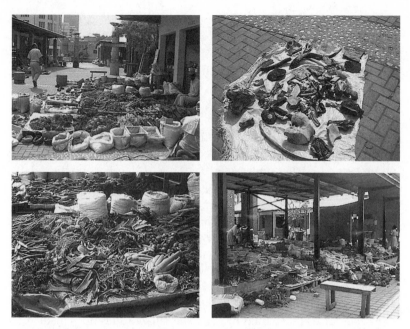

FIGURES 25 a, b, c, d. Faraday market, Johannesburg. Photos taken by the author in 2005.

Xaba (2005) notes that because of increasing violence and hardship (and the inability or unwillingness of the police to manage it), more people turned to indigenous healing to protect themselves from harmful powers or criminal intent or to make themselves attractive to employers (123, 164–83). Others saw indigenous healing as a means of protesting apartheid ideologies and practices.[31] But for many, it was simply normal health practice: "under apartheid . . . people used traditional healers as part of going to the clinic . . . people went first to the traditional healer and then to the clinic."[32] Healers explain that though they needed to be careful about how publicly they advertised their services, the legislation did not keep them from practicing.[33]

Despite the legislation, white populations largely tolerated indigenous healing and recognized it for the important role it played in Africans' sense of culture.

In spite of the development of "White" medical services for Africans, the African belief in the "isangoma" (witchdoctors) [sic] is increasing. (*The Star* 1964)

Witchcraft still has its usefulness in modern medicine among Africans and is strongest where least expected—in the sophisticated townships. (*The Star* 1967)[34]

It was often perceived as more amusing than menacing: "far too many Europeans regard it [witchcraft] as generally useful, slightly comic, and an essentially harmless part of the Romance of Africa" (*The Star* 1965). It is important to note that throughout its long history in South Africa, biomedical healing has been domesticated and rendered intelligible through localized interpretations and practices. Although biomedicine has consistently resisted hybridization, in the cultural lexicons of Africans, its diagnostic codes, illness categories, and therapies have been reinterpreted to fit people's experiences of illness—often by translating them into more familiar, indigenous lenses. In fact, some African doctors and nurses helped to facilitate this process (Vaughan 1991; Digby and Sweet 2002).

In many ways, hybridity was a product of apartheid. Although apartheid institutionalized rigid, spatial segregation, the white population was reliant on African labor—not only in the mines, but also in their homes. Therefore, Africans traversed great spatial divides to work in white spaces, and people of different races (especially in urban areas) interacted on a daily basis—making South Africa, in the words of Alan Paton, "a very strange society" (Drury 1968; quoted in Thornton 2008, 8). Africans' quotidian trajectories, then, were marked by a strange mix of boundaries and transgressions. Hybridity allowed South Africans to navigate this system—spatially, socially, and culturally.

Practicing Hybridity

Indigenous healing is inextricably linked to Africans' sense of identity. Torong once told me that apartheid stole his identity and history from him, and that indigenous healing taught him who he was again. "When I was growing up, I would wish I was a white person. . . . [After apartheid], learning about indigenous knowledge systems and traditional healing . . . broadened my understanding of who I am and where I come from."[35] It is possible, therefore, that embracing one's indigenous identity has become *more* important over time as a means of resisting colonialism, apartheid, and racism.

It's true that after 1994, everybody started searching for indigenous origins. They wanted their identity and they wanted to know where they emanate from. Even those who went toward Western civilization or who went to get educated in the Western way, they came back . . . Because people now started to reclaim who they are. And they wanted to know their origin, their sense of origin, you know.[36]

And yet, indigenous health practices and the role they have played in people's identities have shifted over time.

In fact, indigenous healing has managed to survive colonialism and apartheid through adaptation. "Indeed, the continued vitality of indigenous medicine came about partly from this ability to adapt and reinvent through selective incorporation of aspects of biomedicine within a changing repertoire of practices" (Digby 2006, 371). And it continues to adapt to present-day constraints, not least of which is the AIDS pandemic. Contemporary indigenous beliefs and practices exhibit some etiological traces from previous historical periods (Green 1994 and 1999; Setel, Lewis, and Lyons 1999; Delius and Glaser 2005) and are simultaneously mediated by contemporary social circumstances. Like any paradigm of knowledge, indigenous forms of healing reflect structural (social, economic, and cultural) transformations and inequalities and are, therefore, socially constructed and historically contingent. However, there are certain enduring ontological premises, epistemologies, and customs that characterize indigenous healing and make it amenable to hybridity. As Janzen notes, "therapeutic pluralism" is facilitated by the dynamism of African healing "traditions" (1981).

Aspects of both "tradition" and "modernity" are incorporated and synthesized in indigenous conceptualizations of the body and health.

Traditional healers see this as an opposition of categories that can be combined, but that must be "balanced" in order to achieve well-being for the African person. They seek to incorporate both sets of ideas and knowledge into a single system of healing, while maintaining the opposition of "modern" and "traditional" as separate potentials whose interaction yields power. . . . Achieving the proper balance between the "African" and the "Western" is essential. This makes it possible for healers to remain completely open to Western medical practice while at the same time placing equal value on African healing practices and treatment with herbs. (Thornton 2002)

There are two primary reasons for this accommodation of dualism. First, because illness has many different causes and origins from multiple different domains (including the social, spiritual, and physical), treatments must also be multiple. Illness can enter the body from diverse entry points or can arise from a variety of unhealthy interactions; thus, healing must be performed using equally multiplicative methods (Viljoen et al. 2003, 332). HIV actually brings on *other* diseases. AIDS is a syndrome, which refers to a set of symptoms that only collectively signify disease. The danger of HIV is that it breaks down the immune system, so that the body is at risk from multiple infectious agents or opportunistic infections. Therefore, AIDS is not really *one* disease at all. Many indigenous healers recognize that a hybrid approach to healing, one that combines *both* biomedical and indigenous methods, may be the most effective means of treating a disease as complicated and complex as HIV/AIDS.

In addition, as explained in chapter 1, according to an indigenous ontology, the boundaries of the body (and of subjectivity) are permeable.

Although modern personhood tends to posit an autonomous agent, free from external sources and individualized to an ever-increasing degree . . . "traditional" notions of personhood understand the self as "permeable and partible." They believe their bodies impart substances to and incorporate substances from other bodies. (Niehaus 2002, 189)

Because subjects' selves are contiguous with both the social and ancestral world, the body cannot be healed in isolation; it must be situated within its social, material, and communal context. The individual is deeply embedded in networks of not only living kin, but also in an entire system of ancestral relations. The individual body cannot be extracted from those bonds of kinship if it is to be properly healed. As Dr. Sheila Khama explained it: "In a family when the husband is sick, the whole family is sick. So a traditional health practitioner has to ensure that there's harmony in that family. That's the entry point."[37] Healers are *mediums* between the natural and the social, between the living and the dead, between the individual and the community. As such, indigenous healers occupy multiple social roles (Gumede 1990; Thornton 2009).

African patients use various logics to determine when and how to mix indigenous and biomedical healing (historically and in the contemporary era). For example, there is a certain functional division of labor some people heed. If a person breaks her leg, she may have the bones set by a biomedical doctor,[38] but will go to her *sangoma* to understand *why* she broke her leg. It is very likely that such a mishap is an ancestral message of some kind. "While biomedicine asks what caused the condition and how, traditional healing asks 'who' and 'why'" (Abdool-Karim Ziqubu-Page, and Arendse 1994, 6). In addition, indigenous healers cannot "look inside" the body; therefore, they often ask their patients to go to biomedical facilities to get x-rays or blood work (including CD4 counts), to verify their diagnoses.[39] Africans have often seen biomedical practitioners for what are perceived as "Western diseases" and for surgeries, whereas chronic or psychological ailments are considered the domain of indigenous healers, because they require more individualized forms of care (Digby 2006, 386).

In order to illustrate all of the varied complexities of the hybrid nature of indigenous ontology, but to also show how the fundamental split between "traditionalism"/"modernity" is maintained and yet incorporated within an indigenous paradigm, I would like to provide a case study of one of the healers I met during my research. Rebecca Rogerson is a white, Canadian *sangoma*, trained in Soweto. Dr. Rogerson claims that the indigenous healing community in South Africa has been nothing but supportive of her, in part because they accept the simultaneity of "modernity" and "traditionalism" and in part because they understand subjectivities to be necessarily multiple.

But this idea of being able to have these kinds of simultaneous cultures and backgrounds is embraced by traditional healing. So . . . so my work, ultimately, I've been received well, and that's part of the reason that I do what I do. Because of how exceptional traditional healing is. Because for traditional healers, identity is always, yeah, fluid. And multiple . . . It's like a multiplex hybridity.[40]

She explains that she only faces difficulties surrounding her identity when she is back in "Western" society.

What's been the most challenging for me is going to North America where there isn't that fluidity. Where things are very much left or right, black or white, you know. North Americans think that I'm a contradiction. They think modern health care and being a *sangoma* is like trying to be two races. You know, like totally conflicting ideologies.[41]

According to Dr. Rogerson, then, South African indigenous healers accept contradiction as a lived reality. She mentions that it is a "Western" practice to segregate and isolate different healing paradigms, but also to segregate healing from social networks (of the family and the community), spirituality, and religion. Here is an excerpt from her website, where she describes the different approaches:

When I first returned to Canada from South Africa I was overwhelmed with what I can only describe as a sort of spiritual poverty in the health care industry. . . . I saw dis-connectedness, isolation and fragmentation with regards to health care. The cerebral approach to the industry in general really struck me . . .

Though Western medicine is vital and important to the world at large, there is a real lack of education on this continent on divergent medical systems, and the cultural values or beliefs that sustain them. All too often, vast bodies of knowledge are condensed into marketable courses designed for convenience, with little or no regard for history . . .

In Africa, individual health is the responsibility of everyone—the families, and the community at large. Healing draws heavily on the concept of collectivism, and communal prayer is an integral part of the process. On a similar note, when a person is ill all aspects of their being are taken into consideration: mental, emotional, physical and spiritual. Rather than isolating obvious symptoms, the indigenous view on illness is one of relationships; of finding and restoring an overall connectedness. There is no separation made between mind, body and the spiritual realm . . .

Traditional African medicine is serious, and practitioners assume responsibility for both preserving community wellness and upholding its most sacred cultural values. It is a system based in science—not science as it's known in the West, but a science deeply rooted in rich and ancient ethnomedical knowledge.[42]

Indigenous Healing and HIV/AIDS

In his study of the history of anthropology, Fabian (2002) notes that Time is often used to construct, situate, and study the Other of colonial epistemology. Indigenous healing has often been detemporalized in precisely this way by social scientists who rigidly circumscribe it within a fixed and static past, where it can be comfortably signified as a leftover from the precolonial days of yore. Against this historical tendency, this book seeks to highlight the flexibility of the profession and to recognize the ways in which it has changed over time, especially in response to HIV/AIDS. As I have shown, many researchers note that indigenous healers have long incorporated biomedical explanations and treatments into their own health practices, and my research shows that this has continued in the era of AIDS.[43]

Traditional healing is going to have to change. Because of HIV/AIDS for one thing. We have to change some of our beliefs and practices in order to help prevent its spread and to take better care of people who are infected.[44]

Now, a traditional health practitioner needs to be informed and to be educated on what is going on in the twenty-first century and align ourselves with that, whilst not forgetting where we come from.[45]

Adam Ashforth (2002) has argued that because HIV/AIDS challenges the ontological basis of indigenous healing, it may have more durable and injurious ramifications for the longevity of the profession. The notion of a virus, which is by definition incurable but treatable, is not readily accommodated within an indigenous paradigm of the body because, Ashforth argues, indigenous healing involves the purging and cleansing of pollutants, not teaching the body to live with them. Further, he argues that because indigenous healing locates the causes of disease within the *social* and *ancestral* world, healers should be able to resolve and cure all disorders of the body. My own data suggest that HIV/AIDS has had a much more complex and nuanced impact on South Africa's knowledge systems.

Scholars of African indigenous healing (and healers themselves) have often debated whether certain indigenous "germ theories" help healers make sense of viruses like HIV. For example, Green has argued quite forcibly that "when it comes to diseases that account for greatest morbidity and mortality (i.e., those biomedically classified as infectious and contagious), the indigenous and biomedical etiological models are, in fact, not very different in fundamental and important ways" (1999, 12). Whenever I brought the topic up in focus group discussions or interviews with indigenous healers, they were largely indignant at the insinuation that their ontology was antithetical to viruses:

The idea of a virus *does* exist in traditional healing. It is sometimes referred to as insects, worms, parasites, or microbes, but it is the same idea. And it can be caused from simply environmental factors. It can be caused from pollution, or it can be caused from witchcraft. The causation theories differ, but the idea of germ and that kind of thing doesn't. And HIV is generally understood as one of these "germs"—at least by most of the traditional healers I know. . . . The idea of microbes, for sure it exists. The causation is different than biomedicine, but absolutely . . . And you can have something in your body and still be sick, particularly, and it may manifest, not in a physical problem. So you could have a worm in your body that's caused or related to something that . . . that isn't tangible.[46]

As this healer explains, then, the idea of an asymptomatic virus is also part of an indigenous ontology.

Thornton notes that part of the difficulty healers face with HIV/ AIDS has to do with how its etiology is conceived. "Is AIDS ours, African—from us and within us—or is it foreign, un-African, from without rather than from within?" (Thornton 2008, 150–51). Interpretations of AIDS' belonging have serious implications for how HIV/AIDS (and those infected with it) are treated. In my own research, I have found that many healers attempt to own the disease—by pointing out historical similarities between it and indigenous diseases. For example, there is an indigenous disease, referred to as *makhome* in Sotho, which is sexually transmitted to a man who has had sex with a woman who is recently widowed or has lost a child or had an abortion.

Dr. Tshabalala: If you sleep with a widow or with someone who has had an abortion, you know, it's very dangerous, because that person is still very sick, I mean spiritually, and then now that person is going to contract that disease, *makhome*, because the blood of the woman is dirty.

Dr. Mongoya: Yes, it is dirty because the *isithunzi* (aura) of the dead husband or child is still a part of the woman . . . until she is cleansed. So, if she has not gone through the cleansing ritual, then it is dangerous for anyone to have sex with her. She can pollute a man, and he will contract *makhome*.[47]

Because blood is believed to be exchanged during sexual intercourse, a person who is inhabited by the aura of a recently deceased relative or an unborn child can put a sexual partner into a "dangerous state of heat" (Niehaus 2002, 193). As such, sexual activity is banned for widows, women who have recently had abortions, or even people undergoing divination therapy. In two FGDs held with indigenous healers in Soweto in late 2005, I asked the participants about the relationship between *makhome* and HIV/AIDS, and all agreed that though the diseases were different, the symptoms were the same and both were sexually transmitted. "*Makhome* is not HIV/AIDS—it has always been there, but there are similar symptoms."[48]

In addition to recognizing historical similarities between HIV and indigenous diseases, healers also acknowledge that because the disease is decimating their communities, it must be dealt with within the community. If HIV is incurable but manageable with treatment, then people have to learn to accept it as being part of who they are—as even something that defines them. If it is here to stay, it must be domesticated— no matter its original source.

HIV/AIDS is just as often interpreted as a sign of all that has gone wrong with post-apartheid—proof of what happens when people lose sight of their origins and forget their "traditional" roots and cultural practices. In his research in rural villages in the Limpopo province, Stadler (2003) found that his respondents blamed the post-apartheid era for inaugurating a kind of sexual revolution, which led to the spread of HIV/AIDS. "Villagers recognised the political nature of the AIDS crisis, and linked it to the new freedoms ushered in by the political transformations of the early 1990s. . . . Thus conceptualised, AIDS was not only a public health problem but posed an existential crisis that threatened the social fabric" (124). As many of the quotes included throughout this book have shown, my own respondents also blame many of the forces of post-apartheid for the spread of the disease: traditions have been forgotten or ignored, "modern" rights have destroyed the institution of marriage, the bonds of reciprocity and trust within communities have been shaken so that people willfully infect each other, people are jealous of what others have and "witchcraft" has become rampant. There are many signifiers of the ills of "modernity," which are blamed for the onset and pervasive nature of the disease.

Obviously, a new virus, and especially one whose wrath has been so tremendously incomprehensible and overwhelming, poses serious challenges to the epistemology and ontology of any cosmology—but just as biomedicine has come to define it and treat it, indigenous healers hope to do the same. One of the obstacles healers lament on a regular basis is the fact that they have not had the opportunity to come together, as a knowledge network with dedicated resources at their disposal, to collaborate on treatment protocols.

Female: AIDS—we cannot cure it because we are not given the chance and the space to deal with the problem. [Biomedical professionals] ask us to deal with the symptoms, but there is a bigger problem we could attack. They channel our efforts into certain areas instead of giving us the chance to find the cure.
Male: I want to agree . . . that we haven't faced this challenge head-on, and we are not allowed the opportunity to deal with it. We are dealing with it only one on one—when people come to our separate surgeries.[49]

Despite the constraints, indigenous healers are learning how to manage HIV/AIDS, often by following the tradition of pluralism and incorporating biomedical knowledge and therapeutic strategies into their treatment protocols. Some have gone through trainings on HIV/AIDS, STIs, and TB, sponsored by the Department of Health; some regularly refer their patients to clinics and hospitals for tests and treatments; and increasingly, many have patients who are also using antiretrovirals.

When asked to describe how contemporary hybridity differs from that practiced under apartheid, indigenous healers often suggest it is more common now to *begin* at the clinic and then consult with indigenous healers afterward.[50] Others think hybridity is even more common in the post-apartheid era, in part because of AIDS.[51] Dr. Martha

Mongoya offers an explanation for both of these trends: "One of the reasons for my patients to mix [is] to know whether they are positive, there's no other places but the clinic . . . they have to go there and find out. . . . And then that's where now they make choices after that, whether to continue the clinical way, or to consult with their own traditional health practitioners."[52]

Despite the fact that patients are told not to mix indigenous and biomedical treatments when they are being enrolled in ART, healers have discovered ways to continue to treat their patients taking antiretrovirals:

In the traditional health forums that we attend, one of the things that they encourage people to do—even if they are on ARVs or any biomedical treatment, they are advised that they should give space between the consumption of biomedical medicine and traditional medicine. Also, we are advised that if we deal with people living with HIV/AIDS, we should not give them strong *muthi* to give them diarrhea, but instead something that will boost their immune.[53]

Even if they visit *inyangas*, they need to be consistent in taking their conventional treatments [the ARVs]. Because some people have their own remedies. We told them to be consistent in their biomedical treatment, even if they continue to use other kinds of treatment too.[54]

Antiretrovirals are fine. I have many patients who use them. I only recommend that my patients consult with their ancestors before beginning them. This requires a certain ritual.[55]

Many healers and people living with the disease have found that integrating indigenous and biomedical healing is the best means of addressing the pandemic. Yet the ways in which people living with the virus engage in hybrid health behavior differs greatly.

AIDS and the Contemporary Configuration of the Field

One of the underexplored aspects of Bourdieu's field analysis is the way in which external forces impinge upon internal field dynamics, and this is particularly important in the case of healing and health care, as biomedicine is an international industry that exercises great force over national health systems—especially in the wake of epidemiological crises. Although historians and anthropologists have explored the way in which biomedicine served as a "tool of empire" in the colonial and developmental eras,[56] the ongoing global march of biomedical hegemony under the aegis of neoliberalism has been met with scholarly silence. Or rather, it has been documented and described in detail (for example: Rose 2007; Janes and Corbett 2009; Lock and Nguyen 2010), but the underlying cultural imperialism at work goes largely unquestioned.[57] This is not to suggest that humanitarian, public health, and national efforts should not be aimed at expanding the reach of biomedical health care access to address inequalities in morbidity and mortality rates. Nor is it to ignore the efforts of the World Health Organization to publicly recognize and sanction the usage of indigenous forms of healing throughout the global South (World Health Organization 2007). Rather, it is simply to note that a vast majority of South Africans (like millions of others throughout the world) continue to rely on and value indigenous forms of healing, which are slowly being undermined by the ever-advancing march of the biomedical industry.

And HIV/AIDS has become the newest (and perhaps most unlikely) tool for the expansion of biomedical hegemony. After the early years of the pandemic when it was considered inefficient and even dangerous to provide antiretrovirals to populations living in resource-poor settings, biomedical technologies are once again being heralded as the new beacon of salvation for millions of suffering masses throughout the world. As explained in chapter 3, admonitions against pluralism have been strengthened since antiretrovirals have been rolled out in the public sector. These technological interventions (antiretrovirals, TB and malarial drugs, vaccines, voluntary male circumcision) are meant to replace existing cultural practices and healing methods, but they leave relatively untouched some of the more fundamental causes of ill health, which breed in conditions of systemic inequality.

One of the abiding lessons of health policy in poorer countries, in both the colonial and postcolonial eras, is that technical fixes to health, whether DDT for malaria or vaccinations for smallpox or ARVs for AIDS, tend to leave the social and economic determinants of health, and the socio-spatial relations that underpin them, untroubled. (Hunter 2010, 225)

The erasure of indigenous forms of healing may also further exacerbate these conditions of inequality, as people are left bereft of communal identity and solidarity, vulnerable to ontological insecurities that seriously destabilize bonds of trust and reciprocity (as discussed in chapter 1). Chapters 2 and 3 both noted efforts made by the South African state to formalize indigenous healing within the national field of health and healing, and yet these efforts have largely fallen off under President Zuma—most likely due to his renewed commitment to deploying biomedical solutions to address the AIDS epidemic and his efforts to distance himself from his predecessor's overwhelming doubts.

As such, the field of health and healing is today more bifurcated and hierarchically uneven than ever before in its history. Biomedical healing is invested with economic, social, and symbolic capital from national and international sources, *and* it has secured hegemony in the public health care system. Indigenous healing continues to exist largely as an informal and peripheral health care option for poor Africans. Although indigenous healing occupies a *dominated* position within the field, it employs the largest number of producers of health care and attracts the largest consumer base.

The most often cited statistic is that 80 percent of South Africans use some form of indigenous healing (van der Linde 1997; Campbell 1998; Department of Health 2003); however, this is an estimate at best. There have been no reliable studies on the subject, partially because the breadth and scope of indigenous healing is impossible to measure for several reasons. As explained in chapter 1, "indigenous healing" refers to many different practices and trades. Many South Africans use a combination of these forms of healing, at different times in their lives. Mander and colleagues suggest that the average frequency of South Africans' usage of indigenous medicine is 4.8 times per year (2007, 190).

In addition, it is approximated that there are 300,000 to 350,000 indigenous healers in South Africa (Select Committee on Social Services 1998; Meissner 2004; Liddell, Barrett, and Bydawell 2005)—fifteen times more than biomedical practitioners (Liddell, Barrett, and Bydawell 2005). However, this number does not include prophets or faith healers (Ashforth 2005, 8). It is also likely this number is an underestimation because many indigenous health practitioners practice under the radar of any regulatory mechanism and are very secretive about their practice and clientele. Ashforth estimates that at "least a million African healers are at work outside the formal biomedical system in South Africa" (ibid.). Further, it is estimated that 133,000 people (mostly women) are employed in the informal trade of medicinal herbs and animal products (Mander et al. 2007, 194–95), and that US$75 to $100 billion is spent each year on medicinal plants in South Africa (Mander and Le Breton 2006).[58]

People continue to use indigenous healing despite the availability of antiretrovirals for a number of reasons. In a study conducted between 1999 and 2000 in KwaZulu-Natal, patients' responses to indigenous versus biomedical care were surveyed (Colvin et al. 2001). Indigenous healers were incorporated into a tuberculosis directly observed treatment (DOT) control program. Indigenous healers attended fifty-three patients, and either clinic workers or lay community members supervised 364.

Overall, 89% of those supervised by traditional healers completed treatment, compared with 67% of those supervised by others. . . . The mortality rate among those supervised by traditional healers was 6%, whereas it was 18% for those supervised by others. . . . Interestingly, none of the patients supervised by traditional healers transferred out of the district during treatment, while 5% of those supervised by others did. (Colvin et al. 2001)

The reasons provided for the success of supervision by indigenous healers included the following: patients and indigenous healers have established long relationships of trust, and indigenous healers spend more quality time with their patients and exhibit much greater care and nurturance than biomedical health workers. In addition, indigenous healers live locally and are familiar with the patients' social settings (Colvin et al. 2001). Biomedical health care workers (in part due to human resource constraints) rarely spend time explaining patients' symptoms and treatment options. Indigenous healers not only explain the problem, but do so in a language and conceptual framework the patient can immediately grasp.

Traditional healers have a closer relationship with the people. They talk to them more . . . rather than waiting for two hours on a bench, then finally getting a very dehydrated, tired doctor or nurse, saying "What's wrong with you? Ok, we'll take your blood" . . . and then asking a whole bunch of embarrassing questions instead of engaging. I think . . . people want to be engaged . . . and traditional healers *know* the person and provide counseling . . . they listen. . . . Because one of the things that I think is happening is that medical professionals are under so much pressure, especially in Soweto and other urban areas because you have a hundred people waiting. You can't give specialized attention. . . . You end up not really giving enough time to the person because it's always hurry hurry hurry . . . a traditional healer hasn't got a queue, and because you are going there for different things, no one will identify you as someone with HIV because you go there.[59]

Thornton (2002) and Gumede (1990) also note that indigenous healers' approach is far more comprehensive and holistic than biomedical care. For indigenous healers, treating the body means understanding its social and material embeddedness. Whereas the biomedical approach assumes an autonomous, independent, and mechanistic body, indigenous healing helps *situate* illnesses and recognizes them as composites of cultural, social, environmental, historical, economic, *and* biological factors. The healer also *uses* his or her own body and spirit (as well as insight about the patient's social location and psychological state) in order to heal the patient; thus, healing is an intuitive and empathetic process (Thornton 2002). Overall, indigenous health care is holistic, communal, and takes patients' material and social conditions into account.

In sum, while the hybridity articulated in and through my respondents' health-seeking behavior is reminiscent of and informed by historical patterns of health pluralism, it is also inflected with decidedly *post*colonial expressions. The international politicization of HIV/AIDS and the subsequent increase in attention paid to biopolitics at the global scale makes healing a primary site for hegemonic struggle. In the case of South Africa, this has manifested itself in a prolonged symbolic struggle between treatment activists and state denialists over the signification of AIDS, which has served to (newly) reify a myth of incommensurability, driving an essentialist wedge between different methods of healing. Each side's domination and legitimacy is rooted in its ability if not to squash competing paradigms, at least to wholly and completely dominate, define, and thereby contain them. The myth of incommensurability operates in order to attempt to secure the hegemonic legitimation of one approach, at the wholesale expense of the other. Hybridity renders this legitimacy fragile and unstable.

There is a structural disjuncture between the realities of *consumption* within the field of health and healing and the logic of the field as it is articulated in the symbolic struggle raging in the field of power. Although the field is fundamentally (and unequally) bifurcated, the actions of the majority of South Africans reflect a historical practice of pluralism. The field of health and healing is characterized, therefore, by a simultaneous bifurcation and hybridity—which is reflected in HIV-infected South Africans' beliefs and practices. As the cases provided at the beginning of this chapter show, many HIV-infected South Africans *identify* with one or another healing paradigm—largely because of what they have come to represent in public sphere discourses about HIV/AIDS. When they claim to follow one or another paradigm, they are making a *political* statement about where they stand in a broader debate about healing. But their *practices* reveal a historical and pragmatic hybridity because bodies serve as structural "memory pads" (Bourdieu

2000, 141). The participants in this study are not merely acted upon in this process—they have played a role in configuring the structure of the field, or insuring its unique configuration such that the disjuncture between health production and consumption is maintained.

Toward a Postcolonial Theory of Practice

In this "post-colonial" moment, these transverse, transnational, transcultural movements, which were always inscribed in the history of "colonisation," but carefully overwritten by more binary forms of narrativisation have, of course, emerged in new forms to disrupt the settled relations of domination and resistance. . . . They reposition and dis-place "difference" without, in the Hegelian sense, "overcoming" it. (HALL 1996A, 251)

Articulations of hybridity in the post-apartheid era require new theories of action that can account for disjunction. This is first of all because the layout of the field of health and healing cannot really explain the hybrid health behavior of its consumers. There is a disjuncture, in other words, between the structure of the field and the habitus of its users. Because of the greater capital invested in biomedical care, one might think it is within the best interest of marginalized populations to fully subscribe to its tenets, monotherapy being primary among them, or else risk losing the capital gained from accessing well-resourced health care or from securing biomedical citizenship. Yet, people continue to subscribe to a pluralized health regimen.

The second reason why explaining hybrid health behavior requires a theory of disjunction is due to the fact that new binary oppositions have been imposed on the field. On the one hand, people are slowly losing the knowledge and practices associated with an indigenous cosmology, and the scope of biomedical hegemony is extending, especially as it is increasingly being linked to citizenship rights. On the other hand, there is an effort to combat the slow march of biomedical imperialism with a renewed effort to hold fast to indigenous forms of subjective expression and a need to utilize the full panoply of health care options available in order to combat the mutual pandemics of AIDS and poverty. In other words, the reification of the myth of incommensurability in the era of AIDS is met with resistance. As such, the tension between binary differentiation and the expansion of multiplicity must be kept in play, even within our theories of action. However, sociological theories of action are largely ill equipped to handle such a task. In the rest of this chapter, I engage in a postcolonial refashioning of Bourdieu's notion of habitus in order to explore the effects of disjunction on subjects' trajectories of action and the changing nature of hybridity over the *longue durée*.

Bourdieu first developed the concept of habitus while conducting field research in colonial Algeria (Bourdieu 1962; 1979), and in fact, it was first meant to describe a situation of disjuncture—where subjects' dispositions were necessarily out of sorts with the newly imposed structural conditions:

> It was not by chance that the relationship between structures and habitus was constituted as a theoretical problem in relation to a historical situation in which that problem was in a sense presented by reality itself, in the form of a permanent *discrepancy* between the agents' economic dispositions and the economic world in which they had to act. (Bourdieu 1962, vii)

He wrote that part of the job of the habitus is to synthesize binaries and overcome ontological contradictions (Steinmetz 2006, 582). But in conditions of sustained, systemic disjunction (as in the case of colonialism), Bourdieu suggests that the habitus is unable to synthesize—it remains internally contradictory. As such, the theory of habitus was developed out of reflection of the strange disjunctures the colonial era inaugurated, and should thus be well suited for analyzing their ongoing effects.

In the American academy, the concept of habitus is often interpreted as being overly structuralist and tied explicitly to class positionality (at the expense of other embodied identities).[60] Such an interpretation severely delimits the theoretical capacities of the concept as it was developed over the course of Bourdieu's long career. The habitus *should* be understood as a "strategy-generating principle enabling agents to cope with unforeseen and ever-changing situations" (Bourdieu 1977, 72). In other words, the habitus arms subjects with an innovative capacity to move within and across various fields with differential hierarchies and rules of engagement. In my usage of habitus, I show that it is informed not only by class location, but similarly by gender, race, nationality, educational level, and place of residence. In fact, I argue that the hybrid habitus incorporated by the subjects of post-apartheid *enables* and *shapes* their ability to traverse the many boundaries that circumscribe their daily lives. As John Levi Martin explains, "Like a poet breaking meter for emphasis, players break the rules precisely because they are rules. Accordingly, field theory is well equipped to deal with one of the fundamental weaknesses of mainstream sociological theory, namely its inability to do much with cases in which persons stand somewhat apart from the patterns of regularity upon which sociology focuses" (2003, 31).

I have shown that despite the bifurcated nature of the field of health and healing *and* the powerful biopolitical strategies in circulation in the post-apartheid era, certain members of the African population exhibit a hybrid habitus. There are two concepts within Bourdieu's conceptual apparatus that might explain this disjuncture: dominated taste (a taste for necessity) or hysteresis.

According to Bourdieu, "although all members of the settled field agree on what counts as symbolic capital, the dominated may still hold proudly to a dissonant set of 'values' and even developed a *taste for necessity*, a taste for their own cultural domination" (Steinmetz 2007, 323; my emphasis). The dominated are rooted in their material social conditions, and as such, their "tastes" are oriented toward products and symbols that have a direct correlation to or use-value in the material world (Bourdieu 1984). The "realism" of the working classes in some ways necessitates the development of certain "tastes" to survive, but their refinement also serve to reify their own subjugated class position. Resistance is only possible if the subjugated *recognize* their own domination and engage in a symbolic struggle for legitimacy. In post-apartheid South Africa, one could interpret Africans' insistent usage of indigenous healing as a form of "dominated taste." However, this form of healing is not without its own cultural capital (as I have shown throughout the book, in my review of the various ways in which "traditional" healing gets used to legitimate state power). In addition, the concept of dominated taste would only explain why people might subscribe to an indigenous ontology as opposed to a biomedical one; it cannot account for the reasons why people would *mix* methods in a field bifurcated by the myth of incommensurability.

For Bourdieu, *hysteresis* represents a kind of "structural lag" (1977, 85) between the "exertion of a social force and the deployment of its effects" (Wacquant 2004, 392). Hysteresis occurs when a habitus, which was once fitted to its field, lingers on into a field with a new logic and structure. In other words, there is a delay between the imposition or inculcation of particular structural dispositions and subjects' capacity or willingness to grasp and practice them.

In situations of crisis or sudden change, especially those seen at the time of abrupt encounters between civilizations linked to the colonial situation or too-rapid movements in social space, agents often have difficulty in holding together the dispositions associated with different states or stages, and some of them, often those who are best adapted to the previous state of the game, have difficulty in adjusting to the new established order. Their dispositions become dysfunctional and the efforts they may make to perpetuate them help to plunge them deeper into failure. (Bourdieu 2000, 161)

However, Bourdieu believed this to be a temporary condition. In fact, he claimed that colonialism could not be overcome until the contradictions it left behind in the habitus of its subjects were grasped and then surmounted (Bourdieu and Sayad 2004, 470).

According to this theory, then, those whose habitus are informed by the dual logics of indigenous and biomedical healing represent a certain kind of hysteresis. Because hybridity was required of the subjects of apartheid to navigate their segregated social worlds (and segregated systems of healing), hybridity could be interpreted as simply a leftover from the colonial era—something that should be overcome under post-apartheid. Yet I have also argued that the entrenchment of new binaries and structural inequalities has marked the postcolonial period in South Africa, thereby requiring the adjustment of people's trajectories of healing and strategies of action. Because hybrid health behavior cannot be explained by the layout and structure of the field of health and healing, a form of hysteresis is still in play. This could be a product of the contradictions inherent in the field itself, or it could augur the reconfiguration of a new field in emergence, but I will argue this hysteresis may be permanent as opposed to transitory or developmental.

At the end of his life, Bourdieu described his own habitus as *clivé*, or split—which was an effect of his own contradictory background—embodying the habitus of someone from a poor, rural area in southern France and simultaneously the habitus of a highly distinguished academic (Bourdieu 2007; Wacquant 2004, 382; Steinmetz 2006: 457). Therefore, despite the fact that he kept insisting on the capacity of the habitus to *synthesize* contradiction, Bourdieu did often *recognize* the fact that the habitus was often internally contradictory (Bourdieu et al. 1999), split fundamentally because the subject was coercively forced to straddle two different social systems (Bourdieu 1962; 1979; 2007). There is, then, a tension within the very concept of habitus between integration and fragmentation.

"No matter how often Bourdieu restated his definition of habitus he never seemed to come any closer to explaining how and why this integration occurs, and why it sometimes fails" (Steinmetz 2006, 457). Steinmetz (2006) suggests that Jacques Lacan's theory of imaginary identification can help to make sense of this theoretical contradiction. According to this theory, identity is based on an imaginary identification with a gestalt or whole image of oneself in the mirror, despite the fact that the body and self are experienced as fragmentary and lacking (Lacan 1977). The "repressed memory of a 'body in pieces'" (Steinmetz 2006, 459) haunts the subject throughout his life, thereby fueling the need to constantly identify with the gestalt image again and again. As Stuart Hall notes, identification is more than anything a process of forced reiteration (1996b). Reanalyzing habitus within this analytic paradigm "explains why a 'cloven' habitus is just as likely as a unified one. . . . The Imaginary is forever overcoded by the Symbolic, which pushes against integration and toward fragmentation and difference" (Steinmetz 2006, 458).

When South Africans identify with either "tradition" or "science," and in so doing, attempt to fix the signification of HIV/AIDS, they are engaging in an imaginary identification. The ideal "traditional" or "biomedical" body is simply a fantasy of integration and completion. In fact, people also sometimes identify with a whole social body—they disavow the failure of liberation and choose instead to believe in the post-apartheid imaginary, in the democratic illusion of equality. But AIDS, and its wild chain of signifiers and unruly materiality, disrupts and disallows facile imaginary identifications. As do the material conditions in which people are forced to forge survival tactics and navigate severe structural inequalities. There is a tension, therefore, within the very identities of those living on the edges of the body politic, between integration and disjunction. And this is where an intervention from postcolonial theory is helpful.

Postcolonial theories of hybridity (in part because of their reliance on poststructuralism) help make sense of this tension between difference and multiplicity, between integration and fragmentation. Although colonial discourses attempted to secure the colonized within a "unified" discourse of radical alterity, within a "constitutive outside," the colonized refused "to be fixed in place" and slip "back across the porous or invisible borders to disturb and subvert from the inside" (Hall 2006a, 252). Relying on Derridean poststructuralism, Homi Bhabha suggests that it is the ambivalence inherent in colonial desire that is responsible for creating the hybrid subjects of colonialism. The colonizer wishes for the colonial subject to be both similar and radically different. When the colonized perform the hybridity inculcated within them through the colonial encounter, this ambivalence "terrorizes [colonial] authority with the *ruse* of recognition, its mimicry, its mockery" (Bhabha 1994,

115). The hybrid performances of the colonized, thus, unveil the simultaneous partiality and doubleness of colonial signification.

Both colonizer and colonized are in a process of misrecognition where each point of identification is always a partial and double repetition of the *otherness* of the self—democrat and despot, individual *and* servant, native and child. It is around the *"and"*—that conjunction of infinite repetition—that the ambivalence of civil authority circulates as a *"colonial"* signifier that is *less than one and double.* (Bhabha 1994, 97)

Colonial desire is "less than one" because identification is always only partial (the colonized is *"almost* the same, but not quite"), but it is also "double" because it embodies the ambivalences of power—the subjects of colonization incorporate the contradictions inherent in the system— they are both citizen and subject, both "civilized" and "barbaric," both "modern" and "traditional." As such, hybridity puts the signifiers of colonial authority on display, which ultimately undermines their success. And in fact, the colonized engage in resistance through the strategic manipulation (which may or may not be conscious) of this hybridity.

But one must tread carefully with postcolonial theory. It has been critiqued for essentializing and reifying binary difference. In Paul Gilroy's words, "cultural production is not like mixing cocktails" (1994, 54–55). But it has also been critiqued for ignoring or eliding the ever-deepening schisms of inequality that neoliberal globalization has exacerbated. For Ella Shohat (1992) and Arif Dirlik (1996), the "post"-colonial obsession with "hybridity" and the concordant desire to superimpose a certain multiplicity and in-between-ness over the subaltern experience enacts a misrecognition of the various forms of domination that continue to operate in a global capitalist system. Therefore, as Stuart Hall notes (1996a), we have to be able to theorize the ways in which binaries and structural inequalities continue to be reified, while simultaneously recognizing the proliferation of hybrids: "We have to keep these two ends of the chain in play at the same time—over-determination and difference, condensation and dissemination" (249).

The myth of incommensurability shows that binaries do operate with force in the field of health and healing in post-apartheid South Africa, but even those discourses are fundamentally ambivalent and serve to reinvent mythical tropes that matter, but that are also vulnerable.

In order to understand the productivity of colonial power it is crucial to construct its regime of truth, not to subject its representations to a normalizing judgment.

Only then does it become possible to understand the *productive ambivalence* of the object of colonial discourse—that "otherness" which is at once an object of desire and derision, an articulation of difference contained within the fantasy of origin and identity. (Bhabha 1994, 67; my emphasis)

And yet, it is because the new rearticulation of the myth of incommensurability is emerging out of the mouths of the formally colonized that it is so powerful today. The binary between colonized and colonizer is still relevant, but it is also being reconfigured, and these ambivalent "post"-colonial discourses are an important part of that reconfiguration.

In his rereading of Lévi-Strauss's *bricoleur*, Jacques Derrida (1978) suggests that certain binary oppositions (nature/culture, presence/absence, past/present) can be put in "play" such that their opposition, teleology, and hierarchy are disrupted and undermined. It is this Derridean deconstructionism that inspired Bhabha's theory of hybridity—specifically its capacity to mock and thereby terrorize the colonial significations of difference. As such, rather than a sign of an inability to get with the colonial program (as Bourdieu's concept of hysteresis might imply), hybridity may be a radical form of epistemic *bricolage*—a sign of resistance and subversion as opposed to oppression.

In post-apartheid South Africa, the people whose lives have been hardest hit by the dual pandemics of poverty and HIV/AIDS engage in practices that undermine and contradict the dominant discourses that name and contain the virus, the forms of capital invested in the AIDS industry, and the operations of biopower practiced by international health agencies, health care institutions, and the post-apartheid state. I argue that this disjuncture between the field of health and healing and the habitus of people affected by HIV necessitates the bodily incorporation and preservation of a fundamentally contradictory logic of practice. The combination of rigid structural inequalities and the reinvigoration of the mythical colonial tropes of "modernity" and "tradition" are incorporated, reconfigured, but also undermined in the daily practices and beliefs of those living with HIV/AIDS.

This health hybridity is informed, in a palimpsestual fashion, by apartheid history and the fluid notion of the self inherent in indigenous ontology, but is also distinctly postcolonial, largely because AIDS, neoliberalism, and the cultural *bricolage* made possibly by globalization, have introduced new objective structures, signifying systems, and cultural practices. As Bhabha's theory makes evident, hybridity also has subversive capacities to unveil and mock colonial and neocolonial inscriptions, which render binary difference (and the processes of exclusion they facilitate) insecure. This allows the subjects of postcolonialism to both manage and contest its paradoxes. It also leaves open the possibility for radical reconfiguration. By refusing to abandon their hybridity (sometimes despite themselves), practitioners of hybrid health behavior could serve to transform the field (either through a consciously revolutionary process or slowly, over the *long durée*) especially because of the ways in which hybridity threatens biomedical hegemony.

What effect does a permanently disjointed habitus have on subjects' actions and identities? I would like to suggest that it requires a constant refashioning and reworking of one's identity in the process of action. Practicing hybridity, in this way, is ontoformative—it constantly (re)constitutes social reality in a processual and additive fashion. And thus, it allows those most affected by HIV/AIDS to navigate the symbolic, spiritual, and material boundaries that circumscribe daily life in South Africa's shantytowns.

The Myth of Incommensurability

Terence Ranger has shown that African "tradition" was an invention of colonial rule. Prior to colonization, there was no single "tribal" identity: "most Africans moved in and out of multiple identities. . . . Thus, the boundaries of the 'tribal' polity and the hierarchies of authority within them did *not* define conceptual horizons of Africans" (Ranger 2003, 248). In precisely this way, "tribal authority" was invented and sustained by the apartheid state in order to facilitate indirect rule (Mamdani 1996). Ranger explains, then, that not only was African "tradition" a *product* of modernity, but it was also *what made African modernization possible* (Ranger 2003). Once this "traditionalism" was firmly invented, applied to the Bantustans, and incorporated by chiefs, then the myth of incommensurability served to justify segregation by driving an essentialist wedge between a white, urban population interpellated as modern, and a rural population imprisoned within the spatial confines of Bantustans and the ideological constraints of "traditional authority."[61]

Despite these complications, some historians and social researchers continue to conceptualize "tradition" and "modernity" as teleological stages of social development.[62] Not only was African "tradition" an ideological construction of colonial rule, it was also never wholly embodied by the colonized. Those subjects apartheid most exploited were actually forced to live in both worlds simultaneously. As such, apartheid initiated the coexistence and mutual dependency of various heterogeneous kinds of indigenous and "modern" beliefs. But this hybridity occurred not only in urban settings, where subjects were literally straddling the system of indirect rule, but it was also common in rural settings. Most South Africans (no matter their location) participated in the modern economy and were controlled by modern forms of governance.[63] Therefore, the cultural boundaries established by the apartheid regime between "modernity" and "traditionalism" were necessarily flexible and malleable.

The symbolic struggle between the AIDS denialists and the treatment activists, which consumed the South African public sphere from at least 2000 through 2009, contributed to the reification of what I have termed "the myth of incommensurability": the notion that biomedical and indigenous treatments are irreconcilable and thus cannot (ontologically) and should not (scientifically) be combined. This has been done, in part, by grafting the colonial tropes of "modernity" and "traditionalism" onto health care choices. The users/consumers of healing, then, are asked to *choose* one or the other disposition and are told that a failure to do so could lead to further illness or even death. This perception has been exacerbated by the public provision of antiretrovirals, as patients are told, in no uncertain terms, not to mix the two forms of treatment.

Throughout this book, I have shown the various ways in which post-apartheid leaders have revitalized and reinvented the myth of incommensurability between "modernity" and "traditionalism" in an effort to resolve the paradoxes of postcolonialism. Through his fantasy of African renaissance, Mbeki strove to combine economic modernization with African nationalism, which also entailed a celebration of indigenous knowledge systems and a rejection of biomedical imperialism. Zuma, on the other hand, through his "rags to riches" narrative, attempted to identify with the poor and offer them technocratic developmental interventions, which were often cloaked in a performance of Zulu "indigeneity." He has, however, fully embraced biomedical orthodoxy, and citizenship has been increasingly biomedicalized under his reign. Each of these leaders utilized his own hybridity to strategically deploy the "modern" myth of incommensurability. The more biomedically orthodox players in the symbolic struggle over AIDS (like the Treatment Action Campaign, biomedical health professions, and policy makers), however, never learned to play the hybridity game. They subscribed to the myth of modernization, which is premised on atomizing and bifurcating the "modern" and "traditional" (Latour 1991). The poor sometimes deploy the tropes of "modernity" and "traditionalism" in a polarizing fashion in an effort to resist biomedical hegemony and the imposition of cultural neoimperialism, but they also *use* hybridity to survive increasingly polarized forms of structural inequality.

The tropes of "modernity" and "traditionalism" are constructed, but they operate with political and symbolic force. The subjects of apartheid were forced to live between the "modern" and the "traditional" worlds constructed and policed by the apartheid system—they learned to traverse these divides, but also to strategically deploy the languages and symbolic practices associated with each in order to survive and resist. Under the post-apartheid system, the division between the "modern" and the "traditional" is flexible and constantly shifting, but heavily relies on and (re)inforces historically reified ontological binaries (of race, class, and gender). Yet, the subjects of the post-apartheid system are no less savvy in their strategic navigation of the postcolonial world of binaries. Hybridities, in this analysis, are embodied but also tactically deployed.

Life Strategies

On Saturday, August 20, 2005, I was invited to a community gathering in Sol Plaatjie. Up until this point, I had mainly worked with the HIV/AIDS support group, so Thulani wanted to introduce me to the general population of Sol Plaatjie, tell them about my research, and get their feedback and response. When I arrived, before I even had a chance to get out of my car, a community member I had never met approached me: "My children and I are suffering because there are no jobs and there is no food. I cannot provide my children with an education without money—this is their only means of escaping what I have had to endure. They live in shacks without water and electricity and life is very hard for us." This speech and the expectation that if I was going to conduct research in this community, I should do something to improve it, was repeated again and again throughout the day. One man minced no words: "Do you see this filth that we live in? Do you smell the stink of the sewers and the shit that runs through our streets? Do you see how we live? Should *any* human being be forced to live like this? We don't have water or electricity, we live in shacks, we don't have jobs or money—do you *see* this?" "Yes," I replied. "So?" he said, "Make a plan. What are you going to do about it?"[1]

I tell this story, in part, because the image of the AIDS sufferer in a "Third World" shantytown has become a kind of fetish in the dominant, mainstream, Western media. It is as if the more the story gets told, the easier it becomes to understand inequity as a necessary by-product of the rest of the world's development and progress. One of the most enduring legacies of neoliberalism has been an increasing acceptance of structural inequalities as sad, but inevitable features of the landscape of advanced modernity. As all fetishes do, it allows us to avoid really thinking about the trauma and truth it symbolizes and represents. But lest we forget our own complicity and complaisance, I think these stories must be told in the most realistic and brutal terms possible.

But I also tell this story because of the challenge it presents to academics. Indeed, what *is* our responsibility to the communities we study? In recent years, there have been a number of advances in AIDS activism and research, which have triggered hopeful conjectures (from scientists, academics, and activists alike) that we are finally glimpsing the end of the pandemic. People have celebrated the funding the Western world has given to the continent of Africa for treatment over the past decade; how new discoveries in the world of "treatment as prevention" might finally reverse the trend of two-new-infections-for-every-person-beginning-antiretroviral-treatment; how voluntary male circumcision and new efforts at preventing mother-to-child transmission have halved HIV infection risk; and how new advances in vaccine research may finally augur a "cure." While these predictions are certainly comforting and even seductive, they also reveal an enduring conviction that technocratic biomedical (and neoliberal) interventions will someday bring salvation.

A few weeks before I planned to return to Johannesburg in 2012, I discovered that my friend Thulani, whose story inspired much of my analysis in the book, had died. It happened quite suddenly. He caught pneumonia in March and began antiretroviral therapy immediately. But it was too late. He was plagued with one illness after another and passed away in the middle of the night on April 14, 2012. He was only thirty-five. Thulani had dedicated his life to fighting the injustices his community experienced. He was such an energetic and dynamic person—always busy running from one meeting to the next, from one household to another, to help those in need. It was difficult for me to even imagine him sick, let alone gone. Thulani's life and death are a testament to the failure of this form of technocratic "salvation."

Shit still runs through the streets of Sol Plaatjie. Women and children in Lawley still face the threat of sexual violence, as they walk for miles to attend the closest clinic. So many of the people whose stories were told in this book still go to bed hungry, not sure how they will get through the next day, let alone the next year. And so, one of the primary duties I feel I have to the communities I studied is to unveil the ways in which technocratic interventions and their imperialistic undertones have failed to resolve the crises of neoliberal capitalism.

After ten years of conducting research on HIV/AIDS in South Africa and after having been told tremendously intimate details of people's everyday lives, I feel I have another equally important responsibility to the people whose stories fill the pages of this book. And that is to expand the boundaries of the polis by discussing the political nature of survival. In this era of advanced marginality, people's everyday trajectories—the ways in which they strive and thrive—constitute a radical form of politics in their own right.

For Giorgio Agamben (1998), "bare life"[2] is that which had been *excluded* from political life in the premodern era, but which is increasingly politicized under modernity, as the state begins to concern itself with the reproductive habits, healthiness, and food consumption of its population. Foucault labeled this historical moment the birth of biopower (1990). Theorists of contemporary biopower have argued that since the end of World War II, a whole host of "powerful agencies within states and transnational bodies" have given rise to a "bioethical complex," and the management of life has become the domain of increasingly more nonstate actors in order to increase the human capital of the nation as a whole (Rabinow and Rose 2006, 203). As such, the market, citizenship, and the production of knowledge are all marshaled toward the goal of fostering and capitalizing on life. According to Nikolas Rose, this latest era of biopolitics is marked by a certain biologization of the politics of life: "As human beings come to experience themselves in new ways as biological creatures, as biological selves, their vital existence becomes a focus of government, the target of novel forms of authority and expertise, a highly cathected field of knowledge, an expanding territory for bioeconomic exploitation, an organizing principle of ethics, and that stake in a molecular vital politics" (2007, 4).

Alongside or in response to this effort to govern and control the politics of life, the struggles of the population also unfold on the terrain of life. Sometimes this takes the shape of communities forging bonds over a common biosocial identity (Rose and Novas 2005; Petryna 2002; Nguyen 2010). But this focus on contestations over the "biomedical definition of life" (Comaroff 2007, 206) obscures a much more generalized struggle on the part of those who have been rendered disposable by the neoliberal market. For those on the margins of the new biopolitical social body, the fight is for health care, for water and electricity, for housing, for sustainable livelihoods, but also for spiritual freedom, for cultural autonomy, and for community solidarity. In other words, they do not simply toil to survive, they struggle for their very identities and selves. These are the life strategies[3] of the poor.

As the focus of governance has shifted increasingly to the "political technologies of individuals" to manage and discipline the way people conduct themselves (Foucault 1985; 1988; 1991), resistance is increasingly forged through technologies of the self. For Foucault, it is through these technologies that people "work" on their "ethical substance"—the "raw material of the self" (Foucault 1985, 26; Nguyen 2010, 39). HIV-infected residents of South Africa's squatter camps work daily to navigate structural obstacles, to forge community links and networks, to access healing, to remake and reinterpret their cultural beliefs and practices—they work, in other words, to take care of their selves. Through these life strategies, their subjectivities are constituted and reworked—as individuals and as communities. And these pathways to livelihood are also ontoformative—they reconstruct and remake the social world in which they live.

In making use of the life stories and itineraries of AIDS sufferers living on the periphery of Johannesburg, I redraw the map of the city outlined by the bodies of those who are poor, hunted, suffering, and in search of care. I show how, far from being immobile, the sick body moves and travels. In doing so, it shuttles constantly between private and public spaces, unveiling the city through its movements. I show how the body afflicted with AIDS itself constitutes an archetypal figure in the city of Johannesburg and how, in its search for care and for sanctuary, it acts as a place of mediation and meeting between the public and the private, the official and the unofficial, the here and the elsewhere. (Le Marcis 2004, 454)

Frédéric le Marcis (2004) traces the routes of the "suffering body" in Johannesburg and thus highlights the ways in which people's daily trajectories get caught up in and often reconfigure markets of exchange, circuits of care, and the boundaries of the polis. Inspired by his approach, I have shown, throughout this book, how people deploy various life strategies to navigate structural obstacles, access the means of social reproduction, and thus forge not only new technologies of the self but also new forms of biopolitical resistance.

Pheello was very sick and in and out of the hospital for several months in 2005. When I visited him in the hospital and he could see that I was quite concerned about his condition, he used to say to me,

"Claire, don't you worry. I'm a fighter." And Pheello is a fighter. He wouldn't have survived if he weren't. But Pheello never fights only for his own survival; he fights so that one day, people will not be made to suffer the way he has. Pheello would use the hospital wards to mobilize other patients to oppose the government's denialism and neglect and become activists in the struggle for quality public health care. Often when I visited him, when he wasn't too sick, he would be holding court at another patient's bed. When I asked him what he was discussing, he said that he was trying to inspire hope in them. He was telling them not to give up, but to demand better health care, and together, they could fight for their lives.

With growing inequality, the informalization of the economy, and the devastation wrought by AIDS, people's subjectivities have been destabilized. Through the embodiment of the insecurity that haunts their daily lives, their habitus have been rendered precarious. This has a whole array of effects on their navigation of the post-apartheid health and welfare system, not to mention the constitution of their families and communities. And yet, people continue to "get by," to *ukuphanda* as they say, *and*, in so doing, they forge new senses of belonging and new communities while they struggle for life in South Africa's slums.

Notes

1. Those subjects whose names are used in this study have consented to the use of their names. All other participants' identities remain confidential.
2. Soweto is actually a conglomeration of multiple townships, coined as such by a committee in 1963 to refer to its location vis-à-vis Johannesburg: *South West Townships*. Soweto's population is approximately 1.5 million, and it covers an area of about thirty square miles (Ashforth 2005, 21). Most of modern Soweto was built in the 1950s and 1960s. The Council for Scientific and Industrial Research and the National Building Research Institute produced designs for "low-cost, four-roomed, 40-square-metre houses which were soon to spring up in identical rows all over the Witwatersrand" (Bonner and Segal 1998, 28). These "matchbox" houses still mark Soweto's vast landscape. For more information on the history of Soweto, see Bonner and Segal 1998.
3. Interview with Sibusiso Skhosana and Bongani Sibeko held on June 28, 2009, in Sol Plaatjie.
4. Informal settlement is the official government classification for shack settlements established on open land—as opposed to shacks constructed in occupied buildings or backyard shacks in formal townships.
5. Interview with Thulani Skhosana held on May 30, 2009, in Sol Plaatjie.
6. The Natives Act, No. 67, of 1952, required Africans to carry a "pass book" at all times, which provided the person's name, photograph, place of origin, employment, tax and criminal record. Inability to produce a pass book was a

criminal offense. Further, according to amendments made to the Native Urban Areas Act in the 1950s, Africans were required to obtain a permit to travel from a rural to an urban area, and once arriving in a city, the person had to find employment within seventy-two hours. Without employment, Africans were not permitted to live in urban areas. Therefore, Africans had to violate the "pass laws" in order to secure work, and people living in urban areas were under constant threat of harassment and arrest.

7. Interview with Thulani Skhosana held on June 5, 2006, in Johannesburg.

8. All of this information was provided by Sibusiso Skhosana and Bongani Sibeko in an interview held on June 28, 2009, in Sol Plaatjie.

9. Interview with Bongani Sibeko held on June 28, 2009, in Sol Plaatjie.

10. Interview with Thulani Skhosana held on June 5, 2006, in Johannesburg.

11. Interview with Bongani Sibeko held on June 28, 2009, in Sol Plaatjie.

12. Interview with Thulani Skhosana held on June 25, 2006, in Johannesburg.

13. Interview with Thulani Skhosana held on September 30, 2005, in Sol Plaatjie.

14. Ibid.

15. Field notes, June 9, 2005, Sol Plaatjie.

16. Female participant in a focus group discussion (FGD) held on October 20, 2005, in Lawley.

17. The challenge of AIDS was also mentioned in the Reconstruction and Development Programme (Heywood 2004b, 8). Nattrass suggests that this initial AIDS plan showed early support for a comprehensive and "uniquely effective drive against AIDS," which was quickly undermined by the first signs of denialism, which began to emerge in 1999 (Nattrass 2008a, 158).

18. For further information on the epidemic in its early years, see van der Vliet 1994; Department of Health 2001; Abt. Associates 2000.

19. Nelson Mandela was the leader of the ANC during the anti-apartheid struggle. He was imprisoned on Robben Island for twenty-seven years and was released in 1990. He was the first democratically elected leader of post-apartheid South Africa, and he served only one term, from 1994 through 1999.

20. Annually, from 1990, the Department of Health estimated national HIV prevalence rates based on survey data collected from pregnant women attending antenatal (prenatal) clinics. Because pregnant women attending public clinics represent the population *most* likely to be infected with the disease, there has been vast speculation that the statistics gleaned from these antenatal surveys *over*estimate the prevalence of HIV infection (Zuma 2007). In 2009 the National HIV and Syphilis Sero-Prevalence Survey estimated that 29.4 percent of pregnant women were living with HIV (Department of Health 2009). In 2002, 2005, and 2008, the Human Sciences Research Council (HSRC) conducted national randomized household surveys. The 2008 HSRC survey found that the national HIV prevalence in the population of people two years and older is estimated to

be 10.9 percent (HSRC 2008a). The HSRC study is considered to be a low estimate of HIV prevalence because of the difficulties of collecting blood samples (Levinsohn 2007). Therefore, the actual prevalence rate may be somewhere in between these two percentages. Both surveys indicate that the prevalence rate has stabilized since 2006. See Marais 2005 for further information.

21. *Prevalence* refers to the total number of cases of a disease in a particular population at a particular time. *Incidence* refers to the number of *new* infections occurring in a particular population during a particular time interval.

22. UN-HABITAT has found that South Africa's *cities* have the most unequal distribution of income in the world (2009, 72).

23. The post-apartheid era is often referred to as the "new" South Africa or the "new dispensation."

24. This is a rather vast set of literatures, but see, for example: Nandy 1983; Comaroff and Comaroff 1991; Bhabha 1994; Cooper and Stoler 1997; Chakrabarty 2000.

25. Much scholarship has focused on the reasons for the post-apartheid state's adoption of neoliberalism, citing, to name but a few: the need to address severe economic disparity and uneven development, the crisis of over-accumulation, the rise of finance capital, and the particularities of South Africa's own economic bases. There was widespread fear that capital would flee the country along with the white elite if apartheid should fall. The post-apartheid state accepted the apartheid government's international debt of $20 billion because they were frightened that a refusal of the debt would scare away foreign investment, which South Africa was desperate to attract after the boycott and divestment campaigns of the 1970s and 1980s. In addition, the post-apartheid state wanted to sustain its dominant economic position on the continent. For further information on how the adoption of neoliberalism played an integral role in South Africa's transition to democracy, see Marais 2001 and 2005; Bond 2000 and 2002.

26. Hunter (2010) suggests GEAR was rolled out in 1996 in the wake of rumors circulating about Mandela's poor health, which caused the currency to plummet; however, the foreign investment the ANC so desperately sought to attract never arrived (107).

27. Thabo Mbeki was deputy president under Nelson Mandela, and he became the second democratically elected South African president in 1999. He served for almost two full terms, until he resigned in September 2008 (after having been ousted from the leadership of the ANC in December 2007). The politics of Mbeki's presidency are the topic of chapter 2.

28. Gillian Hart explores this possibility in a complex and detailed way in her 2006 article, while simultaneously illustrating the "slippages, openings and contradictions" that characterize such governmental power (14).

29. I use "fantasy" in a psychoanalytically informed way. Contrary to popular usage, fantasy is *not* simply a cover story for a truth that is too horrifying to face (Žižek 1997, 7). Rather than offering an escape from reality, fantasies are constitutive of it (Žižek 1989). Because they originate at the moment of the subject's constitution, which is experienced as lack, they are inherently contradictory—they elicit both pleasure and antagonism on the part of the subject, toward the object of its desire. Because they are forged through imaginary identifications, they are extremely fragile and are in constant peril, and so must be told again and again, especially when at risk of exposure (ibid.). And yet, as narratives, they attempt to occlude the paradoxes inherent within them (Žižek 1997, 13).

30. Jacob Zuma is the third democratically elected president of South Africa. He was deputy president under Mbeki until June 2005, when he was charged with corruption and asked to resign. In addition to corruption, Zuma was accused of raping an HIV-positive woman who was a long-time family friend. Zuma admitted that he had unprotected sex with the woman but claimed it was consensual. His trial and acquittal of rape took place in May 2006. In December 2007, Zuma beat Mbeki in a race for the leadership of the ANC. In April 2009, he was acquitted of all corruption charges and won the national presidency in a landslide victory. The politics of Zuma's presidency is the topic of chapter 4.

31. See also Bhabha 1990.

32. Interview with Thulani Skhosana held on June 5, 2006, in Johannesburg.

33. Several postcolonial theorists have pointed to the way in which the indigenous are used to build the nation, but are simultaneously an obstacle to successful nation building (Comaroff and Comaroff 1993; Vincent 2006).

34. Interview with Thulani Skhosana held on June 18, 2009, in Sol Plaatjie.

35. Antiretrovirals are the biomedical treatment for HIV. In South Africa, they are often referred to as ARVs or ART (antiretroviral treatment). They are usually taken in combinations of three drugs, from three different *classes* of medications, including: nucleoside reverse transcriptase inhibitors, non-nucleoside reverse transcriptase inhibitors, and protease inhibitors. Combining the drugs in these "cocktails" delays drug resistance and suppresses the virus. The therapy is sometimes referred to as HAART (Highly Active Antiretroviral Therapy).

36. It has been estimated that 365,000 people died as a direct result of denialism (Chigwedere et al. 2008; Dugger 2008).

37. Interview with AIDS Law Project (ALP) activist on November 24, 2005, in the Johannesburg ALP offices.

38. Following other scholars, such as Kleinman 1988; Farmer 1992 and 1999; Biehl 2005.

39. Between 2002 and 2009, I conducted thirty months of ethnographic research in one formal township and two informal settlements outside

of Johannesburg where I participated regularly in community activities and the lives of people living with HIV/AIDS. I conducted focus group discussions with 250 people, including community stakeholders in each community, people living with HIV/AIDS, indigenous healers, and home-based care workers. I conducted multiple in-depth interviews with 165 people in my different research sites, including people living with HIV/AIDS, home-based caregivers, NGO staff, nurses and doctors, indigenous healers, spiritual healers, activists, and government officials.

CHAPTER ONE

1. Interview with Pheello Limapo held on April 15, 2005, in the Johannesburg LPM offices.
2. Field notes, July 16, 2005, Johannesburg.
3. Nevirapine was an antiretroviral drug given to mothers during childbirth (and to the child directly after birth) to reduce the chances of the child contracting HIV. This policy is no longer used in South Africa. See footnote 58 in this chapter.
4. Interview held with Pheello Limapo on August 18, 2005, in Lawley.
5. Interview with Pheello Limapo held on April 15, 2005, in the Johannesburg LPM offices.
6. Interview with Pheello Limapo held on December 8, 2005, in Lawley.
7. Influx controls is the name given to any legal measures the apartheid state used to control the inflow of Africans to urban areas. The pass laws (the primary example of influx controls) were finally abolished by P. W. Botha in 1986.
8. Gauteng is the province in which Johannesburg, Soweto, and both Lawley and Sol Plaatjie are situated. It is also home to the executive (administrative) and de facto national capital of South Africa, Pretoria.
9. These statistics, as well as those used in the descriptions of Lawley and Sol Plaatjie later in the chapter, emerge from a community participatory research (CPR) survey I conducted in both communities in June/July 2009. Five hundred households in each community were surveyed (approximately 10 percent of the population). I use "CPR survey 2009" throughout the book to cite data gathered from this survey.
10. "South Africa is the only country that is ensuring that the poorest of the poor have access to land, and are assisted to get houses," said Strike Ralegoma, Johannesburg Mayoral Committee Member for Housing, on November 29, 2007 (Davie 2007).
11. South Africa has been harshly criticized for its adoption of the "willing seller/willing buyer" approach to land redistribution as well. Land redistribution relies on voluntary transactions through the market, assisted by grants from the state. The World Bank actively promoted this approach as an alternative to state-led land reform. It is this policy that most argue

is responsible for the fact that only 7 percent of the land in South Africa (90 percent of which was owned by white South Africans at the end of apartheid) has been redistributed (Lahiff 2010).

12. Huchzermeyer explains: "This subsidy requires home-ownership of a standardised housing unit, and has been translated into large-scale developments of uniform, free-standing, mostly one-roomed houses with individual freehold title in standardised township layouts located on the urban peripheries" (2001, 306).

13. They are also poorly built, and there have been innumerable complaints of their shoddy construction.

14. This policy was the eventual outcome of a long struggle by slum dwellers. In 2007, the province of KwaZulu-Natal introduced a Slum Elimination Act, which was fiercely resisted by the social movement Abahlali base-Mjondolo (which translates to "Shack Dwellers" in Zulu). This movement argued successfully in Constitutional Court that the act violated citizens' constitutional right to housing, which ultimately prevented the state from eliminating shacks without providing alternative housing (Hunter 2010, 224). For further information on the movement, see http://www.abahlali .org/.

15. As of 2010, it was estimated that one-quarter of Johannesburg's 3.9 million residents lived in informal settlements (Vearey 2010, 40). Given that the population of the city is anticipated to climb to 5.2 million by 2015 (ibid.), the city could be battling an ever-expanding population of shack dwellers, despite its efforts to formalize informal settlements. This problem is discussed later in the chapter.

16. Undermining is simply land that is stripped from mining gold, and dolomite is a mineral that is soluble, so it dissolves over time, producing cave systems and voids in rock (Department of Public Works 2003). Both of these conditions can lead to sinkholes.

17. During the anti-apartheid struggle, the African population engaged in "rent boycotts"—the nonpayment of housing rent and municipal services—to protest the apartheid state's usage of local African authorities to regulate the townships. This form of resistance helped to make townships ungovernable. Once apartheid ended, the post-apartheid state was intent on combating what came to be understood as a growing "culture of nonpayment" among the African population.

18. For further information on the privatization of basic services in South Africa and the social movement response to it, see McDonald and Ruiters 2005; von Schnitzler 2008; McKinley and Veriava 2010.

19. Interview with Thulani Skhosana held on May 30, 2009, in Sol Plaatjie.

20. Interview with local government councilor Alfred Mudau on June 24, 2009.

21. The Soweto Uprising began on June 16, 1976, when school kids throughout Soweto took to the streets to protest the introduction of Afrikaans as

the language of instruction. The riot police were called in and tear gas and live bullets were used against the students. The day is now a national holiday, referred to as Youth Day.

22. The history of Sol Plaatjie was provided in part by Thulani Skhosana in an interview held on June 5, 2006, and by Bongani Sibeko and Sibusiso Skhosana on June 28, 2009. Details were confirmed through a series of archival documents available in the South African History Archives, housed at the William Cullen Library at the University of the Witwatersrand, Collection AL2878, Freedom of Information Programme, Special Projects A6 on South African Migration. Additional information was available at the Centre for Applied Legal Studies (CALS) at the University of the Witwatersrand, which represented the residents of Mandelaville in their court case against the city of Johannesburg.

23. Interview held with Thulani Skhosana on June 5, 2006, in downtown Johannesburg.

24. Interview held with local government councilor Alfred Mudau, on June 24, 2009, in Roodepoort.

25. The reason for the usage of this form of housing (called C-type), which looks like a row of townhouses connected to one another (see the images), is because land was too expensive in Sol Plaatjie to give each person her own stand. This type of housing accommodated more people in less physical space, but the residents see their allotment as an unfair apportionment of their constitutional right to housing.

26. Interview held with Bongani Sibeko on June 28, 2009, in Sol Plaatjie.

27. Interview with local government councilor Alfred Mudau on June 24, 2009, in Roodepoort.

28. Ibid.

29. Ibid.

30. Under apartheid, there were four racial groupings: White (approximately 13 percent of the population), "Indian" (3 percent), "Coloured" (9 percent), and African (75 percent). In 1970, the African population was further segregated by ethnicity.

31. Affidavits, oral testimonies, letters, and court proceedings for a court case in which ten individuals were charged with illegal squatting in Lawley in 1987 were available in the Wits Historical Papers, Collection A2346, "Community Research and Information Network." Box D14 on Informal Settlements.

32. The red ants are what South Africans call the dreaded eviction squad "Wozani Security" because of the red overalls they wear. The red ants are poor South Africans the state hires to carry out the unpopular work of dismantling illegal shack settlements.

33. FGD held in Lawley with community leaders on June 19, 2009.

34. Member of the Executive Council. Each of South Africa's nine provinces has its own legislative and executive governments. The executive govern-

ment is made up of a provincial premier and members of his/her executive council.

35. FGD held in Lawley with community leaders on June 19, 2009.

36. Field notes, April 15, 2005, Johannesburg.

37. FGD with community leaders held on June 19, 2009, in Lawley. This story was essentially corroborated by the local government councilor, Paul Molutsi, in an interview held on June 25, 2009, in Ennerdale.

38. Pheello told me this on a tour of the community on June 2, 2009, and Teboho Mohapi (a local community leader involved in the upgrades) corroborated it in an interview held on June 25, 2009.

39. Interview with Pheello Limapo held on June 2, 2009, in Lawley.

40. Ibid.

41. See, for example, Norman et al. 2010; Vearey et al. 2010; Sanders and Chopra 2006; Shisana et al. 2005; Thomas, Seager, and Mathee 2002.

42. I borrow the term "environmental suffering" from Javier Auyero and Débora Swistun's book *Flammable* (2009).

43. Female participant in FGD held on October 6, 2005, in Lawley.

44. Female participant in FGD held on October 20, 2005, in Lawley.

45. Male participant in FGD held on October 14, 2005, in Sol Plaatjie.

46. Female participant in FGD held on June 10, 2006, in Sol Plaatjie.

47. Male participant in FGD held on June 10, 2006, in Sol Plaatjie.

48. Interview with home-based care worker in Lawley on June 17, 2009.

49. A *veld* is an Afrikaans word meaning "rural plain." This was said in an FGD in Lawley held on June 21, 2009.

50. This was mentioned again and again in FGDs with Lawley residents. I consistently asked why residents would throw trash into their own water supply, and the response was generally that "people don't care about one another," or "some people want to hurt others." I will return to this issue later in the chapter.

51. Male participant in FGD held on October 20, 2005, in Lawley.

52. A *spaza* shop is an informal convenience shop usually operated out of a home. They are also referred to as "tuck" shops.

53. "Bara" is what people call the Chris Hani Baragwanath Hospital in Soweto.

54. Interview with Pheello Limapo on June 2, 2009, in Lawley.

55. Ibid.

56. FGD held on October 14, 2005, in Sol Plaatjie.

57. Female resident of Sol Plaatjie, interview held on June 20, 2009.

58. Due to concerns about the development of drug resistance and the efficacy of the treatment, the World Health Organization provided new guidelines that suggested nevirapine should *not* be used for MTCTP in 2010, but rather should be replaced by enrolling HIV-infected pregnant women on a lifelong ART program. This policy also reduces the chances

of vertical transmission through breast-feeding. As of 2010, this is the new policy in South Africa (WHO 2010b).

59. Field notes, June 6, 2006, Johannesburg. A member of the APF said this after visiting Sol Plaatjie for the first time and being asked of his impressions.

60. "Transactional sex" refers to the cultural expectation that women will receive gifts and/or financial subsistence from the men with whom they are engaged in sexual relations (that are often lasting). This phenomenon will be discussed in detail in chapter 4.

61. Field notes, December 19, 2005, Soweto.

62. Interview held with Thulani Skhosana on May 20, 2006, in Sol Plaatjie.

63. Female respondent in FGD held on June 10, 2009, in Lawley.

64. Interview held with female HIV/AIDS activist on April 15, 2005, in Soweto.

65. This number varies by municipality, but this is the most common threshold point used to define indigence. The term indigent means "lacking the necessities of life," therefore, indigence is not only calculated on the basis of income, but also includes insufficient access to water, sanitation, health care, environmental health, basic energy, and housing. In post-apartheid South Africa, if you are registered by the government as indigent, you have the right to extended free basic services (Department of Provincial and Local Government 2005).

66. A *shebeen* is an unlicensed drinking establishment.

67. Interview with Pheello Limapo on June 2, 2009, in Lawley.

68. Male respondent in FGD held on July 4, 2009, in Sol Plaatjie.

69. Interview with Pheello Limapo on June 21, 2009, in Lawley.

70. Field notes, August 8, 2005, Lawley.

71. Female participant in FGD held on July 3, 2009, in Lawley.

72. Female participant in FGD held on June 10, 2009, in Lawley.

73. Field notes, December 20, 2005, in Sol Plaatjie.

74. Reviews of the vast literature on stigma can be found in Deacon, Stephney, and Prosalendis 2005.

75. I volunteered with a prominent NGO in Soweto from December 1, 2004, to September 30, 2005. During this time I worked extensively with support groups in Zola; Dobsonville; and Orlando East, Soweto.

76. Interview with Thulani Skhosana held on September 30, 2005, in Sol Plaatjie.

77. Field notes, June 15, 2009, Lawley.

78. Female participant in an FGD held on June 10, 2006, in Sol Plaatjie.

79. Female participant in an FGD held on June 10, 2006, in Sol Plaatjie.

80. Interview held with Thulani Skhosana on May 20, 2006, in Sol Plaatjie.

81. FGD held in Lawley on June 10, 2009.

82. This was mentioned by Sibusiso Skhosana and Bongani Sibeko in an interview held on June 29, 2009, by Thulani in an interview on June 5, 2006,

NOTES TO CHAPTER 1

and by the local government councilor, Alfred Mudau, in an interview on June 24, 2009.

83. Inkatha Freedom Party (IFP). During the political struggles against apartheid, there was a lot of violent disagreement between the IFP and the ANC. The ANC accused the National Party (the party responsible for apartheid) of paying the IFP (which was largely made up of Zulus from the KwaZulu-Natal province) to incite intraethnic violence among the African population, as a means of undermining the anti-apartheid struggle as a whole. The ANC labeled this secret state operation the "Third Force." In the Johannesburg region, six thousand people were killed because of this violence between the years of 1990 and 1994 (Ashforth 2005, 269). During the Truth and Reconciliation process, the apartheid state and the IFP refused to admit to this strategy, but most ANC members believe this is the only explanation for the brutal "Black-on-Black" violence that plagued the townships as apartheid was falling.

84. Interview with Teboho Mohapi held on June 25, 2009, in Lawley.

85. I borrow the concept of *habitus* from Pierre Bourdieu (1977, 1990, 2000). It refers to a set of acquired dispositions and strategy-generating skills for guiding social action. It is a subjective reflection of objectified symbolic and material structures. The theory will be explained in further detail in chapter 5.

86. FGD held on June 21, 2009, in Lawley.

87. Participants were always asked in advance if they wanted to conduct the interview in English, or if they would prefer I use an interpreter. Although I speak rudimentary Zulu, the complexity and the sensitivity of the issues being discussed necessitated interpretation. In addition, Zulu is not the primary language of many of my research participants, and Torong is fluent in eleven languages. Although there are certainly drawbacks to relying on interpretation in ethnographic research, I found more often than not that Torong's participation facilitated rather than hindered the research process.

88. Interviews were held in Orlando East, Soweto, on April 8, July 22, August 3, August 17, September 3, December 1, 2005, and July 13, 2009.

89. The ancestors can also intervene in people's lives in protective and beneficial ways. For example, if a person narrowly escapes a misfortune, s/he will usually attribute this to strong ancestral defenses.

90. These include, in addition to divination or knowledge of herbs, communication with Nguni ancestors and/or "foreign" and water spirits, or experience of *ngoma* ("embodied" knowledge) expressed through singing, dancing, and drumming (Thornton 2009, 23–24).

91. Sometimes the distinction between herbalists and diviners is categorized, rather than through the relationship to ancestors, through the relationship to the *ngoma* cult. This was Janzen's (1992) and Ngubane's (1992) means of distinguishing between the two.

92. Another primary difference between *inyangas* and *sangomas* is a gender division. Historically, *sangomas* were women, and *inyangas* were men (Xaba 2005). This has changed over time. I will discuss this further in chapter 5.
93. This was explained to me by Dr. Robert Tshabalala in an interview held on April 18, 2005, in Orlando East, Soweto. For further information, see Thornton 2002 and 2009.
94. I learned this by undergoing a consultation with Dr. Martha Mongoya on December 1, 2005, in Orlando East, Soweto.
95. I learned this means of divination through a consultation with Dr. Robert Tshabalala on December 2, 2005, in Diepkloof, Soweto.
96. Three female participants in an FGD held on June 13, 2005, in Pimville, Soweto.
97. Female indigenous healer in Lawley from an FGD held with healers on June 22, 2009.
98. Female indigenous healer in Lawley from an FGD held with healers on June 22, 2009.
99. Female respondent in FGD held in Lawley on June 21, 2009.
100. Female respondent from FGD held in Sol Plaatjie on June 28, 2009.
101. Male respondent from FGD held in Sol Plaatjie on June 28, 2009.
102. Field notes, July 14, 2009, Johannesburg.
103. Interview with Sibusiso Skhosana on June 28, 2009, in Sol Plaatjie.
104. Faraday market is a place in Johannesburg where *muthi* and animal products are sold.
105. An *imbiza* is an indigenous remedy used to cleanse the blood.
106. Female indigenous healer from an FGD with healers held in Lawley on June 22, 2009.
107. Female participant in FGD held on October 20, 2005, in Lawley.
108. Female participant in FGD held on June 10, 2006, in Sol Plaatjie.
109. It is from this participatory research project I helped to conduct for the Anti-Privatisation Forum that I borrow the phrase "The Struggle for Life"; see APF 2006.
110. It is important to note that these numbers may be low due to the fact that people are not necessarily forthcoming about discussing their usage of indigenous healing, especially with strangers.
111. Interview with Thulani Skhosana held on September 30, 2005, in Sol Plaatjie.
112. Male participant in FGD held on October 14, 2005, in Sol Plaatjie.
113. This occurred in a support group meeting held on Thursday, September 15, 2005, in Lawley, which was before antiretrovirals were readily available in the public health sector.
114. Interview held with Thulani Skhosana on September 30, 2005, in Sol Plaatjie.
115. Female participant in FGD held on October 20, 2005, in Lawley.
116. Female participant in FGD held on June 10, 2006, in Sol Plaatjie.

117. Interview held with Pheello Limapo on August 18, 2005, in Lawley.
118. Interview with Maria Tshukudu held on June 20, 2009, in Sol Plaatjie.
119. "Most funerals appear to cost approximately US$1,500. Compared with an average household income of between US$155 and US$308 per month, households can easily spend an amount comparable to approximately 7 months of income on one funeral" (Collins and Liebbrandt 2007, S77). For an even higher estimate of the cost of funerals, see page 50.
120. Many poor people invest large sums of money (which they could use to cover living expenses) to purchase funeral insurance or join a burial society. Ten million people in South Africa have funeral insurance; eight million belong to an informal burial society (Collins and Liebbrandt 2007, S77). There are approximately eighty to one hundred thousand burial societies in South Africa (ibid).
121. Most burials happen on Saturday—this is now the "fashion," but it also allows family members traveling from afar to attend the ceremony. During the week, the family will gather to figure out the logistics of the burial (scheme coverage, insurance, burial plots, ceremony planning, invitations, furnishing rental, and the purchasing of food). The family will visit the corpse at the mortuary and will bring the clothing the deceased will wear for the burial (as well as any keepsakes that should be placed in the casket). On Friday, before three, the hearse will deliver the casket (with the corpse in it) to the family house—before sunset. The casket will be placed inside the home, and the women will remain around the casket while the men hold vigil outside. The vigil lasts all night. In the morning people will all attend the funeral at the gravesite, followed by two full days of mourning at the homestead, lasting from after the funeral until sunset on Sunday night. (Interview held with Torong Ramela on August 13, 2005, at Avalon Cemetery, Soweto.)
122. Trucks.
123. There are, on average, eight hundred funerals a month at the Avalon cemetery alone (Davie 2009). After fears circulated that Avalon was close to capacity in 2009 (and that twenty-seven of Johannesburg's thirty-six cemeteries had already reached maximum capacity), the city purchased additional land to expand Avalon for R9.9 million (Cele 2011).

CHAPTER TWO

1. Mark Heywood is deputy chairperson of the South African National AIDS Council (SANAC), executive director of the AIDS Law Project (ALP), which is now called Section 27 (http://www.section27.org.za/), and former national treasurer of the Treatment Action Campaign (TAC). The quote is from an interview held on November 24, 2005, in the Johannesburg ALP offices.
2. This was not the only early sign of denialist tendencies within the ANC government. Nkosi Dlamini-Zuma (a former wife of the current president,

Jacob Zuma) was the first minister of health under Mandela. Although trained as a biomedical doctor, she refused to allow the government to dispense AZT and nevirapine to pregnant women to prevent mother-to-child transmission. In addition, she was implicated in the virodene scandal and was the cause of another scandal associated with the funding and promotion of *Sarafina II*, a musical performed on World AIDS Day in 2005. See Thornton (2008, 164–67), and Nattrass (2007, 41), for further details.

3. Virodene was tested outside of the country with financial support from the ANC, but its effectiveness was never established (Nattrass 2007, 43).

4. Myburgh (2012) suggests that "it was the Virodene researchers who introduced . . . President Mbeki to the 'dissident' or 'denialist' view of HIV/AIDS in October 1999. Mbeki seized on this literature to justify the . . . refusal to provide AZT through the public health care system."

5. The minister of health asked the Medicines Control Council (MCC) to review the safety of the drug before its use could be permitted (Heywood 2004b, 9).

6. Mbeki also never expressly stated that HIV did not cause AIDS (Heywood 2004b; Johnson 2005). He did, however, refuse to have an HIV test because it would be tantamount to "confirming a particular paradigm" (Nattrass 2007, 91). He also regularly refuted AIDS death statistics, claiming they were overestimated (Nattrass 2008a, 165; Nattrass 2007, 92–95).

7. The article was first circulated via e-mail, and the Microsoft Word's properties menu originally gave the name Thabo Mbeki in the author field (Thornton 2008, 251n34; Nattrass 2007, 91). Peter Mokaba, who died a year later, most likely from AIDS, is considered to be the coauthor (Thornton 2008, 178).

8. It quotes John le Carré's *Constant Gardener* (2000) directly.

9. It also quotes Herbert Marcuse's *Eros and Civilization* (1962): "in a period when the omnipotent apparatus punishes real nonconformity with ridicule and defeat" (243).

10. Like her predecessor, Tshabalala-Msimang was biomedically trained and initially exhibited a rather orthodox and progressive position on HIV/AIDS. In 1972, she founded the ANC's health department in exile. When she returned to South Africa, she immediately made HIV/AIDS a priority. She worked for the National Progressive Primary Health Care Network and sat on the National AIDS Convention of South Africa, which drew up an initial AIDS plan for the ANC in 1992–93. When she was first appointed minister of health in 1999, she tried to forge a connection between civil society and government in the battle against AIDS (Heywood 2004b, 12; Nattrass 2008a, 158).

11. In addition to Tshabalala-Msimang, Peter Mokaba, Smuts Ngonyama, and Ngoako Ramathlodi often used the venue of *ANC Today* to voice denialist claims once Mbeki stopped speaking publicly on the matter (Heywood 2004b, 15).

12. Information on the Treatment Action Campaign and the politics of international trade agreements are provided in chapter 3. Under the World Trade Organization's Agreement on Trade-Related Intellectual Property Rights (TRIPS), patent rights last twenty years. In order for a country to either generically produce or import a generic drug that is still under a pharmaceutical company's patent, it has to pass national legislation demanding parallel importing or the issuing of a compulsory license (which can only be done under certain conditions and often ends in trade sanctions issued by the United States). Or pharmaceutical companies can be "forced" to issue voluntary licenses—in which they "agree to" sell their drug for a reduced price or allow generic manufacturers to produce the drug. For further information on the Treatment Action Campaign and their struggle for treatment, see also Mbali 2005; Nattrass 2007; Heywood 2008 and 2009.

13. Highly Active Anti-Retroviral Therapy, HAART.

14. This discrepancy between provincial and national policy was made possible by the fact that in the political negotiations that took place between the ANC and the apartheid government preceding the transition, the ANC conceded to the establishment of a "quasi-federal political system to satisfy minority interests," where the control over social spending and policy implementation rests with the provincial government (Johnson 2005, 323; Schneider and Stein 2001).

15. The transmission of HIV from mother to child.

16. In December 2001, the Pretoria High Court ruled in favor of TAC's mother-to-child-transmission-prevention (MTCTP) campaign and ordered the government to implement a policy, but the government appealed the order. Then, in July 2002, the South African Constitutional Court ruled that the government's failure to make nevirapine widely available to pregnant women violated their constitutional right to health, and a single-dose nevirapine policy for women giving birth was rolled out as standard policy in public health clinics (Heywood 2009). As of 2010, this drug is no longer used. Based on new guidelines by the World Health Organization, South Africa now provides HIV-infected pregnant women with full course ART, which is not only safer, but also further reduces the chances of vertical transmission through either birth or breast-feeding (WHO 2010b).

17. For other sources that deconstruct Western representations of "AIDS in Africa," see Treichler 1999; Patton 2002; Comaroff 2007; Fassin 2007b.

18. In fact, the most famous TAC leader of that era, Zackie Achmat, is not white, but is part of the so-called "Indian" population.

19. Isaac Skhosana, Gauteng provincial chairperson of the TAC, admitted this was a popular critique in an interview held on November 9, 2005, in the TAC Johannesburg offices. I often heard this insinuation in my interviews with community activists and people living with HIV.

20. Mark Heywood acknowledged "a tension between the profile of the leadership and the base" (Friedman and Mottiar 2004, 11).

21. This is a topic to which I will return in the next chapter.

22. This bill was the product of twelve years of formulation and consultation, and yet the legislation was almost identical to the Health Professions Act (Act No. 56) of 1974 (Ashforth 2005, 293).

23. Doctors for Life International called the constitutionality of the first act into question on the basis of limited public consultation. Doctors for Life gave evidence in 1998 to the Parliamentary Committee on Health alleging that "primary health care should be *quality* health care and not *primitive* health care," which they asserted was inevitable if indigenous healers were sanctioned because many were "possessed," used toxic treatments and committed "muti murders" (Digby 2006, 437). The organization claims to uphold "sound scientific principles" on the basis of Christian ethics (ibid.; see also http://www.doctorsforlife.co.za/index.php/category/issues/alternative-medicine/). In August 2006, the Constitutional Court ruled in favor of the Doctors for Life. In 2007, parliament reenacted the act, which was assented to by President Mbeki in January 2008 (Republic of South Africa 2007; Doctors for Life 2006; Singh 2008). Despite the proceedings, the act was not much altered between 2005 and 2007.

24. Hunter (2010) makes a similar point when he notes that the "rights"/"tradition" binary is maintained by the ANC government through the constitution and its establishment of separate institutions to protect "modern rights" and "traditional" practices, such as the Human Rights Commission and the House of Traditional Leaders (8–9).

25. Interview with Dr. Sheila Khama held on July 14, 2009, in Johannesburg.

26. Interview held with Dr. Robert Tshabalala on April 8, 2005, in Orlando East, Soweto.

27. The Gauteng Traditional Healer's Task Team was a joint indigenous healing and Gauteng Department of Health (DOH) initiative. The Gauteng DOH invited members from different prominent indigenous healing associations based in Gauteng Province to meet with representatives of the DOH on a regular basis to attempt to build collaborative initiatives and to respond to the needs of the indigenous healing community—in regards to HIV/AIDS, TB, and STIs. I was an active member of the task team for six months in 2005 (from July 1 to December 20) and attended their bimonthly meetings and met with DOH and indigenous healing representatives individually. This provided me an opportunity to observe the relationship between the government and indigenous healers in the province in which I was working. This task team is no longer in existence.

28. Interview with Dr. Martha Mongoya held on July 13, 2009, in Orlando East, Soweto.

29. Dr. Liz Floyd, director of the Intersectoral HIV/AIDS Unit, Gauteng Department of Health, for example, attempted to promote indigenous heal-

ing, and the Gauteng Task Team was her own initiative. But she was a rare example within a much broader public health care system.

30. I was unable to secure interviews with members of Jacob Zuma's Ministry of Health, headed by Dr. Aaron Motsoaledi, about the status of the legislation and the registration and training of indigenous healers at present. It seems, however, that the institutionalization of indigenous healing is no longer a priority (or even a consideration) of the new more biomedically orthodox regime.

31. The specifics of this case (as well as its implications) will be discussed in the next chapter.

32. Interview held with AIDS Law Project (ALP) lawyer and activist on November 22, 2005, in the Johannesburg ALP offices.

33. See the following sources for further information: TAC 2005b; Rath Foundation 2005b.

34. Interview held with Mark Heywood, executive director of the AIDS Law Project, on November 24, 2005, in Johannesburg ALP Offices.

35. Brink told me in an interview that his work on the toxicity of AZT was what caused Mbeki to "order an inquiry into the safety of the drug in Parliament on the 28 October 1999." Interview held on May 20, 2005, in the Rath Foundation offices in Cape Town. James Myburgh also claims that the Vissers (the two scientists who introduced virodene at a cabinet meeting in 1997) brought Brink's papers on AZT to the president's attention (Nattrass 2008a, 160–61; see also Myburgh 2012).

36. In fact, this was a source of controversy. The Medicine Control Council (MCC) started an investigation into the safety of the vitamins Rath was distributing in early 2005, but then the original investigator was removed (Nattrass 2008a, 170). In an interview with a prominent AIDS Law Project advocate, Adila Hassim, I learned that several leaders of the MCC were removed during this era, prompting the TAC to file a lawsuit against the MCC. As Adila Hassim put it: "the old MCC was stopped. The new MCC's going to do whitewash" (interview held on November 14, 2005, in Cape Town ALP offices). Nattrass suggests: "The Health Minister appears to have succeeded in de-clawing the MCC, which now seems incapable of responding to complaints against the illegal trials undertaken by . . . Rath" (2008a, 171).

37. Interview with Rath Foundation spokesperson held on November 16, 2005, in the Rath Foundation offices in Cape Town.

38. Interview with Rath Foundation spokesperson held on May 20, 2005, in the Rath Foundation offices in Cape Town.

39. Ibid.

40. Interview with Anthony Brink held on May 20, 2005, in the Rath Foundation offices in Cape Town.

41. Interview with Anthony Brink held on November 16, 2005, in the Rath Foundation offices in Cape Town.

42. Local government councilors for Lawley and Sol Plaatjie were explicit about the connection between upgrading and the acceptance of prepaid meters. Interviews held with Paul Molutsi on June 25, 2009, in Ennerdale and Alfred Mudau, on June 24, 2009, in Roodepoort.

43. Many South Africans still did not pay their municipal service fees after the end of apartheid. Citizens began to accrue accumulated debt on these unpaid services. It was this accumulated debt that could be erased if citizens were labeled indigent and agreed to the installation of prepaid meters.

44. "Iketsetseng" is Sotho, and "vukuzenzele" is Zulu.

45. Interview with Pheello Limapo held on December 8, 2005, in Lawley.

46. Interview with Thulani Skhosana held on June 11, 2006, in Sol Plaatjie.

47. Hunter points out that the number of South Africans receiving social grants increased from 2.6 million in 1999 to more than 12 million in 2007 (2010, 225n8).

48. Social welfare is not provided on the basis of poverty alone; instead, South Africans qualify for state support if they are elderly, are the primary caregiver to a vulnerable child, or live with a disability.

49. A CD4 count (or T-cell count) measures the number of white blood cells per milliliter of blood. A healthy person has between 800 and 1,600 T-cells per milliliter of blood. According to a female participant in the FGD held on October 20, 2005, in Lawley, the disability grant was not initially linked to a person's CD4 count. She had applied and received a grant, which was then cut, not because her CD4 count went up, but because it was still too high to be eligible under the new cut-off point. This provides evidence to support my argument that the post-apartheid state changed their policies after the National Treatment Plan was passed in 2004.

50. The US government's Department of Health and Human Services HIV Treatment Guidelines recommends that people begin HIV treatment if they are suffering from a serious OI (opportunistic infection), or *before* the T-cell count falls below 350 (DHHS 2008).

51. Female participant in FGD held on June 21, 2009, in Lawley.

52. Female participant in FGD held on October 20, 2005, in Lawley. Emphasis added.

53. Female participant in FGD held on June 10, 2006, in Sol Plaatjie.

54. Interview held with Thulani Skhosana on June 11, 2006, in Sol Plaatjie.

55. Biopower can take two forms: disciplinary (focused at the level of the body) or regulatory (focused at level of the population)—thus modern power is both individualizing and massifying (Foucault 1997, 243). These forms of power often overlap and work in conjunction with each other and with sovereign power (Foucault 1991, 102). They also operate at multiple levels—in and through the state, social and civic institutions, regimes of knowledge and discourse, and through the production and regulation of technologies of the self.

56. Female participant in an FGD held on June 11, 2009, in Sol Plaatjie.
57. Foucault traces several historic shifts in the technologies of powers states use against contaminated populations. For example, in *Discipline and Punish* (1995, chapter 3) and again later in a series of lectures given at the *Collège de France* (Foucault 2003, January 15, 1975), he charts the different biopolitical strategies states used against lepers and then plague victims. Lepers were excluded, whereas an inclusive quarantine was utilized during the plague, which led to the rise of disciplinary practices and eventually, the disciplinary society. I am not suggesting that we are returning to a period of exclusion like the one established during the Middle Ages toward leper communities. Rather, following Foucault (as well as Rose, Deleuze, and Castel), I am suggesting that this new form of marginalization operates according to a certain laissez-faire logic, whereby exclusion operates on the basis of whether one is capable or willing to engage in constant risk calculation and self-entrepreneurialization. The state does not "have to" intervene because previous systems of exclusion and inequality have already rendered these populations precarious and incapable of living up to the demands of the control society (though this is not to say that extraordinary sovereign measures are not still likely, such as criminalizing an entire racial population). But here, the blame is placed on the individuals themselves, and their exclusion is not based on an inherent quality but rather on an incapacity.
58. Interview held with Thulani Skhosana on June 5, 2006, in downtown Johannesburg.
59. Interview held with Thulani Skhosana on May 20, 2006, in Sol Plaatjie.
60. These also tend to escalate around local government elections, so there was a renewed round of these protests in May 2011.
61. In 2005, the South African government pledged to eradicate the bucket system in South Africa. In 2009, the media unveiled that there were still 200,000 bucket toilets in use in municipalities around the country (SABC 2011).
62. For Julia Kristeva (1982), who was influenced by Mary Douglas's work and theory, the identity of the social being is constructed through the act of expulsing that which society deems polluted, that which jeopardizes the purity and sanctity of its integrity. However, these threatening elements (blood, semen, vomit, feces, as well as social acts, such as masturbation, incest, homosexuality, and prostitution) can never be fully annihilated; they continually and constantly threaten to disorder and dissolve the social, in its totality. Abjection demarcates the borders between self and other, and it is always a self that is imminently in danger of extinction, in a state of perpetual danger. Therefore, the abject constitutes a threshold between the internal and external, but because its indeterminacy is threatening, a solid and coherent boundary must be established and con-

stantly policed. Exclusionary rituals, therefore, are necessary to confirm and solidify both the body politic and the physical body.

CHAPTER THREE

1. Because many of its battles have been fought in the courts, the TAC has forged an enduring relationship with the AIDS Law Project (ALP), which was established by Edwin Cameron (who is currently a Supreme Court of Appeals justice) in 1993. The ALP helped to form the Treatment Action Campaign, and the two organizations share a lot of the same leadership (for example, Mark Heywood has held key administrative positions in both organizations). The ALP has served, throughout TAC's history, as its legislative arm; it has recently been incorporated into a new NGO, titled Section 27. See their website for further information: http://www.section27.org.za/.

2. On June 7, 2001, Andrew Natsios, the Bush administration's director of the US Agency for International Development (USAID), stated publicly in both the *Boston Globe* and in testimony before the House International Relations Committee, that antiretrovirals should not be promoted in the African context. "Ask Africans to take their drugs at a certain time of day, said Natsios, and they 'do not know what you are talking about'" (Attaran, Freedberg, and Hirsh 2001).

3. Interview held with ALP lawyer and activist on June 30, 2009, in the Johannesburg ALP offices.

4. The soteriological is concerned with bodily salvation from suffering and death. In general, technology and expertise are the tools of biomedical salvation. I would like to thank Stephanie Rieder for bringing the literature in medical anthropology on the soteriological dimensions of biomedicine to my attention. For further information, see Good 1994.

5. Fifteen people staged a one-day fast on the steps of St. George's Cathedral in Cape Town demanding medical treatment for people living with HIV. By the end of the day, they had collected over a thousand signatures calling for the government to develop an HIV/AIDS treatment plan (Robins 2008a, 116).

6. There is a great deal of scholarship dedicated to chronicling the history and achievements of the Treatment Action Campaign. For further information, see Heywood 2008 and 2009; Mbali 2005; Nattrass 2007; Robins 2008a; Friedman and Mottiar 2004; Achmat 2004; Cameron 2005; Jacobs and Johnson 2007; De Waal 2006. Also, their website: www.tac.org.za.

7. This campaign was also referred to as the Christopher Moraka Defiance Campaign, named after an activist who had died from thrush. Zackie Achmat went to Thailand and illegally smuggled five thousand capsules of generic fluconazole back into South Africa (Robins 2008a, 118).

8. Throughout this chapter, I often refer to TAC in a manner that suggests organizational coherence and homogeneity. There are moments when I try to point out debates among the leadership and differences emerging from different levels of the organizational structure or geographical regions; however, I did find that as a political actor, the organization succeeded in presenting itself as a united front. I conducted interviews with national, provincial, and municipal leaders as well as grassroots members of the organization in both Cape Town and Johannesburg, and I found that when asked about touchy political topics, their responses were surprisingly similar, suggesting a strong central organization and efficient communication of its political and ideological positions on important topics.

9. Prior to 2004, antiretroviral therapy was only available through the private sector and in a few pilot sites where nongovernmental organizations provided the drugs to select populations.

10. Interview with Xolani Kunene on December 12, 2005, in Johannesburg.

11. Interview with Thulani Skhosana on June 18, 2009, in Sol Plaatjie.

12. Interview with Mark Heywood held on November 24, 2005, in the Johannesburg ALP offices.

13. The byline of this newspaper article reads: "Safe-sex advocate who broke his own rules went to traditional healers, shunning new drugs" (*Observer* 2004).

14. Interview held with ALP lawyer and activist on November 22, 2005, in the Johannesburg ALP offices.

15. Interview held with female nurse at the Chris Hani Baragwanath Hospital, Soweto, in January 2003.

16. Interview held with female HIV-infected NGO worker in White City, Soweto, in February 2003.

17. Female participant of FGD held in Lawley on June 21, 2009.

18. Female participant of an FGD held in Sol Plaatjie on June 11, 2009.

19. Female participant of an FGD held in Sol Plaatjie on June 28, 2009.

20. Interview with a home-based caregiver in Lawley, held on June 17, 2009.

21. When HIV reproduces itself in the body, it often mutates (a mistake occurs in the genetic copying of its RNA or DNA). Some mutations are harmless, but certain mutations make HIV resistant to a particular ARV drug, meaning that drug is no longer capable of stopping HIV's replication. Drug resistance is more likely to develop if a person has gone on and off of the drugs, skipped dosages, or taken them singly or doubly, as opposed to in combinations of three or more. Drug resistant HIV is also transmissible.

22. In fact, there have been some historical studies testing toxicity in common indigenous treatments as well; see Digby (2006, 325–27). Digby notes two studies conducted in the early 1990s that found conclusive evidence of toxicity for treatments used during childbirth (Veale 1992; Hutchings and van Staden 1994).

23. In 2009, a group of academics wrote an open letter to the MCC indicating that its failure to regulate "complementary medicines" marketed, advertised, and widely used in South Africa was a violation of the constitution and the Medicines and Related Substances Act (Act 101 of 1965) (TAC 2009b). In fact, the MCC's capacity and commitment had been earlier called into question surrounding its failure to investigate the vitamins distributed by the Rath Foundation (Nattrass 2008a). It was widely believed that the MCC was being "remote controlled by the . . . incompetent Minister of Health, Manto Msimang [sic]" (interview with Isaac Skhosana, TAC's Gauteng provincial chairperson, held on May 18, 2006, in Johannesburg TAC offices). This same sentiment was expressed by an entire cadre of TAC activists and ALP lawyers I interviewed in late 2005 and early 2006, at the height of the Rath Foundation fiasco. In fact, when TAC filed court papers against the Rath Foundation, it simultaneously filed papers against the MCC and the minister of health (in addition to other parties they believed were guilty of collaboration with the Rath Foundation) (Thornton 2008, 187).

24. See Adams 2002 for a fascinating account of the contradictions that emerged when biomedical scientists conducted clinical trials on Tibetan medicines.

25. Interview held with indigenous healer, Dr. Koka, on September 7, 2005, in Noord Wyk, Johannesburg.

26. Female participant in an FGD with indigenous healers held on September 5, 2005, in Soweto.

27. Interview with indigenous healer, Dr. Sheila Khama, on July 14, 2009, in Johannesburg.

28. Interview with ALP lawyer held on November 22, 2005, in Johannesburg ALP offices.

29. Interview held with Phephsile Maseko, acting chair of the THO, on May 15, 2005, in the THO offices in Johannesburg.

30. Jonathan Berger, head of the Law and Treatment Access Unit, AIDS Law Project. Interview held on November 24, 2005, in the Johannesburg ALP Offices.

31. "The government did not have antiretrovirals in mind when it drafted the bill; it was simply hoping to reduce the countries' massive expenditures on drugs" (Hunter 2010, 212–13).

32. For detailed information on the TRIPS agreement and the struggles of countries in the global South (most notably Brazil, Thailand, India, and South Africa) to alter international IP protections for essential medications, see Biehl 2006a; Heimer 2007; Hein 2007; Nattrass 2008b.

33. There is some debate among scholars of global health governance about compulsory licensing, generic production, and the future of ARV provision in the global South. Only some middle-income countries (like Brazil, India, Thailand, and South Africa) are capable of generic medication

production, and the pharmaceutical industry largely sees the developing world as an "unattractive market," in part because of the need to reduce prices and in part because the developing world is plagued with diseases no longer common in the global North (Heimer 2007, 560). In addition, there is concern that the production of generic drugs might, in the long run, undermine the global supply of ARVs because without the promise of profit, pharmaceutical corporations have no incentive to engage in expensive research and development to produce new AIDS drugs, thereby compromising the ability of all counties to provide new drugs, as resistance to the medications grows worldwide (Nattrass 2008b, 575). This is one of the reasons that pharmaceutical corporations have pursued differential pricing whereby drugs sold at reduced rates in the "developing" world are sold at astronomically higher prices in the "developed" world; parallel importing from generic manufacturers in the global South is also disallowed in North American and European countries (Hein 2007). However, there is some speculation that, in fact, supplying drugs to countries in the global South for their large HIV-infected populations could be profitable. Despite the pharmaceutical industry's fears about lowering medication costs in the "Third World," the magnitude of the problem and the amount of drugs states are forced to buy to accommodate their infected publics might eventually make up for the loss of individual costs. In a 2004 pharmaco-economic report on emergent HIV/AIDS pharmaceutical markets (including Brazil, Thailand, India, China, and South Africa), it was estimated that these countries could provide a basic three ARV "cocktail" at 10 percent of the current US price, to 30 percent of the infected population, and the pharmaceutical industry would *still* make an $11.2 billion profit for the year (Biehl 2004, 112). What is clear is that the pharmaceutical corporations and the US trade representative have not given up their battle to retain their right to profit off of essential medicines. Activists at the International AIDS Conference in July 2010 filed a complaint against the United States' policy of imposing trade sanctions on countries on their "Special 301" watch list, who have bypassed twenty-year patents or who produce and export generic medications (Health Gap 2010).

34. Interview with Fatima Hassan of the ALP held on November 14, 2005, in the Cape Town ALP offices.

35. The court case was filed in the name of several HIV-infected South Africans (who were also members of TAC). When the ALP threatened to make GlaxoSmithKline and Boehringher Ingelheim defend their pricing system on drugs, they came to the ALP and agreed to settle out of court for the voluntary licenses. This is the process by which they were won. This information was made clear to me in a series of interviews held with ALP lawyers who were involved in the case, including Jonathan Berger, Fatima Hassan, and Mark Heywood.

36. Interview with Jonathan Berger of the ALP held on November 24, 2005, in the Johannesburg ALP offices.
37. Interview with Mark Heywood of the ALP held on November 24, 2005, in the Johannesburg ALP offices.
38. See Heywood 2004b for a discussion of these accusations.
39. Interview with Mark Heywood of the ALP held on November 24, 2005, in the Johannesburg ALP offices.
40. Interview with Xolani Kunene, Gauteng provincial organizer for TAC, held on December 12, 2005, in Johannesburg.
41. The idea behind the Basic Income Grant campaign is that providing a modest payment of R100 ($12.50) to every South African citizen on a monthly basis, regardless of age or income, would universalize income welfare without stigmatizing poverty or disability. Wealthier South Africans would also receive the grant, but those funds would be recuperated through taxes. For more information, see Ferguson 2007; http://www.big .org.za/.
42. Nguyen uses the term "therapeutic citizenship" (2005; 2010) to index the forms of citizenship that arise when people must rely on an abstract set of international agencies to adjudicate rights-claims or provide treatment and care (Nguyen 2010, 109).
43. In his book (2008a), Steve Robins makes an interesting point that Mbeki's denialism might also arise out of "calls for citizen participation in scientific juries and the adjudication of scientific knowledge" (112). In other words, Mbeki's questioning of scientific truths emerges from the selfsame health citizenship discourses that TAC drew from to argue for the importance of treatment literacy. Robins suggests this is similar to the way in which right-wing politicians in the US used renowned science and technology theorist Bruno Latour's work on the social construction of science to call global warming into question (114; See Latour 2004). Robins does not offer any analysis of the oddity that both sides of the denialist debate were pulling on the same set of social scientific theories.
44. SANAC is currently three-tiered: (1) the plenary makes up the leadership, chaired by the ANC deputy president and the deputy chairperson from civil society and includes representatives from seven government departments and seventeen civil society sectors; (2) the Programme Implementation Committee and the Resource Management Committee, each of whom have representatives from seven governmental departments and seventeen civil society organizations; (3) the seven Sectoral Coordinating Committees. For more information, see their website: www.sanac .org.za.
45. This information was offered by a female ALP lawyer in an interview held on June 30, 2009, in the Johannesburg ALP offices.
46. Ibid.

47. Interview conducted with a male ALP lawyer held on June 30, 2009, in the Johannesburg ALP offices. See also ALP 2010b; TAC 2010; PMG 2010.
48. Ibid. The disability grant is $135 per month.
49. In the political negotiations that took place between the ANC and the apartheid government preceding the transition, the ANC conceded to the establishment of a "quasi-federal political system to satisfy minority interests," where the control over social spending and implementation rests with the provincial government (South Africa has nine provinces) (Johnson 2005, 323; Schneider and Stein 2001). This has resulted in vast discrepancies in AIDS budgets across the provinces, and federal law is translated into policy differently in each province. As such, the policies on the disability grant and best practices for patient compliance with treatment schedules only have a family resemblance to each other at the national level.
50. Interview with HAART nurse at the Zola clinic in Soweto held on June 7, 2006.
51. This information was first provided by a HAART nurse at the Zola clinic in an interview held on June 7, 2006, but then it was confirmed by Pheello Limapo in an interview held on June 2, 2009, in Lawley.
52. The following information was gleaned from Department of Health clinical guidelines and modules available on their website (Department of Health 2010a and 2010b), in addition to interviews with nurses involved in ARV rollout and patients who have gone through the trainings.
53. Interview held with HAART nurse at Zola clinic in Soweto on June 7, 2006.
54. FGD held in Lawley on June 10, 2009.
55. Field notes from first encounter with Pheello Limapo after a three-year absence. May 23, 2009.
56. This is a pseudonym.
57. Female member of an FGD held in Lawley on June 21, 2009.
58. Female member of an FGD held in Sol Plaatjie on June 11, 2009.
59. Helen Joseph Hospital is in downtown Johannesburg, which is where Elizabeth still has to go once a month to get her ARV supplies, even though it is a two-hour taxi ride each way, from Lawley. The Chris Hani Baragwanath Hospital is closer, in Soweto, which is where she was admitted.
60. Interview with Pheello Limapo on June 2, 2009, in Lawley.
61. Interview with Mark Heywood held on November 24, 2005, in the Johannesburg ALP offices.
62. Interview held with Thulani Skhosana on June 11, 2006, in Sol Plaatjie.
63. Interview with ALP lawyer held on November 22, 2005, in the Johannesburg ALP offices.
64. Following T. H. Marshall, I use the term "social citizenship" to indicate a bundle of civic rights including access to health care and education, and

to distinguish it from political or economic citizenship (Marshall and Bottomore 1992).

65. Interview held with Nomachina Makalo on July 1, 2009, in Lawley.
66. Interview with Thulani Skhosana held on June 18, 2009, in Sol Plaatjie.
67. This was particularly true during the Rath scandal, where the choice became one between Rath's vitamins and the TAC's antiretrovirals—or so it seemed in Khayelitsha—the township where Rath set up a clinic and where TAC had its stronghold and partnered with an MSF clinic that dispensed ARVs. I conducted a series of interviews with people living in Khayelitsha on Saturday, November 12, and Friday, November 18, 2005.
68. Female participant in an FGD held on June 21, 2009, in Lawley.
69. Interview with ALP lawyer held on June 30, 2009, in Johannesburg ALP offices.
70. Ibid.
71. Ibid.
72. Interview held with a female nurse in the Dobsonville Clinic in Soweto on June 7, 2006.
73. This has been exacerbated by a number of poor policy decisions. For example, voluntary severance packages were offered to public sector staff in the mid-1990s, so many moved to the private sector or retired. Also in the late 1990s, a number of nursing colleges were closed, and so fewer nurses are graduating into the profession (Coovadia et al. 2009, 830).
74. Interview held with a female nurse working in the HIV Clinic at the Chris Hani Baragwanath Hospital in Soweto on May 25, 2006.
75. Interview held with the head nurse and unit manager of the Critical Care ward at the Chris Hani Baragwanath Hospital in Soweto on May 25, 2006.
76. This information was largely gleaned from ethnographic work with communities, but also with government officials working in different departments. An interview with an ALP lawyer on June 30, 2009, in the Johannesburg ALP offices also confirmed a lot of this information.
77. They have helped to form the Joint Civil Society Monitoring Forum (JCSFM), which is a group of civil society and private sector organizations that meet monthly to monitor the implementation of the ARV rollout by sharing challenges and strategies with one another. See http://www.tac .org.za/community/jcsmf.
78. Interview with Thulani Skhosana held on September 30, 2005, in Sol Plaatjie.
79. Female participant in an FGD (with people living with HIV/AIDS) held on June 10, 2009, in Lawley.
80. Interview with Pheello Limapo held on June 2, 2009, in Lawley.
81. This whole scene occurred during an interview with Pheello Limapo held on June 21, 2009, in Lawley.
82. Female respondent in FGD held on July 4, 2009, in Sol Plaatjie.

83. Female respondent from FGD (with HIV-positive residents) held on June 10, 2009, in Lawley.
84. Interview held with Andiswa Sononophana on July 28, 2012, in Sol Plaatjie.
85. See the introduction, footnote 35, for an explanation of the different classifications of drugs that make up an ARV "cocktail."
86. Interview held with Andiswa Sononophana on July 28, 2012, in Sol Plaatjie.
87. Interview with Sandra Mkhwanazi held on July 1, 2009, in Lawley.

CHAPTER FOUR

1. I borrow this apt phrase from Louise Vincent (2006), who uses it to describe the "revival" of "'ancient' practice[s] . . . after a period of dormancy" (18). Drawing on Chabal and Daloz's (1999) concept of retraditionalization, she examines the practice of virginity testing. I use it here in a broader context to indicate the (re)articulation of the trope of "tradition" in the postcolonial era. Eric Hobsbawm referred to this same practice as *inventing* tradition: "Ancient materials . . . [are used to] construct invented traditions of a novel type for novel purposes," which are usually "readily grafted onto old ones" ([1983] 2003, 6).
2. Mark Hunter (2011) also argues that Mbeki portrayed race as the single dividing line in the country, and Zuma shifts this approach by focusing, instead, on the politics of gender and sexuality (1123).
3. Throughout this chapter, I focus my attention on *hetero*sexuality and do not explore dynamics associated with same-sex relations. While not wishing to contribute to the silence on same-sex relations or the reification of heteronormative assumptions about African sexuality, I am limited by my research design and data. For studies of same-sex relations in South Africa, see Gevisser and Cameron 1995; Donham 1998; Epprecht 2004; Oswin 2007.
4. For reading on the problematic focus on African sexuality, see Packard and Epstein 1991; Vaughan 1991; McClintock 1995; Treichler 1999; Jochelson 2001; Mbembe and Nuttall 2004; Fassin 2007b.
5. Interview held with Jonathan Berger, ALP lawyer, on November 24, 2005, in the Johannesburg ALP offices.
6. Justice Edwin Cameron was one of the first and still remains one of the only high-ranking governmental officials to publicly disclose his HIV status. He is also author of a best-selling book, *Witness to AIDS* (2005).
7. Interview held with Edwin Cameron on December 9, 2005, in Brixton, Johannesburg.
8. Black Economic Empowerment (or BEE) is a certain kind of affirmative action policy implemented by the post-apartheid state to promote Black

leadership in corporate enterprise. It largely benefits a small group of African elite who have close ties to the ANC (Freund 2007).

9. In fact, she was wearing a *kanga*, a "traditional" African cloth worn throughout sub-Saharan Africa, which is widely regarded as a sign of modesty and respectability, but which was sexualized during the trial (Robins 2008a, 150).

10. Zuma's performance of masculinity is also extremely heteronormative. He was embroiled in a scandal in 2002 when he claimed oral sex was "wrong" and "unnatural" in a debate in Parliament concerning sex education (Ratele 2006, 50–51; Maclennan 2002).

11. For an important and detailed critique of simplified versions of Zulu masculinity, see Waetjen 2004.

12. The Recognition of Customary Marriages Act, No. 120 of 1998, legalizes polygamy in South Africa (Republic of South Africa 1998b).

13. Interestingly, Mbeki was also rumored to be a "womanizer," but he never paid *ilobolo*, which made his philandering "less sincere than Zuma's" (Hunter 2011, 27).

14. A number of important postcolonial gender scholars have challenged the ethnocentrism of Western feminism and its assumption of the coherence of gender identity, many of whom have inspired my theoretical approach, including: Mohanty, Russo, and Torres 1991; Narayan 1997; Oyěwùmí 1997.

15. Hunter reflects on the way in which what he refers to as the "crisis of social reproduction" is racialized in the South African context by pointing out the fact that 59 percent of the white population is married and that unemployment rates in the white community are 4.6 percent versus 42.5 percent for Africans (2010, 13).

16. See Hunter 2004 and 2010 for an examination of the historical shifts in idealized definitions of masculinity and femininity in Zulu culture.

17. The literature on transactional sex is vast. For general sources on Africa as a whole, see Luke and Kurz 2002; Luke 2003; Chatterji et al. 2004; Epstein 2002 and 2007; Halperin and Epstein 2004 and 2007; Barnett and Whiteside 2002. For sources on South Africa, in particular, see Hunter 2002, 2004, 2007, 2010; Selikow, Zulu, and Cedras 2002; Wojcicki 2002; Leclerc-Madlala 2003; Dunkle et al. 2004; Kaufman and Stavrou 2004.

18. Interview with Thulani Skhosana held on June 11, 2006, in Sol Plaatjie.

19. Male participant in an FGD held on July 4, 2009, in Sol Plaatjie.

20. Interview held with a female home-based care worker on June 24, 2009, in Sol Plaatjie.

21. A cross-national study conducted by UNAIDS found that men have both lower life expectancy and higher death rates, in part because men are taught that it is unmanly to be ill. This also prevents them from practicing safer sex or seeking treatment (UNAIDS 2000, 21).

22. Interview with Fatima Hassan, advocate for the AIDS Law Project, held on November 14, 2005, in Cape Town.
23. Male participant in an FGD held on June 11, 2009, in Sol Plaatjie.
24. The official employment rate for women in South Africa is 26.6 percent. Of the general population of women, 53.2 percent is economically inactive; however, 13.6 percent of those are discouraged work seekers. Among women who are employed, 65.1 percent are employed in the formal sector, 15.8 percent in the informal sector, 3.7 percent in agriculture, and 15.2 percent in domestic work (Statistics South Africa 2010).
25. Female participant in an FGD held on June 10, 2009, in Lawley.
26. Interview with a female resident of Lawley held on June 20, 2009.
27. According to this study, 21 percent of women attending antenatal clinics in Soweto engaged in sex "for material gain with a man other than a primary partner" (Dunkle et al. 2004, 1588). There is no demographic information that compares the use of "transactional sex" in formal versus informal townships. However, Mark Hunter conducted a comparative ethnographic project (2002), where he found that "transactional sex" is used in both settings, but for different purposes. In formal townships, women engage in transactional sex for cultural capital, where in informal settlements, women were much more likely to use it for economic survival.
28. Interview with a female NGO staff member held on April 6, 2005, in Soweto.
29. Female participant in an FGD held on July 3, 2009, in Lawley.
30. Female participant in an FGD held on July 4, 2009, in Sol Plaatjie.
31. Female participant in an FGD held on July 4, 2009, in Sol Plaatjie.
32. Interview with Nomachina Makalo held on July 1, 2009, in Lawley.
33. Interview held with a female resident of Lawley on October 26, 2005.
34. It is often in these long-term, affectionate relationships where condom use is *least* likely (Hunter 2007, 697n16).
35. Interview with Nomachina Makalo held on July 1, 2009, in Lawley.
36. Female participant in an FGD held on June 10, 2009, in Lawley.
37. Interview with female community member on October 26, 2005, in Lawley.
38. Female participant in an FGD held on June 21, 2009, in Lawley.
39. Interview with female community member on October 26, 2005, in Lawley.
40. Female participant in an FGD held on June 10, 2006, in Sol Plaatjie.
41. Interview with Pheello Limapo held on November 9, 2005, in Johannesburg.
42. Interview held with Nelly Mbiletsa on July 1, 2009, in Lawley.
43. Interview with Nelly Mbiletsa held on July 1, 2009, in Lawley.
44. Female participant in an FGD held on July 3, 2009, in Lawley.
45. Robert Morrell (2001) also distinguishes between "traditional" (or defensive) masculinity, versus masculinities that are accommodating or progressive depending on men's reception of the liberal, gender equity

initiatives introduced in the post-apartheid era, but he includes men from a variety of different class and race positions in each category.

46. Such an analysis builds on other work in masculinity studies highlighting the complex, relational, and processual nature of hegemonic masculinity (Morrell 2001; Xaba 2001; Wyrod 2008).

47. Under apartheid, there were ten homelands, called Bantustans, designated for the African population—similar to Native American reservations. They were organized on the basis of language and ethnic groupings and were used to administer racial segregation and delimit the movement of African populations.

48. Male participant in an FGD held in Lawley on July 3, 2009.

49. Social capital is defined as "the aggregate of the actual and potential resources which are linked to membership in a group" (Bourdieu 1986, 250).

50. This engagement in "transactional sex" for consumption is far more likely among working- or middle-class youth. For further information on this, see Swidler and Watkins 2007; Hunter 2002 and 2010; Motsemme 2007.

51. Interview held with Robert Tshabalala on September 3, 2005, in Orlando East, Soweto; italics are used to highlight important components of his analysis.

52. Interviews with Dr. Mputhi held on July 18, 2005, in Evaton West and Dr. Robert Tshabalala held on August 3, 2005, in Orlando East, Soweto.

53. "Zunami" was a popular expression used to describe the overwhelming support Zuma enjoyed in the 2009 elections after his surprising 2007 defeat of Mbeki. See also Hunter 2011.

54. Hart (2008, 692) makes a similar point about Zuma's new articulation of nationalism having the capacity to fuse "multiple, often contradictory meanings into a complex unity that appeals powerfully to 'common sense' across a broad spectrum."

55. Thulani Skhosana discussed this with me, in an informal conversation held in Sol Plaatjie on June 28, 2009.

56. Interview with Thulani Skhosana held on June 18, 2009, in Sol Plaatjie.

57. Interview with Pheello Limapo held on June 21, 2009, in Lawley.

58. TAC labeled it "one of the most important speeches in the history of AIDS in South Africa" (*Lancet* 2009).

59. Interview with Thulani Skhosana held on June 18, 2009, in Sol Plaatjie.

60. FGD held on June 29, 2012, in Lawley.

CHAPTER FIVE

1. This is a pseudonym. Interviews were held on April 22, August 8, and September 29, 2005, in Alexandra, Johannesburg.

2. Interview held on August 8, 2005, in Alexandra, Johannesburg.

3. I volunteered with this organization (which must remain anonymous to protect the participants' identities) from December 1, 2004, to Septem-

ber 30, 2005. During this time, I worked extensively with support groups in Zola, Dobsonville, and Orlando East, Soweto. "Tebogho" (a pseudonym) was my guide and closest contact during this fieldwork.

4. I conducted interviews with "Tebogho" on April 6 and October 19, 2005; however, she would never talk about herself during an official interview. She told me this in the car, during one of our many trips to and from support groups in the Soweto area. Field notes, February 2, 2005, Soweto.

5. Interview with Pheello Limapo held on October 5, 2005, in Lawley.

6. Field notes, May 17, 2006, Lawley.

7. Interview held with Pheello Limapo on December 8, 2005, in Lawley.

8. All of the quotes from this story are taken from an interview held with Nozipho Dlamini on June 26, 2009, in Sol Plaatjie.

9. The South African equivalent of a Tylenol.

10. FGD held on June 11, 2009, in Sol Plaatjie (with people living with HIV).

11. Field notes, September 16, 2005, Sol Plaatjie.

12. Interviews with female nurses in the maternity ward, critical care wards, and HIV clinics conducted in May 2006 at the Chris Hani Baragwanath Hospital in Soweto.

13. Interviews with residents of Khayelitsha held on November 12 and November 18, 2005, in Mandela Park, Cape Town.

14. Interview with TAC Gauteng chairperson, Isaac Skhosana, held on May 18, 2006, in downtown Johannesburg.

15. Interview held with female *sangoma* on April 20, 2005, in Mapetla Extension, Soweto.

16. Interview held with male *sangoma* on April 13, 2005, in Diepkloof Extension, Soweto.

17. Throughout this chapter, I focus on the historical relationship between African indigenous healing and biomedicine, and I only discuss the medical pluralism practiced by the African populations of South Africa. For historical information on pluralism within the so-called "Indian" and "Coloured" populations of South Africa, see Flint 2001 and 2006; Digby 2005 and 2006.

18. The ANC's 1994 *National Health Plan* (ANC 1994) promised that "traditional healing will become an integral and recognised part of health care in South Africa." Efforts to institute indigenous healing legislation and test and register herbal remedies were described in chapters 2 and 3 respectively.

19. This is a vast topic, but see also Anderson 2006; Arnold 1993; Gordon 2001; Olumwullah 2002; Prakash 1999; Vaughan 1991.

20. In 1862, the secretary for native affairs in the British colony of Natal sent all magistrates a circular prohibiting all healers and rainmakers from practicing in the colonies; this was codified in the 1875 "Native Law" (Flint 2008, 108). The Natal Code of Native Law (no. 19 of 1891) banned

the practice of divination but required all herbalists and midwives to be registered and licensed (Xaba 2005, 63–64; Flint 2008, chapter 4; see also Devenish 2005). The 1886 African Territories Penal Code also legislated against witchcraft, which was then extended to the whole of the Cape Colony under the 1895 Witchcraft Suppression Act (Digby 2006, 319). These colonial laws are revitalized in the apartheid period with the Witchcraft Suppression Act of 1957 and 1970, which I discuss later in the chapter.

21. For information on disease and health care management in mining communities in South Africa, see Packard 1989; Marks and Andersson 1992; Jochelson 2001.

22. The Rand is short for the Witwatersrand—which is where the gold mines and Johannesburg are both located.

23. It is possible that hybridity developed more quickly in urban areas, but the fluidity of movement between rural and urban areas (for both patients and healers) meant the differences would soon even out. The historical record also notes that chiefs and other indigenous leaders drew heavily from "modern" symbolism, cosmology, and governance (Myers 2008), so hybridity may have looked differently in rural and urban areas, but was no less common or pronounced.

24. Some have even argued that health concerns were a primary justification for racial segregationist policies (Swanson 1977).

25. The Witchcraft Suppression Act of 1957 consolidated all previous statutes, acts, laws, ordinances, and proclamations (Xaba 2005, 123–24).

26. As African men increasingly traveled to urban areas to work, women were left to take care of households in the rural regions. To supplement their husbands' income, women would often engage in agricultural development; however, due to difficult weather conditions (like droughts) and other hardships, women were often forced to look for other means of supplementing the household income. Xaba (2005) suggests that trade in herbs became a viable alternative to agricultural production.

27. For further information on the institutionalization and professionalization of *muthi* trading, see Devenish 2003.

28. Afrikaans word for a rural plain.

29. Interview held with Dr. Robert Tshabalala on July 22, 2005, in Orlando East, Soweto.

30. Interview held with Dr. Martha Mongoya on July 22, 2005, in Orlando East, Soweto.

31. Interview with Torong Ramela held on June 10, 2005, in Johannesburg.

32. Interview with nurse Hilda Pheto held on July 14, 2009, in Johannesburg.

33. Interview with Dr. Robert Tshabalala held on July 22, 2005, in Orlando East, Soweto; interview with Dr. Sheila Khama held on July 14, 2009, in Johannesburg.

34. These newspaper articles are part of the Institute for Race Relations archive, housed at the William Cullen Library at the University of the

Witwatersrand, Johannesburg. Wits Historical Papers, 1940–70. Press Clippings on African Healing. Collection: AD1912, Boxes 112–13.

35. Interview held with Torong Ramela on June 10, 2005, in Johannesburg.
36. Interview held with Dr. Martha Mongoya on July 22, 2005, in Orlando East, Soweto.
37. Interview with Dr. Sheila Khama held on July 14, 2009, in Johannesburg.
38. There are "traditional" bonesetters, so not all people heed such a structured division of labor.
39. Many of the healers I interviewed and spoke with in FGDs relied on biomedical technology in this way. This evidence is further supported by Mills 2005, 141–43.
40. Interview with Dr. Rebecca Rogerson held on August 19, 2005, in Johannesburg.
41. Ibid.
42. Dr. Rogerson's website is no longer on the Internet, but she has given me permission to reprint this brief description here.
43. This was obvious from the FGDs I held with 131 indigenous healers in 2005 and 2006. These conclusions are further supported by a number of scholars who work closely with indigenous healers in the contemporary era: Green 1999; Thornton 2002; Mills 2005.
44. Interview with Dr. Martha Mongoya held on September 3, 2005, in Orlando East, Soweto.
45. Interview with Dr. Sheila Khama held on July 14, 2009, in Johannesburg.
46. Interview with Dr. Rebecca Rogerson held on August 19, 2005, in Johannesburg.
47. This exchange took place during an interview on August 17, 2005, in Orlando East, Soweto.
48. Female respondent in an FGD held on September 6, 2005, in Soweto.
49. This exchange took place in an FGD with indigenous healers held on September 6, 2005, in Soweto.
50. Traditional healers Nelly Mabiletsa (interview held on July 1, 2009, in Lawley) and Maria Tshuduku (interview held on June 20, 2009, in Lawley), as well as nurse Hilda Pheto (interview held on July 14, 2009, in Johannesburg) mentioned this.
51. Traditional healers Esther Zwane (interview held on June 24, 2009, in Sol Plaatjie), Martha Mongoya, and Robert Tshabalala (interview held on July 13, 2009 in Soweto), as well as Sheila Khama (interview held on July 14, 2009, in Johannesburg) mentioned this.
52. Interview with Martha Mongoya held on July 13, 2009, in Soweto.
53. Dr. Nelly Mabiletsa, FGD held on June 21, 2009, in Lawley.
54. Male home-based care worker, FGD held on July 3, 2009, in Lawley.
55. Interview held with Sheila Khama on July 14, 2009, in Johannesburg.
56. Footnote 3 in this chapter provides references for analyses of biomedicine serving as a "tool of empire." For analyses of the link between socioeco-

nomic "development" efforts and the establishment of international public health programs, see, for example, Armstrong 1995; Packard 1997 and 2003; Rabinow 2005.

57. Some exceptions include Adams 2002; Anderson 1998 and 2002; King 2002. King (2002) notes that whereas colonialism's goal was *converting* indigenous beliefs and practices into biomedical ones, the postcolonial agenda uses *integration* as its metaphor. "The universality of biomedical ways of knowing and doing is taken for granted, and achieving 'global health' depends upon integrating localities into global networks of commodity and information exchange. Local populations present obstacles not because of incommensurate belief systems of cultural differences, but because of incomplete integration into the modern projects of total surveillance and seamless exchange" (782).

58. For an interesting study on the various uses of herbal remedies, see Cocks and Møller 2002.

59. Interview with nurse Hilda Pheto held on July 14, 2009, in Johannesburg.

60. Loïc Wacquant has suggested that this critique is particularly prevalent in the American academy where only a few of Bourdieu's texts are read with frequency, which leads to a piecemeal interpretation of Bourdieu's theories and "obfuscate[s] the systematic nature and novelty of his enterprise" (1989, 27).

61. Sources on the apartheid state's construction and use of the traditional/ modern binary include Marks 1986; Ashforth 1990; Beinart and Dubow 1995; Mamdani 1996; and Myers 2008.

62. In fact, Mamdani is critiqued for precisely this error. See Cooper 1983 and 1997.

63. For sources that highlight the way in which chiefs were forced to negotiate between the ideological and institutional constraints of both "modernity" and "traditionalism" in their occupations under the apartheid system in South Africa, see Myers 2008.

CODA

1. Field notes, August 20, 2005, Sol Plaatjie.

2. He bases this concept on the Aristotelian notion of *zoē*, natural life.

3. The term "life strategies" is borrowed from Ahmed Veriava, who used the term in his master's thesis at the University of KwaZulu-Natal (2006) to discuss the ways in which the poor have always fought to maintain a commons to secure their own social reproduction. He traces this from the apartheid era rent and service payment boycotts to resistance in the early 2000s against the installation of prepaid water meters. He links the concept, as I do, to Foucault's work on ethics. I borrow the term with his permission.

Glossary

Amakhosi or Amadlozi (Zulu): Ancestors

Bomoloi (Sotho): Witchcraft

Gauteng: the province in which Johannesburg (and this research) is situated. It is also home to the executive (administrative) and de facto national capital of South Africa, Pretoria

Gobela (Zulu): Sangoma who trains initiates to become diviners

Igazi (Zulu): Blood

Iketsetseng (Sotho): Do-it-yourself

Ilobolo (Zulu): Bride wealth

Imbiza (Zulu): An indigenous remedy used to cleanse the blood

Impepo (Zulu): An indigenous plant used to "call the ancestors"

Inyanga (Zulu): Herbalist (indigenous healer)

Isithunzi (Zulu): Aura

Makhome (Sotho): Indigenous disease associated with having sexual relations with a widow or a woman who has recently had an abortion

Mpande (Zulu): A group of diviners who have all been trained by the same *gobela*, and who therefore share treatments and other indigenous knowledge

Muthi (Zulu): Indigenous herbal remedy

Pahla (Zulu): An offering to one's ancestors as a sign of respect

Sangoma (Zulu): Diviner (indigenous healer)

Shebeen (Irish): An unlicensed drinking establishment

Spaza shop (slang): An informal convenience store operated out of a home in a township

Ubuntu (Zulu): Southern African philosophy stressing communal respect and solidarity. It originates from a Zulu maxim, *umuntu ngumuntu ngabantu*, "a person is a person through (other) persons"

Ubuthakathi (Zulu): Witchcraft

Ukubiza (Zulu): The "calling" by the ancestors that initiates the trainership for becoming a *sangoma*

Ukuphanda (Zulu): To get by, to survive

Umjondolo (Zulu): a shack

Umoya (Zulu): Body

Ukuthwasa (Zulu): Training or apprenticeship to become a diviner

Umthwasa (Zulu): An initiate going through the training to become a diviner

Umzimba (Zulu): Spirit

Veld (Afrikaans): Rural plain

Vukuzenzele (Zulu): To wake up and do-it-yourself

References

Abdool-Karim, S. S., T. T. Ziqubu-Page, and R. Arendse. 1994. "Bridging the Gap: Potential for Health Care Partnership between African Traditional Healers and Biomedical Personnel in South Africa." Report of the South African Medical Research Council. *South African Medical Journal* 84 (December insert): s1–s16.

Abt. Associates. 2000. *The Impending Catastrophe: A Resource Book on the Emerging HIV/AIDS Epidemic in South Africa.* Johannesburg: Henry J. Kaiser Foundation.

Achmat, Zackie. 2004. "The Treatment Action Campaign, HIV/AIDS and the Government." *Transformations* 54: 76–84.

Adams, Sheena. 2005. "Health Minister Defiant on ARV Side-Effects." (May 6). *The Star*: 6.

Adams, Vincanne. 2002. "Randomized Controlled Crime: Postcolonial Sciences in Alternative Medicine." *Social Studies of Science* 32 (5/6): 659–90.

African National Congress (ANC). 1994. *A National Health Plan for South Africa.* http://www.anc.org.za/show.php?id=257. Accessed on December 30, 2011.

———. 2001. *A National Guideline on Home-Based Care and Community-Based Care.* Pretoria: African National Congress.

———. 2002. "Castro Hlongwane, Caravans, Cats, Geese, Foot and Mouth, and Statistics: HIV/AIDS and the Struggle for the Humanisation of the African." Unknown author. First posted to the ANC website by Peter Mokaba in March 2002. http://www.virusmyth.com/aids/hiv/ancdoc.htm. Accessed on June 3, 2011.

Agamben, Giorgio. 1998. *Homo Sacer: Sovereign Power and Bare Life.* Translated by Daniel Heller-Roazen. Stanford, CA: Stanford University Press.

AIDS Law Project (ALP). 2010a. Civil Society Consensus Statement: Meeting the Challenges of HIV Treatment and Prevention through Independent Mobilisation and Work through the South African National AIDS Council (SANAC). http://www.section27.org.za/2010/10/14/meeting-challenges-of -hiv/. Accessed on October 14, 2011.

———. 2010b. Submission on the Social Assistance Amendment Bill, 2010. http://www.section27.org.za/2010/05/04/1545/. Accessed on October 19, 2010.

Ajulu, Rok. 2001. "Thabo Mbeki's African Renaissance in a Globalising World Economy: The Struggle for the Soul of the Continent." *Review of African Political Economy* 28 (87): 27–42.

Altman, Miriam, and Gerard Boyce. 2008. Policy Options to Leverage the System of Social Grants for Improved Access to Economic Opportunity. Human Science Research Council. http://www.hsrc.ac.za/Research_Project -898.phtml. Accessed on April 28, 2010.

Ambert, Cecile. 2006. "An HIV and AIDS Lens for Informal Settlement Policy and Practice in South Africa." In *Informal Settlements: A Perpetual Challenge?*, edited by Marie Huchzermeyer and Aly Karam, 146–62. Cape Town: University of Cape Town Press.

American Association for the Advancement of Science (with Physicians for Human Rights). 1998. Human Rights and Health: The Legacy of Apartheid. http://shr.aaas.org/loa/index.htm. Accessed on June 7, 2011.

Anderson, Warwick. 1998. "Where Is the Postcolonial History of Medicine?" *Bulletin of the History of Medicine* 72: 522–30.

———. 2002. "Introduction: Postcolonial Technoscience." *Social Studies of Science* 32 (5/6): 643–58.

———. 2006. *Colonial Pathologies: American Tropical Medicine, Race, and Hygiene in the Philippines*. Durham, NC: Duke University Press.

Annas, George. 2003. "The Right to Health and the Nevirapine Case in South Africa." *New England Journal of Medicine* 348 (February 20): 750–54.

Anti-Privatisation Forum (APF). 2006. "HIV/AIDS and the Struggle for Life." Report of Community Participatory Action Research, conducted in Sol Plaatjie and Phiri, Soweto.

Armstrong, David. 1995. "The Rise of Surveillance Medicine." *Sociology of Health and Illness* 17 (3): 393–404.

Arnold, David. 1993. *Colonizing the Body: State Medicine and Epidemic Disease in Nineteenth-Century India*. Berkeley: University of California Press.

Ashforth, Adam. 1990. *The Politics of Official Discourse*. Oxford: Oxford University Press.

———. 2002. "An Epidemic of Witchcraft? The Implications of AIDS for the Post-Apartheid State." *African Studies* 61 (July): 121–43.

———. 2005. *Witchcraft, Violence, and Democracy in South Africa*. Chicago: University of Chicago Press.

Attaran, Amir, Kenneth Freedberg, and Martin Hirsh. 2001. "Dead Wrong on AIDS." *Washington Post*, June 15: A33.

Auyero, Javier, and Débora Alejandra Swistun. 2009. *Flammable: Environmental Suffering in an Argentine Shantytown*. New York: Oxford University Press.

Baccaro, Lucio, and Konstantinos Papadakis. 2009. "The Downside of Participatory-Deliberative Public Administration." *Socio-Economic Review* 7: 245–76.

Bakker, Isabella, ed. 1994. *The Strategic Silence: Gender and Economic Policy*. London: Zed Books.

Bareng-Batho, K., and M. S'Thembiso. 1998. "Mob Kills Woman for Telling Truth: Health Worker Stoned and Beaten for Confession about HIV." *Sunday Times*, December 27.

Barker, Drucilla, and Susan Feiner. 2004. *Liberating Economics: Feminist Perspectives on Families, Work, and Globalization*. Ann Arbor: University of Michigan Press.

Barnett, Tony, and Alan Whiteside. 2002. *AIDS in the Twenty-First Century: Disease and Globalization*. New York: Palgrave Macmillan.

BBC News. 2005. "South Africa to Have Gay Weddings." December 1. http://news.bbc.co.uk/2/hi/africa/4487756.stm. Accessed on November 13, 2011.

———. 2006. "South Africa Awaits Zuma Verdict." May 8.

———. 2009. "South Africa Zulus to Revive Circumcision to Fight Aids." December 7.

———. 2010. "South African Workers Begin Strike." August 18. http://www.bbc.co.uk/news/world-africa-11008442. Accessed on October 18, 2011.

Berger, Jonathan. 2004. "Re-Sexualising the Epidemic: Desire, Risk, and HIV Prevention." *Development Update* 5 (3): 45–67.

Beinart, William, and Saul Dubow, eds. 1995. *Segregation and Apartheid in Twentieth-Century South Africa*. London: Routledge.

Benería, Lourdes. 2003. *Gender, Development, and Globalization: Economics as If All People Mattered*. New York and London: Routledge.

Bezuidenhout, Andries, and Khayaat Fakier. 2006. "Maria's Burden: Contract Cleaning and the Crisis of Social Reproduction in Post-Apartheid South Africa." *Antipode* 38 (3): 462–85.

Bhabha, Homi K. 1994. *The Location of Culture*. New York: Routledge.

Bhabha, Homi K., ed. 1990. *Nation and Narration*. New York: Routledge.

Biehl, João. 2001. "Vita: Life in a Zone of Social Abandonment." *Social Text* 68 (Fall): 131–49.

———. 2004. "The Activist State: Global Pharmaceuticals, AIDS, and Citizenship in Brazil." *Social Text* 80 (Fall): 105–32.

———. 2005. *Vita: Life in a Zone of Social Abandonment*. Berkeley: University of California Press.

———. 2006a. "Pharmaceutical Governance." In *Global Pharmaceuticals: Ethics, Markets and Practices*, edited by Adriana Petryna, Andrew Lakoff, and Arthur Kleinman, 206–39. Durham, NC: Duke University Press.

———. 2006b. "Will to Live: AIDS Drugs and Local Economies of Survival." *Public Culture* 18 (3): 457–72.

———. 2007. *Will to Live: AIDS Therapies and the Politics of Survival.* Princeton, NJ: Princeton University Press.

Bofelo, Mphutlane Wa. 2010. "Zuma Abuses Zulu Culture." *Sowetan.* February 10.

Bond, Patrick. 2000. *Elite Transition: From Apartheid to Neoliberalism in South Africa.* Pietermaritzburg: University of Natal Press.

———. 2002. *Against Global Apartheid: South Africa Meets the World Bank, IMF, and International Finance.* Cape Town: University of Cape Town Press.

———. 2004. "Can Five Million People with AIDS Celebrate South African Freedom?" *Against the Current* (July/August).

Bonner, Philip, and Lauren Segal. 1998. *Soweto: A History.* Cape Town: Maskew, Miller and Longman.

Booysen, F. le R., M. Bachmann, Z. Matebesi, and J. Meyer. 2004. "The Socio-Economic Impact of HIV/AIDS on Households in South Africa: Pilot Study in Welkom and QwaQwa, Free State Province." Final Report (January). University of the Free State: Centre for Health Systems Research and Development. http://www.sarpn.org.za/documents/d0001489/ P1822-Welkom-study_AIDS_January2004.pdf. Accessed on June 24, 2011.

Boseley, Sarah. 2005. "Discredited Doctor's 'Cure' for Aids Ignites Life-and-Death Struggle in South Africa." *The Guardian.* May 14. http://www .guardian.co.uk/world/2005/may/14/southafrica.internationalaidand development. Accessed on October 10, 2011.

Bourdieu, Pierre. 1962. *The Algerians.* Translated by Alan C. M. Ross. Boston: Beacon Press.

———. 1977. *Outline of a Theory of Practice.* Translated by Richard Nice. Cambridge: Oxford University Press.

———. 1979. *Algeria 1960: The Disenchantment of the World; the Sense of Honour; the Kabyle House or the World Reversed.* Translated by Richard Nice. Cambridge: Cambridge University Press.

———. 1980. "The Production of Belief: Contribution to an Economy of Symbolic Goods." Translated by Richard Nice. *Media, Culture and Society* 2 (July): 261–93.

———. 1984. *Distinction: A Social Critique of the Judgment of Taste.* Translated by Richard Nice. Cambridge, MA: Harvard University Press.

———. 1986. "The Forms of Capital." In *Handbook of Theory and Research for the Sociology of Education,* edited by J. G. Richardson, 241–58. New York: Greenwood Press.

———. 1989. "Social Space and Symbolic Power." *Sociological Theory* 7: 14–25.

———. 1990. *The Logic of Practice.* Translated by Richard Nice. Stanford, CA: Stanford University Press.

———. 1993. *Sociology in Question*. Translated by Richard Nice. Theory, Culture, and Society, vol. 18. London: Sage Publications.

———. 1996a. *The Rules of Art: Genesis and Structure of the Literary Field*. Translated by Susan Emanuel. Stanford, CA: Stanford University Press.

———. 1996b. *The State Nobility: Elite Schools in the Field of Power*. Translated by Lauretta C. Clough. Cambridge: Polity Press.

———. 2000. *Pascalian Meditations*. Translated by Richard Nice. Stanford, CA: Stanford University Press.

———. 2001. *Masculine Domination*. Translated by Richard Nice. Cambridge: Polity Press.

———. 2007. *Sketch for a Self-Analysis*. Chicago: University of Chicago Press.

Bourdieu, Pierre, and Abdelmalek Sayad. 2004. "Colonial Rule and Cultural Sabir." *Ethnography* 5 (December): 544–86.

Bourdieu, Pierre, and Loïc J. D. Wacquant. 1992. *An Invitation to Reflexive Sociology*. Chicago: Chicago University Press.

Bourdieu, Pierre, et al. 1999. *The Weight of the World: Social Suffering in Contemporary Society*. Stanford, CA: Stanford University Press.

Brenner, Neil, and Nik Theodore. 2002. "Cities and the Geographies of 'Actually Existing Neoliberalism.'" *Antipode* 34 (3): 349–79.

Brenner, Neil, Jamie Peck, and Nik Theodore. 2010. "Variegated Neoliberalization: Geographies, Modalities, Pathways." *Global Networks* 10 (2): 182–222.

Brown, David. 2011. "HIV Drugs Sharply Cut Risk of Transmission Study Finds." *Washington Post*. May 12. http://www.washingtonpost.com/national/hiv-drugs-sharply-cut-risk-of-transmission-study-finds/2011/05/12/AFmFdV1G_story.html?hpid=z3. Accessed on May 12, 2011.

Butler, Judith. 1996. "Sexual Inversions." In *Feminist Interpretations of Michel Foucault*, edited by Susan Hekman, 59–75. University Park: Pennsylvania State University Press.

Cabinet, South African Government. 2007. Statement on Cabinet Meeting, May 2. http://www.info.gov.za/speeches/2007/07050311151002.htm. Accessed on June 8, 2011.

Caldwell, John C., Pat Caldwell, and Pat Quiggin. 1989. "The Social Context of AIDS in Sub-Saharan Africa." *Population and Development Review* 15 (2): 185–234.

Cameron, Edwin. 2005. *Witness to AIDS*. Cape Town: Tafelberg.

Campbell, Susan Schuster. 1998. *Called to Heal: Traditional Healing Meets Modern Medicine in Southern Africa Today*. London: Zebra Press.

Campero Lourdes, Cristina Herrera, Tamil Kendall, and Marta Caballero. 2007. "Bridging the Gap between Antiretroviral Access and Adherence in Mexico." *Qualitative Health Research* 17 (5): 599–611.

Casale, D. 2004. "What Has the Feminisation of the Labour Market Bought Women in South Africa? Trends in Labour Force Participation, Employment and Earnings, 1995–2001." Cape Town: Development Policy Research Unit, Working Paper 4, 84.

Casale, D., and D. Posel. 2002. "The Continued Feminisation of the Labour Force in South Africa: An Analysis of Recent Data and Trends." *South African Journal of Economics* 70 (1): 168–95.

Castel, Robert. 1991. "From Dangerousness to Risk." In *The Foucault Effect: Studies in Governmentality*, edited by Graham Burchell, Colin Gordon, and Peter Miller, 281–98. Chicago: University of Chicago Press.

Cele, Nie. 2011. "Avalon Cemetery Expansion Gives Joburg Burial Space for 69 Years." *The Citizen Online*. February 11. http://www.citizen.co.za/citizen/content/en/citizen/local-news?oid=172377&sn=Detail&pid=334&Avalon-cemetery-expansion-gives-Joburg-burial-space-for-69-years. Accessed on April 8, 2011.

Chabal, Patrick, and Jean-Pascal Daloz. 1999. *Africa Works: Disorder as Political Instrument*. Bloomington: Indiana University Press.

Chakrabarty, Dipesh. 2000. *Provincializing Europe: Postcolonial Thought and Historical Difference*. Princeton, NJ: Princeton University Press.

Chatterjee, Partha. 1993. *The Nation and Its Fragments: Colonial and Postcolonial Histories*. Princeton, NJ: Princeton University Press.

Chatterji, Minki, Nancy Murray, David London, and Philip Anglewicz. 2004. "The Factors Influencing Transactional Sex among Young Men and Women in 12 Sub-Saharan African Countries." USAID Policy Project (October).

Chigwedere, Pride, George R. Seage, Sofia Gruskin, Tun-Hou Lee, and M. Essex. 2008. "Estimating the Lost Benefits of Antiretroviral Drug Use in South Africa." *Journal of Acquired Immune Deficiency Syndrome* 49 (4): 410–15.

Cocks, Michelle, and Valerie Møller. 2002. "Use of Indigenous and Indigenised Medicines to Enhance Personal Well-Being: A South African Case Study." *Social Science and Medicine* 54, 3: 387–97.

Cohen, Jon. 2004. "Allegations Raise Fears of Backlash against AIDS Prevention Strategy." *Science* 24 (December 24): 2168–69.

Cohen, Myron, et al. 2011. "Prevention of HIV-1 Infection with Early Antiretroviral Therapy." *New England Journal of Medicine* 365 (August 11): 493–505. http://www.nejm.org/doi/full/10.1056/NEJMoa1105243. Accessed on October 16, 2011.

Collins, Daryl, and Murray Leibbrandt. 2007. "The Financial Impact of HIV/AIDS on Poor Households in South Africa." *AIDS* 21 (suppl. 7): S75–S81.

Colvin, Mark, Lindiwe Gumede, Kate Grimwade, and David Wilkinson. 2001. "Integrating Traditional Healers into a Tuberculosis Control Programme in Hlabisa, South Africa." Medicine Control Council Brief, No. 4 (December). http://www.mrc.ac.za//policybriefs/tbtraditional.pdf. Accessed on June 20, 2011.

Colvin, Christopher, and Steven Robins. 2009. "Positive Men in Hard, Neoliberal Times: Engendering Health Citizenship in South Africa." In *Gender and HIV/AIDS: Critical Perspectives from the Developing World*, edited by Jelke Boesten and Nana Poku, 177–90. Burlington, VT: Ashgate.

Comaroff, Jean. 2007. "Beyond Bare Life: AIDS, (Bio)Politics, and the Neo-liberal Order." *Public Culture* 19 (1): 197–219.

Comaroff, Jean, and John L. Comaroff. 1991. *Of Revelation and Revolution: Christianity. Colonialism, and Consciousness in South Africa*, vol. 1. Chicago: University of Chicago Press.

———. 2000. "Millennial Capitalism: First Thoughts on a Second Coming." *Public Culture* 12 (2): 291–343.

Comaroff, Jean, and John L. Comaroff, eds. 1993. *Modernity and Its Malcontents: Ritual and Power in Post-Colonial Africa*. Chicago: University of Chicago Press.

Commission for Gender Equality. 2000. Annual Report, 2000. http://www.cge.org.za/. Accessed on November 13, 2011.

Connell, Raewyn. 1987. *Gender and Power: Society, the Person, and Sexual Politics*. Stanford, CA: Stanford University Press.

———. 1995. *Masculinities*. 2nd ed. Berkeley: University of California Press.

———. 2005. "Change among the Gatekeepers: Men, Masculinities, and Gender Equality in the Global Arena." *Signs: Journal of Women in Culture and Society* 30 (3): 1801–25.

Cooper, Frederick. 1983. *Struggle for the City: Migrant Labor, Capital, and the State in Urban Africa*. London: Sage Publications.

———. 1997. "The Dialectic of Decolonization: Nationalism and Labor Movements in Postwar French Africa." In *Tensions of Empire: Colonial Cultures in a Bourgeois World*, edited by Frederick Cooper and Ann Laura Stoler, 406–35. Berkeley: University of California Press.

Cooper, Frederick, and Ann Laura Stoler, eds. 1997. *Tensions of Empire: Colonial Cultures in a Bourgeois World*. Berkeley: University of California Press.

Coovadia, Hoosen, and A. Coutsoudis. 2001. "Problems and Advances in Reducing Transmission of HIV-1 through Breast-Feeding in Developing Countries. *AIDScience* 1 (4).

Coovadia, Hoosen, Rachel Jewkes, Peter Barron, David Sanders, and Diane McIntyre. 2009. "The Health and Health System of South Africa: Historical Roots of Current Public Health Challenges." *The Lancet* 374 (September 5): 817–34.

Coronil, Fernando. 1992. "Can Postcoloniality Be Decolonized? Imperial Banality and Postcolonial Power." *Public Culture* 5 (Fall): 99–100.

Courtenay, Will. 2000. "Constructions of Masculinity and Their Influence on Men's Well-Being: A Theory of Gender and Health." *Social Science and Medicine* 50 (10): 1385–401.

Cowell, Alan, and John Eligon. 2011. "Youth Leader Is Disciplined in South Africa." *New York Times*. November 10. http://www.nytimes.com/2011/11/11/world/africa/south-africas-governing-party-disciplines-youth-leader.html?_r=2&hp. Accessed on December 4, 2011.

Crankshaw, Owen. 1993. "Squatting, Apartheid, and Urbanisation on the Southern Witwatersrand." *African Affairs* 92 (366): 31–51.

Cullinan, Kerry. 2000. "Editorial." In *Community Based Care: Update for Health Workers, Planners and Managers*. Health Systems Trust, Issue 58. http://www.hst.org.za/publications/community-based-care. Accessed on June 9, 2011.

———. 2005. "Another Bizarre Year for AIDS Policy." *Health-E News*. December 8. http://www.health-e.org.za/news/article.php?uid=20031658. Accessed on June 8, 2011.

———. 2006. "Manto Muscled Out in Palace Coup." *Sunday Times*. November 5.

———. 2007. "New Strategic Plan: Is AIDS Denialism Dead?" *Health-E News*. June 18. http://www.health-e.org.za/news/article.php?uid=20031694. Accessed on June 8, 2011.

Davie, Lucille. 2007. "Shack Settlements: Not Here to Stay." Part of the city of Johannesburg online housing archive. (November 29). http://www.joburg.org.za/index.php?option=com_content&task=view&id=1949&Itemid=204. Accessed on April 7, 2011.

———. 2008. "Regularising Informal Settlements." Part of the city of Johannesburg online housing archive. (August 15). http://www.joburg.org.za/content/view/2854/266/. Accessed on April 7, 2011.

———. 2009. "Avalon Cemetery Is Almost Full." Part of the city of Johannesburg online news. http://www.joburg.org.za/content/view/3877/266/. Accessed on April 4, 2011.

Davis, Mike. 2006. *Planet of Slums*. New York: Verso.

De Paoli, Marina Manuela, Arne Backer Grønningsæter, and Elizabeth Mills. 2010. *HIV/AIDS, the Disability Grant and ARV Adherence: Summary Report*. Oslo: Fafo.

De Waal, Alex. 2006. *AIDS and Power: Why There Is No Political Crisis—Yet*. New York: Zed Books.

De Wet, Thea, Leila Patel, Marcel Korth, and Chris Forrester. 2008. Johannesburg Poverty and Livelihoods Study. University of the Witwatersrand, Johannesburg, Centre for Social Development in Africa.

Deacon, Harriet, Inez Stephney, and Sandra Prosalendis. 2005. *Understanding HIV/AIDS Stigma: A Theoretical and Methodological Analysis*. Human Science Research Council Social Cohesion and Integration Unit (HSRC SCI), in collaboration with the HSRC's Social Aspects of HIV/AIDS Unit (SAHA). Cape Town: HSRC Press.

Dean, Mitchell. 2002. "Powers of Life and Death beyond Governmentality." *Cultural Values* 6 (1 and 2): 119–38.

Decoteau, Claire. 2008. "The Bio-Politics of HIV/AIDS in Post-Apartheid South Africa." PhD diss., University of Michigan. Proquest (AAT 3343047).

Deleuze, Gilles. 1997. *Negotiations, 1972–1990*. New York: Columbia University Press.

Delius, Peter, and Clive Glaser. 2005. "Sex, Disease, and Stigma in South Africa: Historical Perspectives." *African Journal of AIDS Research* 4 (1): 29–36.

Department of Health, South Africa (DOH). 1996. National Drug Policy. (January). http://www.doh.gov.za/docs/policy/drugsjan1996.pdf. Accessed on October 13, 2011.

———. 2000. HIV/AIDS and STD Strategic Plan for South Africa, 2000–2005. http://data.unaids.org/Topics/NSP-Library/NSP-Africa/nsp_south_africa_2000-2005_en.pdf. Accessed on October 14, 2011.

———. 2001. Summary Report: National HIV Sero-Prevalence Survey of Women Attending Ante-Natal Clinics in South Africa. Pretoria: Directorate of Health Systems Research and Epidemiology.

———. 2003. Operational Plan for Comprehensive HIV and AIDS Care, Management and Treatment for South Africa. November 19. http://www.info.gov.za/otherdocs/2003/aidsplan.pdf. Accessed on March 20, 2008.

———. 2004. National Antiretroviral Treatment Guidelines, 1st ed. http://www.hst.org.za/publications/national-antiretroviral-treatment-guidelines. Accessed on October 17, 2011.

———. 2007. HIV/AIDS and STI Strategic Plan for South Africa, 2007–2011. http://www.safaids.net/files/S.A%20National%20HIVAIDS_STI%20Strategic%20Plan%202007-2011.pdf. Accessed on October 14, 2011.

———. 2009. National HIV and Syphilis Sero-Prevalence Survey, Pretoria. http://www.health-e.org.za/documents/85d3dad6136e8ca9d02cceb7f4a36145.pdf. Accessed on May 18, 2011.

———. 2010a. Clinical Guidelines for the Management of HIV & AIDS in Adults and Adolescents. http://www.doh.gov.za/docs/factsheets/guidelines/adult_art.pdf. Accessed on October 19, 2010.

———. 2010b. Module on Adherence Counselling. http://www.doh.gov.za/docs/misc/hiv/manual/adherence.pdf. Accessed on October 19, 2010.

Department of Health and Human Services, United States (DHHS). 2008. Guidelines for the Use of Antiretroviral Agents in HIV-1-Infected Adults and Adolescents. January 9. Developed by the Panel on Antiretroviral Guidelines for Adults and Adolescents—A Working Group of the Office of AIDS Research Advisory Council (OARAC).

Department of Health, Medical Research Council, and OrcMacro. 2007. South Africa Demographic and Health Survey 2003. Pretoria: Department of Health.

Department of Housing. 1994. White Paper on Housing: A New Housing Policy and Strategy for South Africa. *Government Gazette* 345 (16178) notice 1376 of December 23, 1994.

Department of Labour. 2006. Women in the South African Labour Market, 1995–2005. Pretoria: Republic of South Africa.

Department of Provincial and Local Government. 2005. Guidelines for the Implementation of the National Indigent Policy by Municipalities. (November). http://www.kzncogta.gov.za/Portals/0/Flagships/free_basic_services/Indigent%20Policy%20Implementation%20Guidelines%20DPLG%20Part%201.pdf. Accessed on June 24, 2011.

Department of Public Works. 2003. Appropriate Development of Infrastructure on Dolomite: Guidelines for Consultants. (August). http://www.info.gov .za/view/DownloadFileAction?id=70186. Accessed on July 11, 2011.

Derrida, Jacques. 1978. "Structure, Sign, and Play in the Discourse of the Human Sciences." In *Writing and Difference*, translated by Alan Bass, 278–300. Chicago: University of Chicago Press.

Desai, Ashwin. 2002. *We Are the Poors: Community Struggles in Post-Apartheid South Africa*. New York: Monthly Review Press.

Devenish, Annie. 2003. "Negotiating Healing: The Professionalisation of Traditional Healers in KwaZulu-Natal between 1985 and 2003." Master's thesis, Development Studies, University of Natal, Durban.

———. 2005. "Negotiating Healing: Understanding the Dynamics amongst Traditional Healers in KwaZulu-Natal as they Engage with Professionalisation." *Social Dynamics* 31 (2): 243–84.

Digby, Anne. 2005. "Self-Medication and the Trade in Medicine within a Multi-Ethnic Context: A Case Study of South Africa from the Mid-Nineteenth to Mid-Twentieth Centuries." *Social History of Medicine* 18 (3): 439–57.

———. 2006. *Diversity and Division in Medicine: Health Care in South Africa from the 1800s*. Oxford and Bern: Peter Lang.

Digby, Anne, and Helen Sweet. 2002. "Nurses as Culture Brokers in Twentieth-Century South Africa." In *Plural Medicine, Tradition and Modernity, 1800–2000*, edited by Waltraud Ernst, 113–29. New York: Routledge.

Dirlik, Arif. 1996. "The Postcolonial Aura: Third World Criticism in the Age of Global Capitalism." In *Contemporary Postcolonial Theory: A Reader*, edited by Padmini Mongia, 294–320. New York: Arnold.

Doctors for Life International v Speaker of National Assembly and Others. 2006. http://www.constitutionalcourt.org.za/uhtbin/cgisirsi/xoSXBfgKRp/ MAIN/259070012/9#top. (August 17). Accessed on June 8, 2011.

Donham, Don. 1998. "Freeing South Africa: The 'Modernization' of Male-Male Sexuality in Soweto." *Cultural Anthropology* 13 (1): 3–21.

Douglas, Mary. 2000. *Purity and Danger: An Analysis of Concepts of Pollution and Taboo*. New York: Routledge.

Drury, Allen. 1968. *"A Very Strange Society": A Journey to the Heart of South Africa*. New York: Pocket Books.

Dunkle, Kristin L., Rachel K. Jewkes, Heather C. Brown, Glenda E. Gray, James A. McIntryre, Sióbán D. Harlow. 2004. "Transactional Sex among Women in Soweto, South Africa: Prevalence, Risk Factors, and Association with HIV Infection." *Social Science and Medicine* 59 (8): 1581–92.

Dugger, Celia. 2008. "Study Cites Toll of AIDS Policy in South Africa." *New York Times*. November 25.

———. 2009. "Zuma Rallies S. African to Fight AIDS." *New York Times*. October 31. http://www.nytimes.com/2009/11/01/world/africa/01zuma.html. Accessed on June 1, 2011.

——. 2010a. "In South Africa, an Unlikely Leader on AIDS." *New York Times.* May 14.

——. 2010b. "South Africa Redoubles Efforts against AIDS." *New York Times.* April 25.

Economist. 2010. "A President Who Promotes Tradition: Polygamy in South Africa." 394 (8664) (January 9): 49.

Electoral Institute for the Sustainability of Democracy in Africa (EISA). 2010. EISA Election Observer Mission Report no. 36: National and Provincial Elections, April 22, 2009. Johannesburg. http://www.eisa.org.za/PDF/sou2009eom.pdf. Accessed on January 28, 2012.

El-Khatib, Ziad, and Marlise Richter. 2009. "(ARV-) Free State? The Moratorium's Threat to Patients' Adherence and the Development of Drug-Resistant HIV." *South African Medical Journal* 99 (6): 412–13.

Epprecht, Marc. 2004. *Hungochani: The History of a Dissident Sexuality in Southern Africa.* Montreal: McGill-Queen's University Press.

Epstein, Helen. 2002. "The Hidden Cause of AIDS." *New York Review of Books* 49 (8): 43–49.

——. 2007. *The Invisible Cure: Africa, the West, and the Fight against AIDS.* New York: Farrar, Straus, and Giroux.

Epstein, Steven. 1996. *Impure Science: AIDS, Activism, and the Politics of Knowledge.* Berkeley: University of California Press.

——. 2007. *Inclusion: The Politics of Difference in Medical Research.* Chicago: University of Chicago Press.

Fabian, Johannes. 2002. *Time and the Other: How Anthropology Makes Its Object.* New York: Columbia University Press.

Fakier, Khayaat, and Jacklyn Cock. 2009. "A Gendered Analysis of the Crisis of Social Reproduction in Contemporary South Africa." *International Feminist Journal of Politics* 11 (3): 353–71.

Farmer, Paul. 1992. *AIDS and Accusation: Haiti and the Geography of Blame.* Berkeley: University of California Press.

——. 1999. *Infections and Inequalities: The Modern Plagues.* Berkeley: University of California Press.

——. 2002. "Introducing ARVs in Resource-Poor Settings." Plenary Speech, Partners in Health. http://www.hawaii.edu/hivandaids/Introducing _ARVs_in_Resource-Poor_Settings_Challenges.pdf. Accessed on October 4, 2011.

Fassin, Didier. 2007a. "Humanitarianism as a Politics of Life." *Public Culture* 19 (3): 499–520.

——. 2007b. *When Bodies Remember: Experiences and Politics of AIDS in South Africa.* Berkeley: University of California Press.

——. 2011. *Humanitarian Reason: A Moral History of the Present.* Berkeley: University of California Press

Fennell, C. W., K. L. Lindsey, L. J. McGaw, S. G. Sparg, G. I. Stafford, E. E. Elgorashi, O. M. Grace, and J. van Staden. 2004. "Assessing African Medicinal

Plants for Efficacy and Safety: Pharmacological Screening and Toxicology." *Journal of Ethnopharmacology* 94: 205–17.

Ferguson, James. 1999. *Expectations of Modernity: Myths and Meanings of Urban Life on the Zambian Copperbelt.* Berkeley: University of California Press.

———. 2007. "Formalities of Poverty: Thinking about Social Assistance in Neoliberal South Africa." *African Studies Review* 50 (September): 71–86.

Ferguson, James, and Akhil Gupta. 2002. "Spatializing States: Toward an Ethnography of Neoliberal Governmentality." *American Ethnologist* 29 (November): 981–1002.

Fihlani, Pumza. 2011. "Could South Africa's Freedom Fighters Return to the Streets?" *BBC News*, July 18. http://www.bbc.co.uk/news/world-africa -13761287. Accessed on July 28, 2011.

Flint, Karen E. 2001. "Competition, Race, and Professionalization: African Healers and White Medical Practitioners in Natal, South Africa in the Early Twentieth Century." *Social History of Medicine* 14 (2): 199–221.

———. 2006. Indian-African Encounters: Polyculturalism and African Therapeutics in Natal, South Africa, 1886–1950s. *Journal of Southern African Studies* 32 (2): 367–85.

———. 2008. *Healing Traditions: African Medicine, Cultural Exchange, and Competition in South Africa, 1820–1948.* Athens: Ohio University Press.

Food and Agriculture Organization, United Nations. 2011. "Global Information and Early Warning System, on Food and Agriculture." www.fao.org/giews/ pricetool2/. Accessed on May 11, 2011.

Forrest, Drew, and Barry Streek. 2001. "Mbeki in Bizarre AIDS Outburst." *Mail and Guardian*, October 26–November 1.

Foster, G., C. Levi, and J. Williamson, eds. 2005. *A Generation at Risk: The Global Impact of HIV/AIDS on Orphans and Vulnerable Children.* Cambridge: Cambridge University Press.

Foucault, Michel. 1972. *The Archaeology of Knowledge and the Discourse on Language.* New York: Pantheon Books.

———. 1985. *The Use of Pleasure.* Vol. 2 of the *History of Sexuality.* New York: Vintage Books.

———. 1988. *Technologies of the Self: A Seminar with Michel Foucault,* edited by Luther Martin, Huck Gutman, and Patrick Hutton. Amherst: University of Massachusetts Press.

———. 1990. *History of Sexuality,* vol. 1. New York: Vintage Books.

———. 1991. "Governmentality." In *The Foucault Effect: Studies in Governmentality,* edited by Graham Burchell, Colin Gordon, and Peter Miller, 87–104. Chicago: University of Chicago Press.

———. 1995. *Discipline and Punish: The Birth of the Prison.* New York: Vintage Books.

———. 1997. *"Society Must Be Defended": Lectures at the Collège de France, 1975–1976.* New York: Picador.

———. 2000. "The Political Technology of Individuals." In *Power: Essential Works of Foucault, 1954–1984*, vol. 3, edited by Paul Rabinow, 403–17. New York: New Press.

———. 2003. *Abnormal: Lectures at the Collège de France, 1974–1975*. Translated by Graham Burchell. New York: Picador.

———. 2007. *Security, Territory, Population: Lectures at the Collège de France, 1977–1978*. Translated by Graham Burchell. New York: Picador.

———. 2008. *The Birth of Biopolitics: Lectures at the Collège de France, 1978–79*. Translated by Graham Burchell. New York: Palgrave Macmillan.

Fraser, Nancy. 1997. *Justice Interruptus: Critical Reflections on the "Postsocialist" Condition*. New York: Routledge.

———. 2003. "From Discipline to Flexibilization? Rereading Foucault in the Shadow of Globalization." *Constellations* 10 (2): 160–71.

Freund, Bill. 2007. "South Africa: The End of Apartheid and the Emergence of the 'BEE Elite.'" *Review of African Political Economy* 34 (114): 661–78.

Friedman, Steven, and Shauna Mottiar. 2004. "Rewarding Engagement?: The Treatment Action Campaign and the Politics of HIV/AIDS." *Centre for Civil Society*: 1–42. http://ccs.ukzn.ac.za/files/FRIEDMAN%20MOTTIER%20A% 20MORAL%20TO%20THE%20TALE%20LONG%20VERSION.PDF. Accessed on June 7, 2011.

Gauteng Department of Health and Social Development. 2010. Service Transformation Plan, 2010–2020. (October). www.healthandsocdev.gpg.gov.za/ Documents/Draft3STP041010.doc. Accessed on March 20, 2012.

Gevisser, Mark, and Edwin Cameron. 1995. *Defiant Desire: Gay and Lesbian Lives in South Africa*. London: Routledge.

Gilroy, Paul. 1994. "Black Cultural Politics: An Interview with Paul Gilroy by Timmy Lott." *Found Object* 4: 46–81.

Gonzalez, Laura Lopez. 2011. "Delayed Drug Registration Could Affect Region." February 2. http://allafrica.com/stories/201102030267.html. Accessed on March 28, 2011.

Good, Byron. 1994. *Medicine, Rationality, and Experience: An Anthropological Perspective*. Cambridge: Cambridge University Press.

Gordon, David. 2001. "A Sword of Empire?: Medicine and Colonialism in King William's Town, Xhosaland, 1856–1891." *African Studies* 60 (2): 165–83.

Govender, Peroshni. 2011. "Zuma Back in the Driving Seat." *Mail and Guardian* online, January 25. http://mg.co.za/article/2011-01-25-zuma-back-in-the -driving-seat. Accessed on December 4, 2011.

GRAIN. 2001. "'TRIPS-Plus' through the Back Door: How Bilateral Treaties Impose Much Stronger Rules for IPRs on Life Than the WTO." http://www .grain.org/article/entries/5-trips-plus-through-the-back-door#_edn1. Accessed on October 9, 2011.

Green, Edward. 1994. *AIDS and STDs in Africa: Bridging the Gap between Traditional Healing and Modern Medicine*. Boulder, CO: Westview Press.

———. 1999. *Indigenous Theories of Contagious Disease*. London: AltaMira.

Greenberg, Stephen. 2004. "Post-Apartheid Development, Landlessness, and the Reproduction of Exclusion in South Africa." Centre for Civil Society Research Report No. 17. Durban: University of KwaZulu-Natal. http://ccs .ukzn.ac.za/files/RR17.pdf. Accessed on May 30, 2011.

Guest, Emma. 2001. *Children of AIDS: Africa's Orphan Crisis*. Pietermaritzburg: University of Natal Press.

Gumede, M. V. 1990. *Traditional Healers: A Medical Practitioner's Perspective*. Cape Town: Blackshaws.

Gumede, William Mervin. 2005. *Thabo Mbeki and the Battle for the Soul of the ANC*. Cape Town: Zebra Press.

——. 2008. "South Africa: Jacob Zuma and the Difficulties of Consolidating South Africa's Democracy." *African Affairs* 107 (427): 261–71.

Gunner, Liz. 2008. "Jacob Zuma, the Social Body, and the Unruly Power of Song." *African Affairs* 108 (430): 27–48.

Hall, Stuart. 1996a. "When Was 'The Post-Colonial'? Thinking at the Limit." In *The Post-Colonial Question: Common Skies, Divided Horizons*, edited by Iain Chambers and Lidia Curti, 242–60. New York: Routledge.

——. 1996b. "Who Needs Identity?" In *The Question of Cultural Identity*, edited by Stuart Hall and Paul DuGuy, 1017. London: Sage.

Halperin, Daniel T., and Helen Epstein. 2004. "Concurrent Sexual Partnerships Help to Explain Africa's High HIV Prevalence: Implications for Prevention." *Lancet* 364 (9,428): 4–6.

——. 2007. "Why Is HIV Prevalence So Severe in Southern Africa?" *Southern African Journal of HIV Medicine* 26 (March): 19–25.

Hammond-Tooke, W. D. 1974. *The Bantu-Speaking Peoples of Southern Africa*. Boston: Routledge and K. Paul.

——. 1981. *Boundaries and Belief: The Structure of a Sotho Worldview*. Johannesburg: University of Witwatersrand Press.

Hardy, Chloe, and Marlise Richter. 2006. "Disability Grants or Antiretrovirals? A Quandary for People with HIV/AIDS in South Africa." *African Journal of AIDS Research* 5 (1): 85–96.

Harrison, P. 1992. "The Policies and Politics of Informal Settlement in South Africa: A Historical Perspective." *Africa Insight* 22 (1): 14–22.

Hart, Gillian. 2006. "Post-Apartheid Developments in Historical and Comparative Perspective." In *The Development Decade? Economic and Social Change in South Africa, 1994–2004*, edited by Vishnu Padayachee, 13–32. Cape Town: Human Science Research Council Press.

——. 2008. "The Provocations of Neoliberalism: Contesting the Nation and Liberation after Apartheid." *Antipode* 40 (4): 678–705.

Hassim, Shireen. 2005. "Gender, Welfare and the Developmental State in South Africa." United Nations Research Institute for Social Development (UNRISD). http://www.sarpn.org/documents/d0001335/index.php. Accessed on October 28, 2011.

———. 2006. *Women's Organizations and Democracy in South Africa: Contesting Authority.* Madison: University of Wisconsin Press.

Health Gap (Global Access Project). 2010. "AIDS Activists Launch United Nations Complaint." http://www.healthgap.org/UNcomplaint.htm. Accessed on October 19, 2010.

Heimer, Carol. 2007. "Old Inequalities, New Disease: HIV/AIDS in Sub-Saharan Africa." *Annual Review of Sociology* 33: 551–77.

Hein, Wolfgang. 2007. "Global Health Governance and WTO/TRIPS: Conflicts between 'Global Market-Creation' and 'Global Social Rights.'" In *Global Health Governance and the Fight against HIV/AIDS*, edited by Wolfgang Hein, Sonja Bartsch, and Lars Kohlmorgen, 38–66. New York: Palgrave Macmillan.

Henderson, Patricia. 2005. "A Gift without Shortcomings: Healers Negotiating the Intersection of the Local and Global in the Context of HIV/AIDS." *Social Text* 31 (2): 24–54.

Herwitz, Daniel. 2006. "Understanding AIDS in South Africa." *Journal of the International Institute* 13 (Winter): 2 and 4.

Heywood, Mark. 2003. "Preventing Mother to Child HIV Transmission in South Africa: Background, Strategies and Outcomes of the TAC Case Against the Minister of Health." *South African Journal on Human Rights* 19: 278–315.

———. 2004a. "Condemn the Threats by NAPWA against AIDS Activists." *TAC Newsletter* 30 (March 30). http://www.tac.org.za/newsletter/2004/ns30_03_2004.htm. Accessed on June 7, 2011.

———. 2004b. "Price of Denial," *Development Update* 5: 3. www.tac.org.za/Documents/PriceOfDenial.doc. Accessed on June 3, 2011.

———. 2008. "Politics of Health." Online book about the TAC. http://www.tac.org.za/community/heywood. Accessed on June 15, 2011.

———. 2009. "South Africa's Treatment Action Campaign: Combining Law and Social Mobilization to Realize the Right to Health." *Journal of Human Rights Practice* 1 (March): 14–36.

Hobsbawm, Eric. [1983] 2003. "Introduction: Inventing Traditions." In *The Invention of Tradition*, edited by Eric Hobsbawm and Terence Ranger, 1–14. Cambridge: Cambridge University Press.

Huchzermeyer, Marie. 1999. "The Exploration of Appropriate Informal Settlement Intervention in South Africa: Contributions from a Comparison with Brazil." PhD thesis, University of Cape Town, South Africa.

———. 2001. "Housing for the Poor? Negotiated Housing Policy in South Africa." *Habitat International* 25 (September): 303–31.

———. 2006. "The New Instrument for Upgrading Informal Settlements in South Africa: Contributions and Constraints." In *Informal Settlements: A Perpetual Challenge?*, edited by Marie Huchzermeyer and Aly Karam, 41–61. Cape Town: University of Cape Town Press.

Huchzermeyer, Marie, and Aly Karam. 2006. "The Continuing Challenge of Informal Settlements: An Introduction." In *Informal Settlements: A Perpetual Challenge?*, edited by Marie Huchzermeyer and Aly Karam, 1–16. Cape Town: University of Cape Town Press.

Hull, Jonah. 2010. "Whoonga Is the Cruelest High." *Al Jazeera*. October 22. http://blogs.aljazeera.net/africa/2010/10/22/whoonga-cruelest-high. Accessed on October 18, 2011.

Human Rights Committee of South Africa. 2002. Press Release: "Forced Removals in Mandelaville: Chilling Echoes of Apartheid." (January 15). Braamfontein, Johannesburg.

Human Sciences Research Council (HSRC). 2005. Fact Sheet: National HIV Prevalence in South Africa—the Graphics. http://www.hsrc.ac.za/Factsheet-40.phtml. Accessed on April 20, 2009.

———. 2008a. *South African National HIV Prevalence, Incidence, Behaviour, and Communication Survey, 2008*. Cape Town: HSRC Press.

———. 2008b. *Violence and Xenophobia in South Africa: Developing Consensus, Moving to Action*. Cape Town: HSRC Press. http://www.hsrc.ac.za/Document-2994.phtml. Accessed on June 25, 2011.

Hunter, Mark. 2002. "The Materiality of Everyday Sex: Thinking beyond 'Prostitution.'" *African Studies* 61 (1): 99–120.

———. 2004. "Masculinities, Multiple-Sexual-Partners, and AIDS: The Making and Unmaking of *Isoka* in KwaZulu-Natal." *Transformation* 54: 123–53.

———. 2006. "Informal Settlements as Spaces of Health Inequality: The Changing Economic and Spatial Roots of the Aids Pandemic, from Apartheid to Neoliberalism." *Centre for Civil Society Research Report* 1 (44): 143–66.

———. 2007. "The Changing Political Economy of Sex in South Africa: The Significance of Unemployment and Inequalities to the Scale of the AIDS Pandemic." *Social Science and Medicine* 64 (3): 689–700.

———. 2010. *Love in the Time of AIDS: Inequality, Gender, and Rights in South Africa*. Bloomington: Indiana University Press.

———. 2011. "Beneath the 'Zunami': Jacob Zuma and the Gendered Politics of Social Reproduction in South Africa." *Antipode* 43 (4): 1102–26.

Hutchings, A., and J. van Staden. 1994. "Plants Used for Stress-Related Ailments in Traditional Zulu, Xhosa, and Sotho Medicines. Part 1. Plants Used for Headaches." *Journal of Ethnopharmacy* 43: 89–124.

Hutnyk, John. 2005. "Hybridity." *Ethnic and Racial Studies* 28 (4): 79–102.

Iliff, P. J., E. Piwoz, N. Tavengwa, C. Zunguza, and E. Marinda. 2005. "Early Exclusive Breastfeeding Reduces the Risk of Postnatal HIV-1 Transmission and Increases HIV-Free Survival." *AIDS* 19: 699–708.

Independent Online. 2001. "AIDS Is South Africa's New Apartheid, Says Tutu." October 7. http://www.iol.co.za/index.php?sf=2813&set_id=&sf=2813&click_id=13&art_id=qw1002460681991B232&set_id=1. Accessed on May 27, 2011.

Irwin, Alan. 1995. *Citizen Science: A Study of People, Expertise, and Sustainable Development*. New York: Routledge.

Jacobs, Sean, and Richard Calland, eds. 2002. *Thabo Mbeki's World: The Politics and Ideology of the South African President*. Durban: University of Natal Press.

Jacobs, Sean, and Krista Johnson. 2007. "Media, Social Movements, and the State: Competing Images of HIV/AIDS in South Africa." *African Studies Quarterly* 9 (Fall). http://www.africa.ufl.edu/asq/v9/v9i4a8.htm. Accessed on June 7, 2011.

Janes, Craig R., and Kitty K. Corbett. 2009. "Anthropology and Global Health." *Annual Review of Anthropology* 38 (167): 183.

Janzen, John M. 1981. "The Need for a Taxonomy of Health in the Study of African Therapeutics." *Social Science and Medicine* 15B (3): 185–94.

———. 1992. *Ngoma Discourses of Healing in Central and Southern Africa*. Berkeley: University of California Press.

Jochelson, Karen. 2001. *The Colour of Disease: Syphilis and Racism in South Africa, 1880–1950*. New York: Palgrave.

Johnson, Krista. 2004. "The Politics of AIDS Policy Development and Implementation in Postapartheid South Africa." *Africa Today* 51 (Winter): 107–28.

———. 2005. "Globalization, Social Policy, and the State: An Analysis of HIV/AIDS in South Africa." *New Political Science* 27 (3): 309–29.

Johnson-Hanks, Jennifer. 2006. *Uncertain Honor: Modern Motherhood in an African Crisis*. Chicago: University of Chicago Press.

Junod, Henri. 1962. *The Life of a South African Tribe*. New Hyde Park, NY: University Books.

Kandiyoti, Deniz. 1991. "Identity and Its Discontents: Women and the Nation." *Millennium: Journal of International Studies* 20 (March): 429–43.

Kapp, Clare. 2009. "Aaron Motsoaledi: South African Minister of Health." *The Lancet* 374 (September 5): 776.

Katz, Alison. 2002. "AIDS, Individual Behaviour, and the Unexplained Remaining Variation." *African Journal of AIDS Research* 1: 125–42.

Kaufman, Carol, and Stavros Stavrou. 2004. "'Bus Fare Please': The Economics of Sex and Gifts among Young People in Urban South Africa." *Culture, Health, and Sexuality* 6 (5): 377–91.

Kimmel, Michael. 1987. "The Contemporary 'Crisis' of Masculinity in Historical Perspective." In *The Making of Masculinities: The New Men's Studies*, edited by Harry Brod, 121–53. Boston: Allen and Unwin.

King, Nicholas B. 2002. "Security, Disease, Commerce: Ideologies of Postcolonial Global Health." *Social Studies of Science* 32 (5/6): 763–89.

Kleinman, Arthur. 1988. *The Illness Narratives: Suffering, Healing, and the Human Condition*. New York: Basic Books.

Kondlo, Kwandiwe. 2010. "Introduction: Political and Governance Challenges." In *The Zuma Administration: Critical Challenges*, edited by

Kwandiwe Kondlo and Mashupye Maserumule, 1–14. Cape Town: HSRC Press.

Krige, Eileen Jenson. 1950. *The Social System of the Zulus*. Pietermaritzburg: Shuter and Shuter.

Kristeva, Julia. 1982. *Powers of Horror: An Essay on Abjection*. New York: Columbia University Press.

Lacan, Jacques. 1977. *Écrits: A Selection*. New York: Norton.

Lahiff, Edward. 2010. Interview on PBS regarding the *Promised Land* documentary. http://www.pbs.org/pov/promisedland/land_reform.php. Accessed on May 23, 2011.

Lancet. 2009. "HIV/AIDS: A New South Africa Takes Responsibility." 374 (December 5): 1867.

Latour, Bruno. 1991. *We Have Never Been Modern*. Translated by Catherine Porter. Cambridge, MA: Harvard University Press.

———. 2004. "Why Has Critique Run Out of Steam? From Matters of Fact to Matters of Concern." *Critical Inquiry* 30 (Winter): 225–48.

Le Carré, John. 2000. *The Constant Gardener*. New York: Scribner.

Le Marcis, Frédéric. 2004. "The Suffering Body of the City." Translated by Judith Inggs. *Public Culture* 16 (3): 453–77.

Leclerc-Madlala, Suzanne. 1997. "'Infect One Infect All': Zulu Youth Responses to the AIDS Epidemic in South Africa." *Medical Anthropology* 17: 363–80.

———. 2001a. "Chasing King Cash Could Prove to Be Our Undoing." *Mail and Guardian*, June 15, 2005.

———. 2001b. "Virginity Testing: Managing Sexuality in a Maturing HIV/AIDS Epidemic." *Medical Anthropology Quarterly* 15 (4): 533–52.

———. 2002. "Youth, HIV/AIDS and the Importance of Sexual Culture and Context. *Social Dynamics* 28 (1): 20–41.

———. 2003. "Transactional Sex and the Pursuit of Modernity." *Social Dynamics* 29 (2): 213–33.

Legassick, Martin, and Harold Wolpe. 1976. "The Bantustans and Capital Accumulation in South Africa." *Review of African Political Economy* 7: 87–107.

Lévi-Strauss, Claude. 1966. *The Savage Mind*. Chicago: University of Chicago Press.

Levinsohn, James. 2007. "Estimating Correct HIV Prevalence Rates: The Case of Botswana." Presentation for the "Appraisal and Action: HIV/AIDS in Southern Africa" conference held at the University of Michigan, Ann Arbor, on November 29–30, 2007.

Liddell, C., L. Barrett, and M. Bydawell. 2005. "Indigenous Representations of Illness and AIDS in Sub-Saharan Africa." *Social Science and Medicine* 60: 691–700.

Light, M. E., S. G. Sparg, G. I. Stafford, and J. van Staden. 2005. "Riding the Wave: South Africa's Contribution to Ethnopharmacological Research over the Last 25 Years." *Journal of Ethnopharmacology* 100 (1–2): 127–30.

Lindow, Megan. 2009. "South Africa's Outraged Poor Threaten President." *Time World.* July 24. http://www.time.com/time/world/article/0,8599,1912479,00 .html#ixzz1cS3tJQWY. Accessed on December 3, 2011.

Lock, Margaret, and Vinh-Kim Nguyen. 2010. *An Anthropology of Biomedicine.* Malden, MA: Wiley-Blackwell.

Love, James. 2005. "Closing the Access Gap: The Equitable Access License." Consumer Project on Technology. www.essentialmedicine.org/EALPrimer .pdf. Accessed on October 10, 2011.

Luke, Nancy. 2003. "Age and Economic Asymmetries in the Sexual Relationships of Adolescent Girls in Sub-Saharan Africa." *Studies in Family Planning* 34 (2): 67–86.

Luke, Nancy, and Kathleen Kurz. 2002. "Cross Generational and Transactional Sexual Relations in Sub-Saharan Africa: Prevalence of Behavior and Implications for Negotiating Safer Sexual Practices." USAID, Africa Bureau: AIDSMark project (September).

Maclennan, B. 2002. "Zuma Says He's Not Prepared to Talk about Oral Sex." *The Herald.* June 13. http://www.theherald.co.za/herald/2002/06/13/news/ n09_13062002.htm. Accessed on November 8, 2011.

Mail and Guardian. 2002. "ANC Will Deal with AIDS, Says Mbeki." December 16. http://mg.co.za/article/2002-12-16-anc-will-deal-with-aids-says -mbeki. Accessed on June 8, 2011.

———. 2006a. "The Rise of South Africa's Shacks." January 6.

———. 2006b. "South African Government Ends Aids Denialism." October 28. http://www.mg.co.za/articlePage.aspx?articleid=288029&area=/ breaking_news/breaking_news_nation/.

———. 2007a . "In the Firing Line." June 15.

———. 2007b. "The Strike Is Over." June 28.

———. 2007c. "Wages: State May Go It Alone." June 15.

———. 2008. "Xenophobia: Special Report." http://mg.co.za/specialreport/ xenophobia. Accessed on June 25, 2011.

———. 2010. "Public-Sector Unions Accept Govt Wage Offer." October 20. http://mg.co.za/article/2010-10-20-publicsector-unions-accept-govt-wage -offer. Accessed on October 18, 2011.

Mamdani, Mahmood. 1996. *Citizen and Subject: Contemporary Africa and the Legacy of Late Colonialism.* Princeton, NJ: Princeton University Press.

Mander, M., and G. Le Breton. 2006. "Overview of the Medicinal Plant Industry in Southern Africa." In *Commercialising Medicinal Plants*, edited by N. Diederichs, 43–52. Stellenbosch: Sun Press.

Mander, Myles, Lungile Ntuli, Nicci Diederichs, and Khulile Mavundla. 2007. "Economics of the Traditional Medicine Trade in South Africa." In *South African Health Review*, edited by S. Harrison, R. Bhana, and A. Ntuli, 189–99. Durban: Health Systems Trust.

Manicom, Linzi. 2005. "Constituting 'Women' as Citizens: Ambiguities in the Making of Gendered Political Subjects in Post-Apartheid South Africa." In *(Un)thinking Citizenship: Feminist Debates in Contemporary South Africa*, edited by A Gouws, 21–52. Cape Town: University of Cape Town Press.

Marais, Hein. 2001. *Limits to Change: The Political Economy of Transition.* New York: Zed Books.

———. 2005. *Buckling: The Impact of AIDS in South Africa.* Pretoria: University of Pretoria Press.

———. 2011. *South Africa Pushed to the Limit: The Political Economy of Change.* New York: Zed Books.

Marcuse, Herbert. 1962. *Eros and Civilization: A Philosophical Inquiry into Freud.* New York: Vintage Books.

Marks, Shula. 1986. *The Ambiguities of Dependence in South Africa.* Baltimore: Johns Hopkins University Press.

Marks, Shula, and Neil Andersson. 1992. "Industrialization, Rural Health, and the 1944 National Health Services Commission in South Africa." In *The Social Basis of Health and Healing in Africa*, edited by Steven Feierman and John M. Janzen, 131–61. Berkeley: University of California Press.

Marshall, T. H., and T. Bottomore. 1992. *Citizenship and Social Class.* Concord, MA: Pluto.

Martin, John Levi. 2003. "What Is Field Theory?" *American Journal of Sociology* 109 (1): 1–49.

Marwaha, Alka. 2008. "Getting High on HIV Drugs in South Africa." *BBC News.* December 8. http://news.bbc.co.uk/2/hi/africa/7768059.stm. Accessed on October 18, 2011.

Mashigo, Polly. 2010. "Socio-Economic Development and Poverty Reduction in South Africa." In *The Zuma Administration: Critical Challenges*, edited by Kwandiwe Kondlo and Mashupye Maserumule, 107–44. Cape Town: HSRC Press.

Masondo, Amos. 2008. Statement by the Executive Mayor of Johannesburg, at a Media Briefing on the Formalisation and Regularisation of Informal Settlements. Metropolitan Centre, Mayoral Parlour, Braamfontein, Johannesburg. Part of the city of Johannesburg online housing archive. http://www.joburg.org.za/content/view/4142/114/. Accessed on April 7, 2011.

Mavimbela, Vusi. 1997. "The African Renaissance: A Workable Dream." Roundtable Discussion. Johannesburg: Foundation for Global Dialogue.

Mazrui, Ali A. 1975. "The Resurrection of the Warrior Tradition in African Political Culture." *Journal of Modern African Studies* 13 (1): 67–84.

Mbali, Mandisa. 2002. "Mbeki's Denialism and the Ghosts of Apartheid and Colonialism for Post-Apartheid AIDS Policy-Making." Paper presented at the Public Health Journal Club Seminar on May 3, 2002. Durban: University of Natal.

———. 2003. "HIV/AIDS Policy-Making in Post-Apartheid South Africa" In *State of the Nation, 2003–2004*, edited by John Daniel, Adam Habib, and Roger Southall, 312–29. Johannesburg: Human Sciences Research Council.

———. 2004. "AIDS Discourses and the South African State: Government Denialism and Post-Apartheid AIDS Policy-Making." *Transformation* 54: 104–22.

———. 2005. "The Treatment Action Campaign and the History of Rights-Based, Patient-Driven HIV/AIDS Activism in South Africa." Research Report #9. Centre for Civil Society, University of KwaZulu-Natal, South Africa. www.nu.ac.za/ccs/files/RReport_29.pdf. Accessed on June 10, 2011.

Mbeki, Thabo. 1996. "I Am an African." Statement of Deputy President TM Mbeki, on Behalf of the African National Congress, on the Occasion of the Adoption by the Constitutional Assembly of "The Republic of South Africa Constitutional Bill 1996." Cape Town, May 8.

———. 1998a. "The African Renaissance." Statement of Deputy President, Thabo Mbeki, SABC, Gallager Estate, Johannesburg, August 13. http://www.dfa.gov.za/docs/speeches/1998/mbek0813.htm. Accessed on July 26, 2011.

———. 1998b. "The African Renaissance, South Africa and the World." Speech at the United Nations University, April 9. http://www.dfa.gov.za/docs/speeches/1998/mbek0409.htm. Accessed on July 26, 2011.

———. 1998c. Speech by Thabo Mbeki at the Opening of the Ministerial Meeting at the XII Summit Meeting of Heads of State and Government of the Countries of the Non-Aligned Movement, Durban, August 31. http://www.dfa.gov.za/docs/speeches/1998/mbek0831.htm. Accessed on July 26, 2011.

———. 1998d. Statement of Deputy President Thabo Mbeki at the Opening of the Debate in the National Assembly, on "Reconciliation and Nation Building," National Assembly Cape Town, May 29, 1998. http://www.dfa.gov.za/docs/speeches/1998/mbek0529.htm. Accessed on June 8, 2011.

———. 1999a. "Address to the National Council of Provinces," Cape Town, October 28, 1999.

———. 1999b. Speech Given in Parliament. "Debates of the National Assembly." *Hansard*, November 16, 1999.

———. 2000. Speech of the President of South Africa at the Opening Session of the 13th International AIDS Conference, Durban, South Africa.

———. 2001. Address of the President of South Africa, Thabo Mbeki, at the Third African Renaissance Festival, Durban, March 31. http://www.dfa.gov.za/docs/speeches/2001/mbek0331.htm. Accessed on July 26, 2011.

———. 2002. "Speech at the Funeral of Sarah Bartmann." Department of International Relations and Cooperation, August 9, 2002. http://www.dfa.gov.za/docs/speeches/2002/mbek0809.htm. Accessed on June 7, 2011.

———. 2003. Media Briefing by President Thabo Mbeki Following the Cabinet Lekgotla, Union Buildings, Pretoria, July 29. http://www.info.gov.za/speeches/2003/03080511461001.htm. Accessed on October 22, 2010.

———. 2004a. "Nevirapine, Drugs, and African Guinea Pigs." *ANC Today* 4, 50 (December 17). http://www.anc.org.za/docs/anctoday/2004/at50.htm#art1. Accessed on June 7, 2011.

————. 2004b. Speech Given to a Group of Faith Leaders at the AGS Tabernacle in Kimberly, Northern Cape. "Mbeki Meets Up with Faith Leaders." *SABC News*. March 30, 2004.

————. 2004c. "When Is Good News Bad News?" *ANC Today* 4, 39 (October). http://www.anc.org.za/docs/anctoday/2004/at39.htm. Accessed in December 2011.

Mbembe, Achille. 2001. *On the Postcolony*. Berkeley: University of California Press.

————. 2003. "Necropolitics." *Public Culture* 15 (1): 11–40.

Mbembe, Achille, and Sarah Nuttall. 2004. "Writing the World from an African Metropolis." *Public Culture* 16 (3): 347–72.

McClintock, Anne. 1992. "The Angel of Progress: Pitfalls of the Term 'Post-Colonialism.'" *Social Text* 10 (Spring): 84–98.

————. 1995. *Imperial Leather: Race, Gender, Sexuality, and the Colonial Contest*. New York: Routledge.

McDonald, David, and Greg Ruiters. 2005. *The Age of Commodity: Water Privatization in South Africa*. Earthscan Publications.

McGrane, Michelle. 2006. "Khabzela: The Life and Times of a South African by Liz McGregor." *The New Review*. http://www.laurahird.com/newreview/khabzela.html. Accessed on October 10, 2011.

McGregor, Liz. 2005. *Khabzela: The Life and Times of a South African*. Johannesburg: Jacana Media.

McIntyre, J. 2007. "Antiretrovirals for Reducing the Risk of Mother-to-Child Transmission of HIV Infection: RHL Commentary." Last revised August 22, 2007. *The WHO Reproductive Health Library*. Geneva: World Health Organization.

McKinley, Dale, and Ahmed Veriava. 2010. *Arresting Dissent: State Repression and Post-Apartheid Social Movements*. Lambert Academic Publishing.

McNeil, Donald, Jr. 1998. "Neighbors Kill an H.I.V.-Positive AIDS Activist in South Africa." *New York Times*. December 28.

Medical Research Council (MRC), South Africa. 2002. A Toxicity Study of *Sutherlandia* Leaf Powder (*Sutherlandia microphylla*) Consumption. (April). http://www.sahealthinfo.org/traditionalmeds/firststudy.htm. Accessed on October 13, 2011.

————. 2003. National Reference Centre for African Traditional Medicines: A South African Model. http://www.mrc.ac.za/traditionalmedicines/national.htm. Accessed on October 11, 2011.

————. 2004. A Toxicity Study of LEAF Consumption. http://www.mrc.ac.za/iks/iksleaf1.pdf. Accessed on October 13, 2011.

Meissner, Ortrum. 2004. "The Traditional Healer as Part of the Primary Health Care Team?" *South African Journal of Medicine* 94 (11): 901–2.

Mills, Elizabeth. 2005. "HIV Illness Meanings and Collaborative Healing Strategies in South Africa." *Social Text* 31 (2): 126–60.

Mmila, Puleng. 2009. "Do Not Blame Culture for Vice." *Sowetan*. February 5.

Mohanty, Chandra Talpade, Ann Russo, and Lourdes Torres. 1991. *Third World Women and the Politics of Feminism*. Bloomington: Indiana University Press.

Mohlala, Thabo. 2002. "Down in the Dumps." *Mail and Guardian*. April 5–11.

Morrell, Robert. 2001. "The Times of Change: Men and Masculinity in South Africa." In *Changing Men in Southern Africa*, edited by Robert Morrell, 3–37. New York: Zed Books.

Morris, M., and M. Kretzschmar. 1997. "Concurrent Partnerships and the Spread of HIV." *AIDS* 11 (5): 641–48.

Motsemme, Nthabiseng. 2007. "'Loving in a Time of Hopelessness': On Township Women's Subjectivities in a Time of HIV/AIDS." In *Women in South African History*, edited by Nomboniso Gasa, 369–95. Pretoria: Human Science Research Council Press.

Mpye, Siphiwe. 1999a. "Department Ignores Order." *Sowetan*. October 12.

———. 1999b. "Lawley Residents Fume." *Sowetan*. October 15.

———. 1999c. "Lawley Squatters Face More Evictions." *Sowetan*. October 21.

———. 1999d. "Lawley Squatters' Goods Returned." *Sowetan*. October 19.

Murray, Martin. 2008. *Taming the Disorderly City: The Spatial Landscape of Johannesburg after Apartheid*. Ithaca, NY: Cornell University Press.

Myburgh, James. 2007. "The Virodene Affair, Parts I and II." Politicsweb. (September). http://www.politicsweb.co.za/politicsweb/view/politicsweb/en/page71619?oid=83156&sn=Detail. Accessed on June 3, 2011.

———. 2012. "Virodene, Transformation, and the Constitution." Politicsweb. (March 19). http://www.politicsweb.co.za/politicsweb/view/politicsweb/en/page71619?oid=287176&sn=Detail&pid=71616. Accessed on March 20, 2012.

Myers, J. C. 2008. *Indirect Rule in South Africa: Tradition, Modernity, and the Costuming of Political Power*. Rochester, NY: University of Rochester Press.

Naidoo, Prishani. 2010. "Indigent Management: A Strategic Response to the Struggles of the Poor in Post-Apartheid South Africa." In *New South African Review 2010: Development or Decline?*, edited by John Daniel, Prishani Naidoo, Devan Pillay, and Rogers Southall, 184–204. Johannesburg: Wits University Press.

Naidu, Veni, and Geoff Harris. 2006. "The Cost of HIV/AIDS Related Morbidity and Mortality to Households: Preliminary Estimates for Soweto." *South African Journal of Economic and Management Sciences* 9 (3): 384–91.

Nandy, Ashis. 1983. *The Intimate Enemy: Loss and Recovery of Self under Colonialism*. Delhi: Oxford University Press.

Narayan, Uma. 1997. *Dislocating Cultures: Identities, Traditions, and Third World Feminism*. New York: Routledge.

Nattrass, Nicoli. 2003. *The Moral Economy of AIDS in South Africa*. Cambridge: Cambridge University Press.

———. 2006. "Disability and Welfare in South Africa's Era of Unemployment and AIDS." Centre for Social Science Research Working Paper, no. 147. Cape Town: University of Cape Town. http://www.sarpn.org.za/documents/d0001936/index.php. Accessed on January 13, 2011.

———. 2007. *Mortal Combat: AIDS Denialism and the Struggle for Antiretrovirals in South Africa*. Durban: University of KwaZulu-Natal Press.

———. 2008a. "AIDS and the Scientific Governance of Medicine in Post-Apartheid South Africa." *African Affairs* 107/427: 157–76.

———. 2008b. "The (Political) Economics of Antiretroviral Treatment in Developing Countries." *Trends in Microbiology* 16 (12): 574–79.

Ngubane, Harriet. 1992. "Clinical Practice and Organization of Indigenous Healers in South Africa." In *The Social Basis of Health and Healing in Africa*, edited by Steven Feierman and J. M. Janzen, 366–75. Berkeley: University of California Press.

Nguyen, Vinh-Kim. 2005. "Antiretroviral Globalism, Biopolitics, and Therapeutic Citizenship." In *Global Assemblages: Technology, Politics, and Ethics as Anthropological Problems*, edited by Aihwa Ong and Stephen J. Collier, 124–44. Malden, MA: Blackwell.

———. 2010. *The Republic of Therapy: Triage and Sovereignty in West Africa's Time of AIDS*. Durham, NC: Duke University Press.

Nicodemus, A. 1999. "Africa Still Stigmatises HIV-Positive People." *Mail and Guardian*. May 7.

Niehaus, Isak. 2000. "Towards a Dubious Liberation: Masculinity, Sexuality, and Power in South African Lowveld Schools, 1953–1999." *Journal of Southern African Studies* 26 (3): 387–407.

———. 2002. "Bodies, Heat, and Taboos: Conceptualizing Modern Personhood in the South African Lowveld." *Ethnology* 43 (Summer): 189–208.

Norman, Rosana, Debbie Bradshaw, Simon Lewin, Eugene Cairncross, Nadine Nannan, Theo Vos, and the South African Comparative Risk Assessment Collaborating Group. 2010. "Estimating the Burden of Disease Attributable to Four Selected Environmental Risk Factors in South Africa." *Reviews on Environmental Health* 25 (2): 87–120.

Norman, Rosana, Debbie Bradshaw, Michelle Schneider, Rachel Jewkes, Shanaaz Matthews, Naeemah Abrahams, Richard Matzopoulos, Theo Vos, and the South African Comparative Risk Assessment Collaborating Group. 2007. "Estimating the Burden of Disease Attributable to Interpersonal Violence in South Africa in 2000." *South African Medical Journal* 97 (8): 653–56.

Nullis, Clare. 2006. "Same-Sex Marriage Law Takes Effect in S. Africa." *Washington Post*, A20. December 1. http://www.washingtonpost.com/wp-dyn/content/article/2006/11/30/AR2006113001370.html. Accessed on November 13, 2011.

Nuttall, Sarah. 2004. "Stylizing the Self: The Y Generation in Rosebank, Johannesburg." *Public Culture* 16 (3): 430–52.

Nyanzi, S., R. Pool, and J. Kinsman. 2001. "The Negotiation of Sexual Relationships among School Pupils in South-Western Uganda." *AIDS Care* 13 (1): 83–98.

Observer. 2004. "AIDS Death of DJ Highlights Anguish of South Africa." February 29. http://observer.guardian.co.uk/international/story/0,6903, 1158701,00.html. Accessed on October 10, 2011.

Olumwullah, Osaak A. 2002. *Dis-Ease in the Colonial State: Medicine, Society, and Social Change among the AbaNyole of Western Kenya.* Westport, CT: Greenwood Press.

Ong, Aihwa. 1988. "Colonialism and Modernity: Feminist Re-Presentations of Women in Non-Western Societies." *Inscriptions* 3/4: 79–93.

———. 2006. *Neoliberalism as Exception: Mutations in Citizenship and Sovereignty.* Durham, NC: Duke University Press.

Oswin, Natalie. 2007. "Producing Homonormativity in Neoliberal South Africa: Recognition, Redistribution, and the Equality Project." *Signs: Journal of Women in Culture and Society* 32 (3): 649–69.

Oxfam. 2001. "Priced out of Reach: How WTO Patent Policies Will Reduce Access to Medicines in the Developing World." (October). http://policy-practice .oxfam.org.uk/publications/priced-out-of-reach-how-wto-patent-policies-will-reduce-access-to-medicines-in-114571. Accessed on October 9, 2011.

Oyěwùmí, Oyèrónké. 1997. *The Invention of Women: Making an African Sense of Western Gender Discourse.* Minneapolis: University of Minnesota Press.

Packard, Randall. 1989. *White Plague, Black Labor: Tuberculosis and the Political Economy of Health and Disease in South Africa.* Berkeley: University of California Press.

———. 1997. "Visions of Postwar Health and Development and Their Impact on Public Health Intervention in the Developing World." In *International Development and the Social Sciences: Essays on the History and Politics of Knowledge,* edited by Frederick Cooper and Randall Packard, 93–115. Berkeley: University of California Press.

———. 2003. "Postcolonial Medicine." In *Companion to Medicine in the Twentieth Century,* edited by Roger Cooter and John Pickstone, 97–112. New York: Routledge.

Packard, Randall, and Paul Epstein. 1991. "Epidemiologists, Social Scientists, and the Structure of Medical Research on AIDS in Africa." *Social Science and Medicine* 33 (7): 771–94.

Parliamentary Monitoring Group (PMG). 2010. Public Hearings: Social Assistance Amendment Bill [B5-2010]. (April 21). http://www.pmg.org.za/ report/20100421-public-hearings-social-assistance-amendment-bill-b5 -2010-day-2. Accessed on October 14, 2011.

Patton, Cindy. 2002. *Globalizing AIDS.* Theory Out of Bounds, vol. 2. Minneapolis: University of Minnesota Press.

Peck, Jamie, and Adam Tickell. 2002. "Neoliberalizing Space." *Antipode* 34 (3): 380–404.

Perry, Alex. 2010. "South African Strike Poses a Dilemma for Zuma." *Time World,* August 20. http://www.time.com/time/world/article/0,8599, 2012003,00.html#ixzz1fZSNOQbe. Accessed on December 4, 2011.

Petryna, Adriana. 2002. *Life Exposed: Biological Citizens after Chernobyl.* Princeton, NJ: Princeton University Press.

Porter, Doug, and David Craig. 2004. "The Third Way and the Third World: Poverty Reduction and Social Inclusion in the Rise of 'Inclusive' Liberalism." *Review of International Political Economy* 11 (May): 387–423.

Posel, Deborah. 2005. "Sex, Death, and the Fate of the Nation: Reflections on the Politicization of Sexuality in Post-Apartheid South Africa." *Africa* 75 (2): 125–53.

Prakash, Gyan. 1999. *Another Reason: Science and the Imagination of Modern India.* Princeton, NJ: Princeton University Press.

Rabinow, Paul. 2005. "Midst Anthropology's Problems." In *Global Assemblages: Technology, Politics, and Ethics as Anthropological Problems,* edited by Aihwa Ong and Stephen J. Collier, 40–54. Malden, MA: Blackwell.

Rabinow, Paul, and Nikolas Rose. 2006. "Biopower Today." *BioSocieties* 1 (2): 195–217.

Ranger, Terence. 2003. "The Invention of Tradition in Colonial Africa." In *The Invention of Tradition,* edited by Eric Hobsbawm and Terence Ranger, 211–62. Cambridge: Cambridge University Press.

Ratele, Kopano. 2006. "Ruling Masculinity and Sexuality." *Feminist Africa* 6: 48–64.

Rath Foundation. 2005a. Advertisement. "No Censorship of Life-Saving Natural Health Information!" *Sowetan.* January 25. http://www.dr-rath -foundation.org.za/. Accessed on November 2005.

———. 2005b. http://www.dr-rath-foundation.org.za/ and http://www4 .dr-rath-foundation.org/Accessed on November 2005.

Rehle, Thomas, Olive Shisana, Victoria Pillay, Khangelani Zuma, Adrian Puren, and Warren Parker. 2007. "National HIV Incidence Measures—New Insights into the South African Epidemic." *South African Medical Journal* 97 (3): 194–99.

Republic of South Africa. 1996a. Choice on Termination of Pregnancy Act, no. 2. http://www.info.gov.za/acts/1996/a92–96.pdf. Accessed on November 13, 2011.

———. 1996b. Constitution of the Republic of South Africa, no. 108. http:// www.info.gov.za/documents/constitution/1996/a108-96.pdf. Accessed on January 29, 2012.

———. 1997. Medicines and Related Substances Control Amendment Act, no. 90. Government Gazette. Volume 390, Number 18505. December 12, 1997. http://www.info.gov.za/view/DownloadFileAction?id=70836. Accessed on October 13, 2011.

———. 1998a. Employment Equity Act, no. 1323. Government Gazette. Volume 400, Number 19370. October 19, 1998. http://www.info.gov.za/view/ DownloadFileAction?id=70714. Accessed on November 13, 2011.

———. 1998b. Recognition of Customary Marriages Act, no. 120 of 1998. Amended in 2001. http://www.justice.gov.za/legislation/acts/1998-120 .pdf. Accessed on November 14, 2011.

———. 1998c. South African Medicines and Medical Devices Regulatory Authority Act, no. 132. http://www.info.gov.za/view/DownloadFile Action?id=71294. Accessed on October 13, 2011.

———. 2005. The Traditional Health Practitioners Act, 2004. Cape Town: Government Gazette. Volume 476, Number 27275. February 11, 2005. http://www.doh.gov.za/docs/bills/thb.html. Accessed on June 8, 2011.

———. 2007. Traditional Health Practitioners Act 22, 2007. Cape Town: Government Gazette. Volume 511, Number 42. January 10, 2008. http://www.info.gov.za/view/DownloadFileAction?id=77788. Accessed on June 8, 2011.

———. 2009. "Key Messages for World AIDS Day 2009." December 1. http://www.info.gov.za/issues/hiv/aidsday2009.htm. Accessed on December 3, 2011.

———. 2010. National Treasury, Budget Review. February 17, 2010. http://www.treasury.gov.za/documents/national%20budget/2010/review/Budget%20Review.pdf. Accessed on April 28, 2010.

Robins, Steven L. 2004. "'Long Live Zackie, Long Live': AIDS Activism, Science, and Citizenship after Apartheid." *Journal of Southern African Studies* 30 (3): 651–72.

———. 2006. "From 'Rights' to 'Rituals': AIDS Activism in South Africa." *American Anthropologist* 108 (2): 312–23.

———. 2008a. *From Revolution to Rights in South Africa: Social Movements, NGOs, and Popular Politics after Apartheid.* Durban: University of KwaZulu-Natal Press.

———. 2008b. "Sexual Politics and the Zuma Rape Trial." *Journal of Southern African Studies* 34 (June): 411–27.

Robinson, Vicki, Rapule Tabane, and Ferial Haffajee. 2006. "23 Days That Shook Our World." *Mail and Guardian.* April 28.

Rose, Nikolas. 1999. *Powers of Freedom: Reframing Political Thought.* Cambridge: Cambridge University Press.

———. 2007. *The Politics of Life Itself: Biomedicine, Power, and Subjectivity in the Twenty-First Century.* Princeton, NJ: Princeton University Press.

Rose, Nikolas, and Carlos Novas. 2005. "Biological Citizenship." In *Global Assemblages: Technology, Politics, and Ethics as Anthropological Problems,* edited by Aihwa Ong and Stephen J. Collier, 439–63. Malden, MA: Blackwell.

Rosen, Sydney, Mpefe Ketlhapile, Ian Sanne, and Mary Bachman DeSilva. 2007. "Cost to Patients of Obtaining Treatment from HIV/AIDS in South Africa." *South African Medical Journal* 97 (3): 194–99.

Rossouw, Mandy. 2011. "Zuma Gets Behind Patel's New Growth Plan." *Mail and Guardian* online. January 8. http://mg.co.za/article/2011-01-08-zuma-gets-behind-patels-new-growth-path. Accessed on December 4, 2011.

Sanders, David, and Mickey Chopra. 2006. "Key Challenges to Achieving Health for All in an Inequitable Society: The Case of South Africa." *American Journal of Public Health* 96 (January): 73–78.

Sassen, Saskia. 1998. "Toward a *Feminist* Analytics of the Global Economy." In *Globalization and Its Discontents*, 81–109. New York: New Press.

Scheper-Hughes, Nancy. 2005. "The Last Commodity: Post-Human Ethics and the Global Traffic in 'Fresh' Organs." In *Global Assemblages: Technology, Politics, and Ethics as Anthropological Problems*, edited by Aihwa Ong and Stephen J. Collier, 145–67. Malden, MA: Blackwell.

Schmitt, Carl. 2005. *Political Theology: Four Chapters on the Concept of Sovereignty.* Chicago: University of Chicago Press.

Schneider, Helen, and David Coetzee. 2003. "Strengthening the Health System and Ensuring Equity in the Widescale Implementation of an Antiretroviral Therapy Programme in South Africa." *South African Medical Journal (SAMJ)* 93 (10): 772–73.

Schneider, Helen, and Jo Stein. 2001. "Implementing AIDS Policy in Post-Apartheid South Africa." *Social Science and Medicine* 52: 723–31.

Schneider, Michelle, Rosana Norman, Charles Parry, Debbie Bradshaw, and Andreas Plüddemann, and the South African Comparative Risk Assessment Collaborating Group. 2007. "Estimating the Burden of Disease Attributable to Alcohol Use in South Africa in 2000." *South African Medical Journal* 97 (8): 664–72.

Seekings, Jeremy, and Nicoli Nattrass. 2006. *Class, Race, and Inequality in South Africa.* Scottsville: University of KwaZulu-Natal Press.

Select Committee on Social Services. 1998. Report of the Select Committee on Social Services on Traditional Healers. No. 144-1998. August 4. Parliament of the Republic of South Africa, Cape Town. Hansard.

Selikow, T., B. Zulu, and E. Cedras. 2002. "The Ingagara, the Regte, and the Cherry: HIV/AIDS and Youth Culture in Contemporary Urban Townships." *Agenda* 53: 22–32.

Selva, Meera. 2005. "Apartheid's 'Dr Death' Faces Retrial on Poisoning Claims." *The Independent.* September 10. http://www.independent.co.uk/news/world/africa/apartheids-dr-death-faces-retrial-on-poisoning-claims-506208.html. Accessed on June 7, 2011.

Setel, Philip, Milton Lewis, and Maryinez Lyons, eds. 1999. *Histories of Sexually Transmitted Diseases and HIV/AIDS in Sub-Saharan Africa.* Westport, CT: Greenwood Press.

Sesanti, Simphiwe. 2010. "Africans Do Colonials' Dirty Work." *The Star.* February 5.

Shisana, O., T. Rehle, L. Simbayi, W. Parker, K. Zuma, and A. Bhana. 2005. *South African National HIV Prevalence, HIV Incidence, Behaviour and Communication Survey.* Cape Town: Human Sciences Research Council.

Shohat, Ella. 1992. "Notes on the 'Post-Colonial.'" *Social Text* 10 (Spring): 99–113.

Sideris, Tina. 2005. "'You Have to Change and You Don't Know How!': Contesting What It Means to Be a Man in a Rural Area of South Africa." In *Men*

Behaving Differently, edited by Graeme Reid and Liz Walker, 111–27. Cape Town: Double Storey.

Sidibé, Michel. 2009. "Speech by Director General of UNAIDS on the Commemoration of World AIDS Day." Pretoria Showgrounds, December 1. http://data.unaids.org/pub/SpeechEXD/2009/20091201_ms_speech _wad09_en.pdf. Accessed on June 1, 2011.

Silberschmidt, Margrethe. 2004. "Men, Male Sexuality, and HIV/AIDS: Reflections from Studies in Rural and Urban East Africa." *Transformation* 54: 42–58.

———. 2005. "Poverty, Male Disempowerment, and Male Sexuality: Rethinking Men and Masculinities in Rural and Urban East Africa." In *African Masculinities: Men in Africa from the Late 19th Century to the Present*, edited by Lahouchine Ouzgane and Robert Morrell, 189–203. New York: Palgrave Macmillan.

Singh, Jerome. 2008. "The Ethics and Legality of Traditional Healers Performing HIV Testing." *Southern African Journal of Medicine* (Spring): 6–10.

Sisulu, Lindiwe. 2004. "Speech by the Minister of Housing on the Occasion of the Tabling of the Budget Vote for the Department of Housing for the 2004–2005 Financial Year." June 10. National Assembly, Cape Town. Pretoria: Department of Housing.

Smit, Warren. 2006. "Understanding the Complexities of Informal Settlements: Insights from Cape Town." In *Informal Settlements: A Perpetual Challenge?*, edited by Marie Huchzermeyer and Aly Karam, 103–25. Cape Town: University of Cape Town Press.

Smith, Charlene. 2005. "Voices Being Raised against Baby Rape." *Sunday Independent*. March 6.

Snow, Rachel. 2007. "Who Is Testing for HIV?: A Look at Demographic and Health Surveys from Africa." Presentation for the "Appraisal and Action: HIV/AIDS in Southern Africa" conference held at the University of Michigan, Ann Arbor, on November 29–30, 2007.

Social Housing Foundation. 2010. "A Programme to Formalise Informal Settlements." In *Social Housing Trends*, 2–3. Social Housing Foundation Publication, March edition. Houghton: South Africa.

Soros, Eugene. 2006. "Zuma Trial Heightens Rape Awareness." *Worldpress*. April 29.

South African Broadcasting Company (SABC). 2011. "Bucket System Still a Huge Problem." May 3. http://www.sabc.co.za/wps/portal/news/pages/ details?id=6addf68046b8f027a4dafdaf5ec458d0&page=VoterInfo.Group1. Accessed on July 27, 2011.

South African Cities Network. 2011. State of the Cities Report. http://www .sacities.net/what/strategy/reporting/projects/607-towards-resilient-cities. Accessed on May 17, 2011.

South African Institute of Race Relations (SAIRR). 2010a. South Africa Survey, 2009–2010: Crime and Security. http://www.sairr.org.za/services/

publications/south-africa-survey/south-africa-survey-online-2009-2010. Accessed on March 14, 2011.

———. 2010b. South Africa Survey, 2009–2010: Health and Welfare. http:// www.sairr.org.za/services/publications/south-africa-survey/south-africa -survey-online-2009-2010. Accessed on March 14, 2011.

South African National AIDS Council (SANAC). 2010. "About SANAC." www .sanac.org.za. Accessed on March 15, 2011.

South African Press Association. 2006. "Government 'Balanced' on HIV/ AIDS." (August 26). http://www.news24.com/SouthAfrica/AidsFocus/Govt -balanced-on-HIVAids-20060825. Accessed on June 8, 2011.

South African Social Security Association (SASSA). 2011. "You and Your Grants, 2011/2012." http://www.sassa.gov.za/Portals/1/Documents/ d54e383b-7e3d-4c96-8aa2-4cc7d32bc78f.pdf. Accessed on January 29, 2012.

Specter, Michael. 2007. "The Denialists: The Dangerous Attacks on the Consensus about HIV and AIDS." *The New Yorker*. March 12. http://www .newyorker.com/reporting/2007/03/12/070312fa_fact_specter. Accessed on June 3, 2011.

Stadler, Jonathan. 2003. "The Young, the Rich, and the Beautiful: Secrecy, Suspicion, and Discourses of AIDS in the South African Lowveld." *African Journal of Aids Research* 2 (2): 123–35.

The Star. 1964. "Witchdoctors Still Popular." March 21. From Institute of Race Relations Archive, Wits Historical Papers, 1940–1970, Press Clippings on African Healing. William Cullen Library, University of Witwatersrand, Johannesburg.

———. 1965. "Nganga, Your Day Is Done." January 27. By Alan Campling. From Institute of Race Relations Archive, Wits Historical Papers, 1940– 1970, Press Clippings on African Healing. William Cullen Library, University of Witwatersrand, Johannesburg.

———. 1967. "Magic Ritual in Townships." April 19. From Institute of Race Relations Archive, Wits Historical Papers, 1940–1970, Press Clippings on African Healing. William Cullen Library, University of Witwatersrand, Johannesburg.

———. 2009. "So Why Do We Pay So Much in the Supermarket?" June 3.

Statistics South Africa. 2007a. Community Survey 2007. October 24, 2007. http://www.statssa.gov.za/publications/P0301/P0301.pdf. Accessed on January 29, 2012.

———. 2007b. A National Poverty Line for South Africa. February 21, 2007. http://www.treasury.gov.za/publications/other/povertyline/Treasury%20 StatsSA%20poverty%20line%20discussion%20paper.pdf. Accessed on June 24, 2011.

———. 2008a. Mortality and Causes of Death: Findings from Death Notification. (Published November 18). http://www.statssa.gov.za/publications/ P03093/P030932008.pdf. Accessed on March 14, 2011.

———. 2008b. Non-Financial Census of Municipalities for the Year Ended June 2008. http://www.statssa.gov.za/publications/statsdownload.asp? PPN=p9115&SCH=4460. Accessed on April 21, 2011.

———. 2010. Quarterly Labour Force Statistics, Quarter 4. Pretoria. www .statssa.gov.za. Accessed on November 21, 2012.

———. 2011. Quarterly Labour Force Survey, Quarter 1, 2011 (published on May 3). http://www.statssa.gov.za/publications/P0211/P02111stQuarter 2011.pdf. Accessed on May 25, 2011.

Staugard, F. 1985. *Traditional Healers: Traditional Medicine in Botswana*. Gaborone: Ipelegeng.

Steinberg, Jonny. 2009. "A Suspiciously Speedy Plunge to Ignominy of 'National Ogre.'" *Business Day*. December 9. http://www.businessday.co.za/ Articles/Content.aspx?id=89104. Accessed on December 4, 2011.

Steinberg, Malcolm, Saul Johnson, Gill Schierhout, David Ndegwa, Katherine Hall, Bev Russell, and Jonathan Morgan. 2002. "Hitting Home: How Households Cope with the Impact of the HIV/AIDS Epidemic." Washington, DC: Henry J. Kaiser Family Foundation. http://www .kff.org/southafrica/loader.cfm?url=/commonspot/security/getfile .cfm&PageID=14028. Accessed on March 17, 2008.

Steinmetz, George. 2006. "Bourdieu's Disavowal of Lacan: Psychoanalytic Theory and the Concepts of 'Habitus' and 'Symbolic Capital.'" *Constellations* 13 (4): 445–64.

———. 2007. "American Sociology before and after World War II: The (Temporary) Settling of a Disciplinary Field." In *Sociology in America: A History*, edited by Craig Calhoun, 314–66. Chicago: University of Chicago Press.

Stewart, M. J., Vanessa Steenkamp, and Michele Zuckerman. 1998. "The Toxicology of African Herbal Remedies." *Therapeutic Drug Monitoring* 20 (5): 510–16.

Stewart, M. J., J. J. Moar, P. Steenkamp, and M. Kokot. 1999. "Findings in Fatal Cases of Poisoning Attributed to Traditional Remedies in South Africa." *Forensic Science International* 101 (3): 177–83.

Stewart, Michael, Jack Moar, James Mwesigwa, and Michael Kokot. 2000. "Forensic Toxicology in Urban South Africa." *Journal of Toxicology—Clinical Toxicology* 38 (June): 415–19.

Sunday Independent. 2004. "Deputy Minister Sees Traditional Healers Helping to Find a Cure for Aids." November 7.

Sunday Times. 1999. "Child Rape: A Taboo within the AIDS Taboo." April 4.

Susser, Ida. 2009. *AIDS, Sex, and Culture: Global Politics and Survival in Southern Africa*. Malden, MA: Wiley-Blackwell.

Suttner, Raymond. 2009. "The Jacob Zuma Rape Trial: Power and African National Congress (ANC) Masculinities." *Nordic Journal of Feminist and Gender Research* 17 (September): 222–36.

Swanson, Maynard W. 1977. "The Sanitation Syndrome: Bubonic Plague and Urban Native Policy in the Cape Colony, 1900–1909." *Journal of African History* 18 (3): 387–410.

Swidler, Ann, and Susan Cotts Watkins. 2007. "Ties of Dependence: AIDS and Transactional Sex in Rural Malawi." *Studies in Family Planning* 38 (September): 147–62.

Terreblanche, Christelle. 2006. "Women the Losers in Zuma Rape Case." *Sunday Argus*. April 13.

't Hoen, Ellen. 2002. "TRIPS, Pharmaceutical Patents, and Access to Essential Medicines: A Long Way from Seattle to Doha." *Chicago Journal of International Law* 3 (Spring): 27–46.

THO Siyavuma News. 2004. The Journal of the Traditional Healers Organisation. Volume 5, Edition 1 (Spring).

Thom, Anso. 2010. "MCC Blocking Access to Lifesaving Meds—HIV Clinicians." *Health-E News*. March 4. http://allafrica.com/stories/201003040847 .html. Accessed on March 28, 2011.

Thomas, Elizabeth, J. R. Seager, and A. Mathee. 2002. "Environmental Health Challenges in South Africa: Policy Lessons from Case Studies." *Health and Place* 8 (December): 251–61.

Thornton, Robert. 2002. "Traditional Healers and the Biomedical Health System in South Africa: Summary Report—December 2002." Medical Care Development International (MCDI) for the Margaret Sanger Institute. Johannesburg: University of the Witswatersrand.

———. 2008. *Unimagined Community: Sex, Networks, and AIDS in Uganda and South Africa*. Berkeley: University of California Press.

———. 2009. "The Transmission of Knowledge in South African Traditional Healing." *Africa* 79 (1): 17–34.

Timberg, Craig. 2005. "S. Africa's Top Court Blesses Gay Marriage." *Washington Post*, A16. December 2. http://www.washingtonpost.com/wp-dyn/content/ article/2005/12/01/AR2005120100583.html. Accessed on November 13, 2011.

Treatment Action Campaign (TAC). 2000. "Defiance Campaign: Questions and Answers." http://www.tac.org.za/Documents/DefianceCampaign/Q_A _ImportBrazil.htm. Accessed on June 15, 2011.

———. 2004. "Electronic Newsletter concerning the THO." November 24, 2004. http://www.tac.org.za/newsletter/2004/ns23_11_2004.htm. Accessed on October 13, 2011.

———. 2005a. "Health Workers Speak Out." *Equal Treatment Newsletter* 18 (December). http://www.tac.org.za/documents/et18.pdf. Accessed on October 18, 2011.

———. 2005b. "TAC Briefing: The Harmful Activities of Matthias Rath" and other documents. (April 18). http://www.tac.org.za/community/rath. Accessed on June 15, 2011.

———. 2005c. "Traditional Healers and Public Health." *Equal Treatment Newsletter* 15 (May). www.tac.org.za/ET/EqualTreatmentMay2005Issue15.pdf. Accessed on October 13, 2011.

———. 2008. "Health Minister Barbara Hogan Delivers Landmark Speech at HIV Vaccine Conference." (October 16). http://www.tac.org.za/community/node/2421. Accessed on June 14, 2011.

———. 2009a. "The End of the Matthias Rath Affair?" (March 16). http://www.tac.org.za/community/node/2507. Accessed on June 9, 2011.

———. 2009b. "An Open Letter to the Medicines Control Council from Concerned Academics and Others." (April 16). http://www.tac.org.za/community/node/2532. Accessed on March 28, 2011.

———. 2009c. TAC Annual Report, 1 March 2008 to 28 February 2009. http://www.tac.org.za/community/files/file/AnnualReports/TACAnnualReport2009.pdf. Accessed on October 10, 2011.

———. 2010. Submission on the Social Assistance Amendment Bill, 2010. (April 23). www.pmg.org.za/files/docs/100421tac.doc. Accessed on October 19 2010.

Treichler, Paula A. 1999. How to Have Theory in an Epidemic: Cultural Chronicles of AIDS. Durham, NC: Duke University Press.

Tshabalala-Msimang, Manto. 2003. "Speech by the Minister of Health during a Visit to Soweto Home and Community-Based Care Projects." August 21, 2003. http://www.info.gov.za/speeches/2003/1008.htm. Accessed on June 9, 2011.

Tutu, Desmond. 2011. "An End to AIDS Is Within Our Reach." Washington Post. September 20. http://www.washingtonpost.com/opinions/an-end-to-aids-is-within-our-reach/2011/09/18/gIQABABbGjK_story.html. Accessed on October 16, 2011.

UNAIDS (Joint United Nations Programme on HIV/AIDS). 2000. Men and AIDS: A Gendered Approach. 2000 World AIDS Campaign. Geneva: UNAIDS.

UN-HABITAT. 2009. State of the World's Cities, 2008/2009: Harmonious Cities. London: Earthscan.

UNICEF (United Nation's Children's Fund). 2008. Review of the Child Support Grant: Uses, Implementation and Obstacles. (June). http://www.unicef.org/southafrica/SAF_resources_childsupport.pdf. Accessed on January 29, 2012.

UN Integrated Regional Information Networks (UN IRIN). 2005. "South Africa: Men Falling through the Cracks." (July 25, 2005). http://www.aegis.com/news/irin/2005/IR050766.html. Accessed on November 15, 2011.

United Nations (UN). 2010. Millennium Development Goals Report. http://www.un.org/millenniumgoals/pdf/MDG%20Report%202010%20En%20r15%20-low%20res%2020100615%20-.pdf. Accessed on July 11, 2011.

United Nations Development Programme (UNDP). 2007. Human Development Report, 2007/2008. New York: Palgrave Macmillan.

———. 2009. "Economy and Inequality," Human Development Report 2009. http://hdrstats.undp.org/en/indicators/161.html. Accessed on July 29, 2011.

————. 2010. "The Real Wealth of Nations: Pathways to Human Development." http://hdr.undp.org/en/reports/global/hdr2010/chapters/en/. Accessed on July 29, 2011.

United Nations General Assembly Special Session on HIV/AIDS (UNGASS). 2010. "Country Progress Report on the Declaration of Commitment on HIV/AIDS—South Africa." (March 31). http://www.unaids.org/en/dataanalysis/monitoringcountryprogress/2010progressreportssubmittedby countries/southafrica_2010_country_progress_report_en.pdf. Accessed on October 13, 2011.

Vale, Peter, and Sipho Maseko. 1998. "South Africa and the African Renaissance." *International Affairs* 74 (April): 271–87.

van der Linde, I. 1997. "Western and African Medicines Meet." *South African Medical Journal* 87: 268–70.

van der Vliet, Virginia. 1994. "Apartheid and the Politics of AIDS." In *Global AIDS Policy,* edited by Douglas A. Feldman, 107–28. Westport, CT: Bergin and Garvey.

Vaughan, Megan. 1991. *Curing Their Ills: Colonial Power and African Illness.* Stanford, CA: Stanford University Press.

Veale, D. J. H. 1992. "South African Traditional Herbal Medicines Used during Childbirth." *Journal of Ethnopharmacy* 36: 185–91.

Vearey, Joanna. 2010. "Hidden Spaces and Urban Health: Exploring the Tactics of Rural Migrants Navigating the City of Gold." *Urban Forum* 21: 37–53.

Vearey, Joanna, Ingrid Palmary, Liz Thomas, Lorena Nunez, and Scott Drimie. 2010. "Urban Health in Johannesburg: The Importance of Place in Understanding Intra-Urban Inequalities in a Context of Migration and HIV." *Health and Place* 16 (July): 694–702.

Veriava, Ahmed. 2006. "The Restructuring of Basic Service Delivery in Soweto: Life Strategies and the Problem of Primitive Accumulation." Master's thesis, University of KwaZulu-Natal, Centre for Civil Society.

Vetten, Lisa. 2007. "Violence against Women in South Africa." In *State of the Nation, South Africa 2007,* edited by S. Buhlungu, J. Daniel, R. Southall, and J. Luchman, 425–47. Cape Town: HSRC Press.

Viljoen, M., A. Panzer, K. L. Roos, and W. Bodemer. 2003. "Psychoneuroimmunology: From Philosophy, Intuition, and Folklore to a Recognized Science." *South African Journal of Science* 99: 332–36.

Vincent, Louise. 2006. "Virginity Testing in South Africa: Re-Traditioning the Postcolony." *Culture, Health and Sexuality* 8 (January–February): 17–30.

Von Schnitzler, Antina. 2008. "Citizenship Prepaid: Water, Calculability, and Techno-Politics in South Africa." *Journal of Southern African Studies* 34 (December): 899–917.

Wacquant, Loïc. 1989. "Toward a Reflexive Sociology: A Workshop with Pierre Bourdieu." *Sociological Theory* 7: 26–63.

———. 1999. "How Penal Common Sense Comes to Europeans: Notes on the Transatlantic Diffusion of the Neoliberal *Doxa.*" *European Societies* 1: 319–52.

———. 2004. "Following Pierre Bourdieu into the Field." *Ethnography* 5 (December): 387–414.

Waetjen, Thembisa. 2004. *Workers and Warriors: Masculinity and the Struggle for Nation in South Africa.* Urbana: University of Illinois Press.

Walker, Liz. 2005. "Men Behaving Differently: South African Men since 1994." *Culture, Health and Sexuality* 7 (3): 225–38.

Webb, D. 1992. *HIV and AIDS in Africa.* London: Pluto Press.

Wight, Daniel, Mary L. Plummer, Gerry Mshana, Joyce Wamoyi, Zachayo S. Shigongo, and David A. Ross. 2006. "Contradictory Sexual Norms and Expectations for Young People in Rural Northern Tanzania." *Social Science and Medicine* 62 (4): 987–97.

Wilson, Stuart. 2003. "Out of Site, Out of Mind: Relocation and Access to Schools in Sol Plaatjie." Research Report, Centre for Applied Legal Studies, CALS, Johannesburg.

Wojcicki, Janet Maia. 2002. "Commercial Sex Work or *Ukuphanda*? Sex-for-Money Exchange in Soweto and Hammanskraal Area, South Africa." *Culture, Medicine, and Psychiatry* 26: 339–70.

Wojcicki, Janet Maia, and J. Malala. 2001. "Condom Use, Power, and HIV/AIDS Risk: Sex-Workers Bargain for Survival in Hillbrow/Joubert Park/Berea, Johannesburg." *Social Science and Medicine* 53 (1): 99–121.

Wolpe, Harold. 1972. "Capitalism and Cheap Labour-Power in South Africa: From Segregation to Apartheid." *Economy and Society* 1 (4): 425–56.

World Health Organization (WHO). 2007. Health of Indigenous Peoples. Fact Sheet, #326. http://www.who.int/mediacentre/factsheets/fs326/en/index .html. Accessed on December 27, 2011.

———. 2009. World Health Statistics. http://www.who.int/whosis/whostat/ EN_WHS09_Full.pdf. Accessed on October 18, 2011.

———. 2010a. Global Price Reporting Mechanism. http://www.who.int/hiv/ amds/gprm/en/ Accessed on October 19, 2010.

———. 2010a. New Guidance on Prevention of Mother-to-Child Transmission of HIV and Infant Feeding in the Context of HIV. July 20, 2010. http:// www.who.int/hiv/pub/mtct/PMTCTfactsheet/en/index.html. Accessed on February 10, 2012.

Wyrod, Robert. 2008. "Between Women's Rights and Men's Authority: Masculinity and Shifting Discourses of Gender Difference in Urban Uganda." *Gender and Society* 22 (6): 799–823.

Xaba, Thokozani. 2001. "Masculinity and Its Malcontents: The Confrontation between 'Struggle Masculinity' and 'Post-Struggle Masculinity' (1990–1997)." In *Changing Men in Southern Africa*, edited by Robert Morrell, 105–24. New York: Zed Books.

————. 2002. "The Transformation of Indigenous Medical Practice in South Africa (1985 to 2000)." In *Bodies and Politics: Healing Rituals in the Democratic South Africa*, edited by Véronique Faure, 23–39. Johannesburg: *Les Cahiers de l'IFAS*, Number 2 (February).

————. 2005. "Witchcraft, Sorcery, or Medical Practice? The Demand, Supply, and Regulation of Indigenous Medicines in Durban, South Africa." PhD diss., University of California, Berkeley.

Zachariah, R., N. Ford, M. Philips, S. Lynch, M. Massaquoi, V. Janssens, and A. D. Harries. 2009. "Task Shifting in HIV/AIDS: Opportunities, Challenges, and Proposed Actions for Sub-Saharan Africa." *Transactions of the Royal Society and Tropical Medicine and Hygiene* 103 (6): 549–58.

Žižek, Slavoj. 1989. *The Sublime Object of Ideology*. New York: Verso.

————. 1997. *The Plague of Fantasies*. New York: Verso.

————. 2011. "Freedom in the Clouds: What Is Possible and What Is Impossible Today." Stanley Fish Lecture, October 21, 2011, University of Illinois at Chicago.

Zuma, Jacob. 2009. "Address by President Jacob Zuma on the Occasion of World AIDS Day." Pretoria Showgrounds, December 1. http://www.info .gov.za/speeches/2009/09120112151001.htm. Accessed on December 3, 2011.

Zuma, Khangelani. 2007. "What Do the Numbers Reveal? Obstacles to Effective Monitoring and Appraisal." Presentation for the "Appraisal and Action: HIV/AIDS in Southern Africa" conference held at the University of Michigan, Ann Arbor, on November 29–30, 2007.

Index

Page numbers followed by *f* indicate figures; those with *t* indicate tables.

Martin, John Levi, 227–28
masculinity, 163–65, 267n10, 267n21;
impact of HIV/AIDS on, 177; material economy of, 174–78; modern vs.
traditional interpretations of, 183–85,
268–69nn45–46; presidential performances of, 162–63, 168–70. *See also*
gender
Maseko, Phephsile, 128
Mavimbela, Vusi, 85
Mbeki, Thabo, 191–92, 243n27, 267n13;
African renaissance discourse of, 13,
84–87, 104, 129, 168–69, 192, 234;
electoral loss in 2007 of, 16–17, 82–83,
150–51, 198; GEAR reforms of, 10,
196; "I Am an African" speech of, 84;
leadership style of, 83, 193; masculinity and, 165, 167–69; on modernity
and traditionalism, 21, 86–87, 163–64,
170–73, 234, 255n24; national treatment plans for HIV/AIDS and STDs
of, 82–83; neoliberal economics of,
98–103, 195; on race and sexuality,
86, 89–90, 96–97, 266n2; rights-based
gender policies of, 163–64, 166–69; on
structural vulnerabilities in poverty,
80, 94–96; thanatopolitics of, 104–6;
Third Way politics of, 10–11, 99–100,
243n28. *See also* denialism
Mbembe, Achille, 89–90
McGregor, Liz, 121
Médecins sans Frontières (MSF), 83, 118
Medical Research Council (MRC), 124–25
medicine. *See* biomedicine; indigenous
healing
Medicines and Related Substances Control Amendment Act, 131, 261n23,
261nn31
Medicines Control Council (MCC), 79,
253n5, 256n36; investigation of indigenous healing by, 124, 127; regulation of
indigenous remedies by, 124, 261n23
methods (research), 244n39, 245n9,
250n88
migration: to mining communities for,
174, 178, 186, 209; to urban areas,
26–27, 178. *See also* squatter camps
millennial capitalism, 13
mining compounds, 30
"miracle" cures, 72–73, 251n114
Mkhwanazi, Sandra, 158–59

Mlambo-Ngcuka, Phumzile, 82
modernity/traditionalism binary, xiii, 7–8,
21, 232–35; as colonial construct, xiii,
233–34; deindustrialization and, 12;
in gender constructs, 163–73, 183–85,
191, 198; in healing paradigms, 7–8,
18–19, 91–93, 123, 129–30, 214–17,
255n24, 256n30; in postcolonial narratives of independence, 12–14, 129–30,
163–64, 244n29. *See also* hybridity
Mongoya, Martha, 62, 220–21
Moraka, Christopher, 259n7
Mostoaledi, Aaron, 193
mother-to-child-transmission-prevention
(MTCTP) campaign, 79, 97, 117, 254n16
Motlanthe, Kgalema, 169
Motsemme, Nthabiseng, 180–81
Motsoaledi, Aaron, 256n30
muthi (herbal substance), 61, 67–68;
biomedical testing of, 124–29, 260n22;
informal economy in, 211–13, 271n26;
traders in, 64; for witchcraft, 67, 71
Myburgh, James, 253n4
myth of incommensurability, 8, 13, 18,
225–26; Mbeki's use of, 19–20, 94, 114,
123–30, 231–35, 273n57; in rollout of
ARVS, 123–24; Zuma's use of, 193
myth of modernization. *See* modernity/
traditionalism binary

Natal Code of Native Law, 270n20
National AIDS Convention of South Africa,
5–6
National Association of People with AIDS
(NAPWA), 90
National Drug Policy, 124
National Health Plan for South Africa of
1994, 5–6
national imagining, 8, 13, 86, 147, 192. *See
also* fantasies of independence
National Party. *See* apartheid
national treatment plans: HIV/AIDS Strate-
gic Plan for South Africa, 2000–2005,
139; HIV/AIDS Strategic Plan for South
Africa, 2007–2011, 82–83, 139–40;
Operational Plan for Comprehensive
HIV/AIDS and AIDS Care, 18, 81–83,
117–118, 260n9
Native Law, 270n20
Natives Act of 1952, 241n6
Natsios, Andrew, 114, 259n2